Third International Visual Field Symposium

Documenta Ophthalmologica
Proceedings Series volume 19

Editor H.E. Henkes

Dr. W. Junk bv Publishers The Hague-Boston-London 1979

Third International Visual Field Symposium
Tokyo, May 3-6, 1978

Edited by E. L. Greve

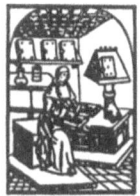

Dr. W. Junk bv Publishers The Hague-Boston-London 1979

Cover design: Max Velthuijs

ISBN-13:978-90-6193-160-7   e-ISBN-13:978-94-009-9611-3
DOI: 10.1007/978-94-009-9611-3

CONTENTS

E.L. Greve: Introduction   1

Session I.   Neuro-ophthalmology
Chairman: H. Bynke
L. Frisén: Funduscopic correlates of visual field defects due to lesions
of the anterior visual pathway   5
Y. Tagami: Correlations between atrophy of maculopapillar bundles
and visual functions in cases of optic neuropathies   17
Y. Isayama: Visual field defects due to tumors of the sellar region. .   27
F. Dannheim, D. Luedecke & D. Kuehne: Visual fields before and
after transnasal removal of a pituitary tumor   43
S.S. Hayreh & P. Podhajsky: Visual field defects in anterior ischemic
optic neuropathy   53
E. Aulhorn & M. Tanzil: Comparison of visual field defects in glaucoma
and in acute anterior ischemic optic neuropathy   73
L. Frisén: Visual field defects due to hypoplasia of the optic nerve .   81
H. Bynke & L. Vestergren-Brenner: Visual field defects in congenital
hydrocephalus   87
T. Otori, T. Hohki & Y. Nakao: Central critical fusion frequency in
neuro-ophthalmological practice   95
Discussion of the session on Neuro-ophthalmology   101
H. Bynke: Summary of session I: Neuro-ophthalmology   109

Session II.   Glaucoma
Chairman: S.M. Drance
P.R. Lichter & C.L. Standardi: Early glaucomatous visual field defects
and their significance to clinical ophthalmology   111
S.M. Drance, M. Fairclough, B. Thomas, G.R. Douglas & R Susanna:
The early visual field defects in glaucoma and the significance of
nasal steps   119
E.L. Greve, F. Furuno & W.M. Verduin: A critical phase in the development of glaucomatous visual field defects   127
J.M. Enoch & E.C. Campos: Analysis of patients with open-angle
glaucoma using perimetric techniques reflecting receptive field-
like properties   137
F. Dannheim: Liminal and supraliminal stimuli in the perimetry of
chronic simple glaucoma   151
R. Lakowski & S.M. Drance: Acquired dyschromatopsias the earliest
functional losses in glaucoma   159

N. Endo: The relation between depression in the Bjerrum area and nasal step in early glaucoma (DBA & NS) 167

M.F. Armaly: Reversibility of glaucomatous defects of the visual field 177

C.D. Phelps: Visual field defects in open-angle glaucoma: progression and regression 187

E.L. Greve, F. Furuno & W.M. Verduin: The clinical significance of reversibility of glaucomatous visual field defects 197

J.T. Ernest: Recovery of visual function during elevation of the intra-ocular pressure 205

Y. Kitazawa, O. Takahashi & Y. Ohiwa: The mode of development and progression of field defects in early glaucoma – A follow-up study 211

E.B. Werner: Peripheral nasal field defects in glaucoma 223

I. Iinuma: Reversibility of visual field defects in simple glaucoma . . 229

K. Iwata: Reversible cupping and reversible field defect in glaucoma . 233

K. Mizokami, Y. Tagami & Y. Isayama: The reversibility of visual field defects in the juvenile glaucoma cases 241

F. Furuno & H. Matsuo: Early stage progression in glaucomatous visual field changes 247

H. Kosaki: The earliest visual field defect (IIa Stage) in glaucoma by kinetic perimetry 255

S. Yamazi, K. Yamasowa & I. Azuma: Relationship between IOP level and visual field in open-angle glaucoma (Study for critical pressure in glaucoma) 261

A.I. Friedman: The relationship between visual field changes and intra-ocular pressure 263

T. Aoyama: Visual field change examined by pupillography in glaucoma 265

M. Zingirian, G. Calabria & E. Gandolfo: The nasal step: An early glaucomatous defect? 273

Discussion of the session on Glaucoma 279

S.M. Drance: Summary of Session II: Glaucoma 292

Session III. Automation
        Chairman: H. Matsuo

F. Fankhauser & H. Bebie: Threshold fluctuations, interpolations and spatial resolution in perimetry 295

S. Hamazaki, T. Yokota, H. Mieno, S. Koike, M. Taga, J. Hamazaki, G. Kikuchi & H. Matsuo: Semi-automatic campimeter with graphic display 311

H. Bynke, A. Heijl & C. Holmin: Automatic computerized perimetry in neuro-ophthalmology 319

M. Zingirian, V. Tagliasco & E. Gandolfo: Automated perimetry: Minicomputers or microprocessors? 327

Discussion of the session on Automation 333

H. Matsuo: Summary of session III: Automation 340

Session IV. Methodology
Chairman: H. Matsuo

K. Kani & Y. Ogita: Fundus controlled perimetry 341

Y. Ohta, T. Miyamoto & K. Harasawa: Experimental fundus photo perimeter and its application 351

A. Inatomi: A simple fundus perimetry with fundus camera. . . . 359

E. Aulhorn, H. Harms & H. Karmeyer: The influence of spontaneous eye-rotation on the perimetric determination of small scotomas . 363

R. Suzuki & M. Tomonaga: Analysis of angioscotoma testing with Friedmann visual field analyser and Tübinger perimeter 369

E.L. Greve: Comparative examinations of visual function and fluorescein angiography in early stages of senile disciform macular degeneration 371

J.M. Enoch, C.R. Fitzgerald & E.C. Campos: The relationship between fundus lesions and areas of functional change 381

K. Matsudaira & R. Suzuki: Visual field changes after photocoagulation in retinal branch vein occlusion 395

T. Hara: Visual field changes in mesopic and scotopic conditions using Friedmann visual field analyser 403

L. Frisén & G. Schöldström: Relationship between perimetric eccentricity and retinal locus in a human eye 409

R. Lakowski & P. Dunn: A new interpretation of the relative central scotoma for blue stimuli under photopic conditions 411

Discussion of the session on Methodology. 417

H. Matsuo: Summary of session IV: Methodology 421

Session V. Free Papers
Chairman: J.M. Enoch

A. Dubois-Poulsen: The enlargement of the blind spot in binocular vision 423

M. Frisén: Evaluation of perimetric procedures a statistical approch . 427

Y. Honda, A. Negi & M. Miki: Eye movements during peripheral field tests monitored by electro-oculogram 433

H. Kitahara, K. Kitahara & H. Matsuzaki: Trial of a color perimeter . 439

S. Kubota: Videopupillographic perimetry perimetric findings with rabbit eyes 447

E. Shinzato & H. Matsuo: Clinical experiences with a new multiple dot plate 453

T. Maruo: Electroencephalographic perimetry clinical applications of vertex potentials elicited by focal retinal stimulation 461

T. Ogawa & R. Suzuki: Relation between central and peripheral visual field changes with kinetic perimetry 469

Discussion on the free papers session 475

Report of the IPS research group on standards 481

G. Verriest: Report on colour perimetry 483

A. Dubois-Poulsen: Closing speech 485

List of contributors 488

Docum. Ophthal. Proc. Series, Vol. 19

INTRODUCTION

ERIK L. GREVE

The 3rd International Visual Field Symposium was held on the 4th till the 6th of May 1978 in Tokyo for the members and guests of the International Perimetric Society.

The Proceedings of this symposium follow the general lines of the programme with some minor alterations.

This symposium was a so-called topic-symposium where selected topics were introduced by experts in the field.

These topics were:

Neuro-ophthalmology.

1. Funduscopic correlates of visual field defects.
2. Visual field defects due to tumors of the sellar region.

Glaucoma.

1. The earliest visual field defects in glaucoma.
2. The reversibility of glaucomatous visual field defects.

Methodology.

1. Automation.
2. The relation between the position of a lesion in the fundus and in the visual field.

Apart from the introductory papers, free papers were given on the topics and also some non-topic free papers.

Much attention has been given to the discussion. Most of the discussion remarks in this Proceedings are the original taped remarks of the discussion-speakers. We have choosen this form of presentation to take to the reader the athmosphere of the discussion and to preserve originality.

The chairman of the sessions have presented a summary or even better an interpretation of the trends in their topics.

This introduction gives a short overview of the main themes of the symposium.

In the first section on Neuro-ophthalmology Frisen gave an introduction about fundoscopic correlates of visual field defects (V.F.D.) in lesions of the anterior visual pathway. Visible defects in the retinal nerve fiber layer (R.N.L.) were shown to exist in several diseases. Local R.N.L. defects usually show a good correspondence with V.F.D. while a generalized reduction of the R.N.L. may not be accompanied by a detectable V.F.D. More data are needed to clarify their discrepancy.

Similar correlations were presented by Tagami who studies the papillomacular bundle in optic nerve disease by fundus controlled maculometry. They found a correlation between visual acuity, visual field and the visible atrophy of the papillomacular bundle, and use their method to predict the prognosis of optic nerve disease.

Isayama introduced the topic of chiasmal defects and showed in complete correspondence between the V.F.D. and the location of tumors. It was stressed again that often chiasmal V.F.D. do not show the typical bitemporal pattern and are frequently misdiagnosed as optic neuritis. Similar findings were presented by Dannheim who used supraliminal stimuli. He found early V.F.D. changes also when a pituitary tumor was intrasellar.

Aulhorn and Hayreh presented their results on VFD in anterior ischaemic optic neurophthy (AION). The type of defect is the same as in glaucoma but the distribution is different. These defects show a considerable reversibility. Further research should clarify why nerve fiber bundle defects (NFBD) in AION show a behaviour different from glaucomatous NFBD.

A highly interesting *Glaumcoma* session discussed the topics of early VFD and reversibility. We have to differentiate the VFD as found by our present methods and those shown by new experimental methods.

The now classical method of combined kinetic and static perimetry dealing with NFBD was introduced by Lichter, Drance, Greve and Endo.

It was agreed that early manifestation of NFBD can be relative defects in the paracentral VF or peripheral nasal steps. These relative defects should preferably be demonstrated in the course of the NF. It is not sure that every glaucomatous defect goes through a stage of relative defects. Early defects have to exceed the normal variation of thresholds. Nasal steps of more than 5 degrees are rare in the normal population.

The investigation of glaucomatous VFD should be divided in a first detection phase and a second assessment phase which provides the basis for accurate follow-up. The best way for the detection of early defects seems to be the presentation of a sufficient number of evenly distributed stimuli in the paracentral field, the nasal field and some in the temporal field. The presentation should be static. The nasal periphery can also be examined by means of kinetic perimetry.

Other possibilities of examination were shown by Dannheim: supraliminal stimuli, and Enoch: Westheimer functions and wind-mill target, and Lakowski: colour vision.

The future may show that these techniques detect glaucomatous VFD in an even earlier stages than present methods and may also show that the N.F.B.D. is not the only significant defect in glaucoma.

Reversibility of G.V.F.D. was introduced by Armaly, Phelps, Greve and Ernest. It was shown that reversibility does exist be it not as frequent as deterioration. It occurs specialy in the early stages of GVFD, in younger patients and after large reductions of IOP. Changes of GVFD have to be larger than the pathological variation of thresholds in defects. This pathological variation can be considerably larger than the normal variation.

Interesting papers on this subject were also given by Iwata and Mizokami. Iwata demonstrated that in the presence of visible RNFL defects reversibility of the corresponding VFD is unlikely to occur. These papers showed again that before the occurence of actual nerve fiber death, the nerve fibers may go through a stage of reversible loss of function, which has interesting implications concerning the pathogenesis of glaucomatous VFD.

Automation of perimetry was introduced by Fankhauser. Several aspects of this important contribution to perimetry were highlighted by Hamazaki, Bynke, Aulhorn and Zingirian. Threshold fluctuations and stimulus density are important factors both in the detection phase and the assessment phase.

It is expected that an automated detection phase will soon be available for routine-examination. The problems of a well-programmed assessment phase have not yet been solved to everyones satisfaction. Programmes for the assessment phase will require most of our attention in the near future.

A new and fasinating area of research is provided by *Fundus-controlled perimetry*. This method originally proposed by Aulhorn was introduced by Kani and further presented by Ohta. The stimulus can be exactly positioned on the fundus due to a combination of a fundus camera, a built-in stimulus presentation device and a simultaneous display of fundus and stimulus. This still experimental method allows exact studies of the correlation between ophthalmoscopic lesions and functional defects.
Much is expected from this type of research once the present technical problems have been overcome.

Similar correlations between fundus lesions and perimetry were presented by Enoch and by Greve using different methods.

Greve demonstrated again that differential mesopic-photopic perimetry was very usefull in macular diseases and specifically in the early stages of Senile disciform macular degeneration.

This 3rd Int. V.F. Symposium showed that the old method of perimetry is very much alive and has many branches of new developments that will enrich our range of diagnostic possibilities to the benefit of the patient.

Miss Kayoho Adachi in Tokyo and Miss Els Mutsaerts and Mr. Bill Miller in Amsterdam gave excellent assistance for the preparation of the symposium.

The local organization was in the capable hands of Professor Ted Matsuo and his staff. We wish to express our gratitude for their accurate and hospitable organization. It is difficult to name the many staff-members of the eye clinic of Tokyo Medical College hospital who have contributed to the success of this symposium. If we specialy thank Dr. Hamazaki it is because he stands for all of them.

The Proceedings are out now thanks to the tremendous work of Miss. Els Mutsaerts to whom we express our gratefullness. The cooperation with Dr. W. Junk bv, the publishers, was efficient and pleasant as ever.

FUNDUSCOPIC CORRELATES OF VISUAL FIELD DEFECTS
DUE TO LESIONS OF THE ANTERIOR VISUAL PATHWAY

LARS FRISÉN

(Göteborg, Sweden)

ABSTRACT

Ophthalmoscopy of the peripapillary retinal nerve fiber layer can give important information on the state of the anterior visual pathway. This information can be used to predict visual field defects, and the extent of recovery that may be possible with treatment. Under certain circumstances, it may even allow a rough timing of destructive events. Examination of the peripapillary retinal nerve fiber layer, by ophthalmoscopy or fundus photography, is therefore a very useful complement to perimetry.

Lesions of the anterior visual pathway may be associated with fundus abnormalities in several ways but most commonly through interference with axoplasmic transport mechanisms and through descending degeneration of axons. Funduscopic signs of these latter abnormalities, and their perimetric correlates, are the subjects of this mini review.

The anterior visual pathway is unique amongst neural pathways in that its axons are accessible to visual evaluation. This is due to the peculiar arrangement of the axons within the eye: from their origins, the retinal ganglion cells, the axons course towards the optic disc in the innermost layer of the retina. Individual axons cannot be resolved by present ophthalmoscopic or photographic techniques, but their convergence on the optic disc causes the formation of increasingly thick bundles, and bundles of nerve fibers can normally be fairly easily visualized in the peripapillary area, particularly above and below the optic disc (Fig. 1 A). Normal bundles of retinal nerve fibers appear as superficial, opaque striae of a pale grey color, with very fine radial striations. Such bundles obscure detail in the underlying retinal structures and blur small retinal vessels. Nerve fiber bundles are much more difficult to see within the optic disc itself because of the poor contrast against the supporting tissues of the optic nervehead. The structural state of the anterior visual pathway is therefore best assessed by ophthalmoscopy of the peripapillary area. Pioneer studies in this field have been made by Vogt, Ito, Hoyt, and Lundström, and their coworkers. The reader is referred to their reports (cited below) for excellent photographs of the appearance of the retinal nerve fiber layer in health and disease. A very complete review of the literature has recently been given by Lundström (Lundström 1977).

Simple inspection of bundles of axons gives little insight into the complex axoplasmic transport phenomena that occur in normal axons. Various transport mechanisms ensure continuous movement of different axoplasmic constituents at different rates both in anterograde and retrograde directions. Disturbances of transport mechanisms may result in a local accumulation of axoplasm. So-called cotton-wool spots in the retina are tell-tale signs of localized blocks (McLeod, Marshall, Kohner & Bird 1977). In retrobulbar disease, signs of interrupted axoplasmic flow are conspicuous only when the optic nervehead is the site of interference, as in papilledema from increased intracranial pressure. In this condition axonal flow is impaired at the level of the optic disc, with the production of a greyish reticulated halo of swollen axons at the disc border, and swelling of the nervehead itself. Hyperemia, venous dilatation, hemorrhages, and cotton-wood spots occur as secondary phenomena (Hayreh 1977). Stasis of axonal flow does not necessarily impair axonal conduction. The increased size of the blind spot in papilledema is probably primarily a reflection of a pre-receptor filtering of light through thickened axons in combination with disalignment of the photoreceptors. The brief obscurations of vision that patients with increased intracranial pressure sometimes complain about, are more likely to be reflections of

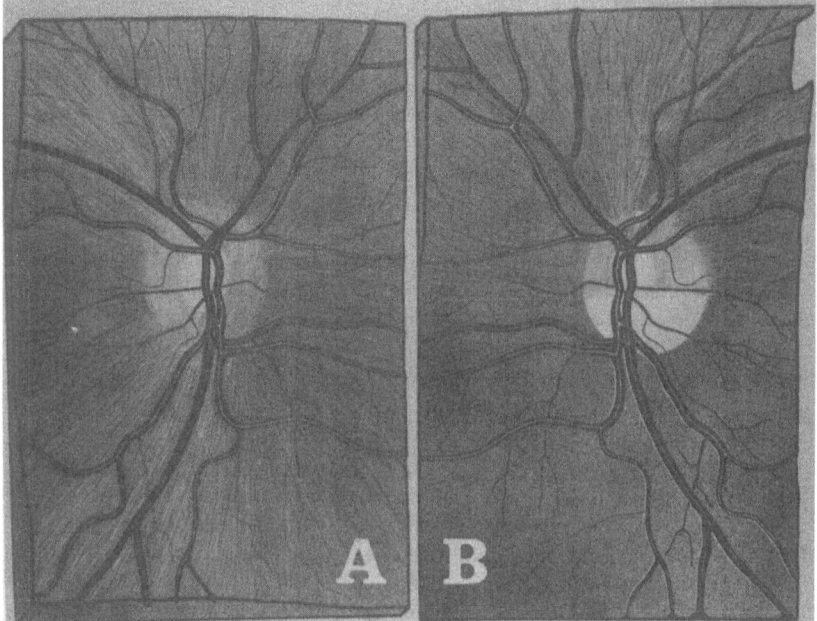

Fig. 1. Schematic representations of normal and abnormal retinal nerve fiber layers. A. Normal eye. B. Eye with complete lower altitudinal atrophy combined with an upper temporal sector defect.

conduction disturbances. Their cause is not known.

Axonal distension has also been described as a feature of optic neuritis, anterior ischemic optic neuropathy, and constrictive optic neuropathy (Hoyt 1976, Ito, Ozawa, Suga & Mizuno 1969, Lundström 1974). It is also seen in the early phase of Leber's acute optic neuropathy, together with hyperemia of the nerve fiber layer (Smith, Hoyt & Susac 1973). What causes axonal distension, and later axonal atrophy, in Leber's disease is as yet unknown. The same clinical picture with central scotomata and hyperemic axonal swelling is characteristic also of the acute phase of so-called tobacco-alcohol amblyopia (unpublished observations).

ATROPHY OF NERVE FIBRES

Damage to axons of the anterior visual pathway somewhere posterior to the eye may lead to both anterograde and retrograde axonal degeneration (Anderson 1973). Degeneration produces pallor of the optic disc and loss of retinal nerve fibers. A circumscript lesion may produce localized pallor and localized wasting of nerve fibers. Recent studies suggest that disc pallor primarily is caused by changes in light transmission and light reflection properties with loss of nerve fibers (Quigley & Anderson 1977). Pallor is an indirect sign of loss of nerve fibers. Its poor reliability in diagnosis requires no comment here. The essential hallmark of optic atrophy, viz. loss of axons, can be better evaluated by ophthalmoscopic examination of the peripapillary retina as the nerve fibers of the anterior visual pathway all have to pass through the peripapillary area to reach the optic disc. They are easier to visualize against the background of the retina and the choroid than against the background of the disc supporting tissues. Admittedly, funduscopic evaluation of nerve fiber bundles requires training: this is why this structure has escaped serious attention for so many years (Lundström 1977, Vannas, Raitta & Lemberg 1977).

Diffuse loss of axons

Complete loss of the retinal nerve fiber layer is easily recognized because of the resulting exposure of retinal and choroidal detail: small vessels can be seen unobscured by overlying nerve fiber bundles throughout their course, and minute detail characterizes also other retinal and choroidal structures. The denuded retina has a finely mottled appearance. The optic disc margin, of course, becomes very sharply defined with loss of overlying nerve fibers (Hoyt, Frisén & Newman 1973, Lundström & Frisén 1975, 1976) (Fig. 1 B).

A partial loss of nerve fibers, uniformly distributed across the optic nerve, is much more difficult to identify with present techniques, particularly if it is bilateral. Cases with unilateral lesions, or asymmetrical bilateral lesions, are best identified by juxta-positioning well focused fundus photographs, and looking for differences between the two eyes with regard to the relative prominence of nerve fiber opacity, and the definition of small detail. Experience with many such cases forces the conclusion that contemporary techniques for visual field evaluation leave much to be desired. Perimetry seems to be quite insensitive to a moderate loss of axons, if the loss is diffusely distributed. This suggests that small demands are put upon the visual system when it is put to the task of identifying an achromatic light spot on a neutral background. It is likely that better functional correlates of a diffuse drop-out of axons could be obtained by asking for resolution instead of mere detection. It is known that peripheral visual acuity is determined primarily by the density of working retinal ganglion cells (Frisén & Frisén 1976). Acuity should therefore drop with a drop in axonal density.

Chronic papilledema from raised intracranial pressure is an example of a disorder that appears to produce a predominantly diffuse loss of nerve fiber bundles. This contrasts with the classical view that this disorder first produces nasal visual field defects. It appears that the discrepancy may be instrumental rather than biological in that only the nasal periphery of the visual field is easily accessible to perimetric definition. True upper, lower, and temporal field limits can be obtained only by the use of eccentric fixation marks, and retraction of the eyelids (Frisén 1978) (Fig. 2). It is likely that the use of such precautions in the examination of patients with chronic, atrophic papilledema would show that the contraction of the visual field is truly concentric instead of primarily nasal, at least in the early stage.

Focal loss of nerve fibers

Focal loss denotes loss of nerve fibers within a circumscript region of the anterior visual pathway and the corresponding part of the retinal nerve fiber layer. The appearances of such defects depend on their depth, width, and position in relation to the circumference of the optic disc (Hoyt, Frisén & Newman 1973, Lundström & Frisén 1976). Full thickness defects are easiest to recognize, particularly within the arcuate bundles (Fig. 1 B). Partial thickness defects are more difficult to define but shallow grooves are often multiple, and tend to give the nerve fiber layer a raked appearance (Frisén & Hoyt 1974, Hoyt 1976, Hoyt, Frisén & Newman 1973, Lundström 1974). Focal defects are always bounded by curves conforming with the curvilinear arrangement of the nerve fiber bundles, and they always taper towards the optic disc. Narrow defects are usually best seen one to three disc diameters from the disc margin and fade from view both more peripherally, with decreasing thickness of the nerve fiber layer, and more centripetally, in the crowding of bundles at the disc margin. Broader, wedge-shaped defects may be followed for longer distances, sometimes all the way down to the disc margin. Focal defects are perhaps easiest to visualize in the atrophic stage of focal ischemic optic neuropathy, and in so-called low-tension glaucoma (Lundström 1974). Chronic glaucoma is considerably more difficult to evaluate as this appears to be a disease with a predominantly diffuse loss of axons: any focal defects are hard to appreciate ophthalmoscopically because of the poor contrast against the surrounding, diffusely wasted areas of the retinal nerve fiber layer (Hoyt, Frisén & Newman 1973, Iwata, Yaoeda &

8

Sofue 1975, Sommer, Miller, Pollack, Maumenee & George 1977).

The distribution of focal nerve fiber defects depends on the site of the lesion within the anterior visual pathway, and it is practical to subdivide the subject into optic nerve, chiasmal, and retrochiasmal lesions.

Optic nerve lesions

Focal nerve fiber defects are often encountered in optic nerve lesions of various types although a majority of such lesions certainly may be capable of producing also a diffuse attrition of axons. Irrespective of the actual mechanism of axonal damage, it will, if irreversible, result in descending degeneration of axons. The appearance of the nerve fiber layer therefore

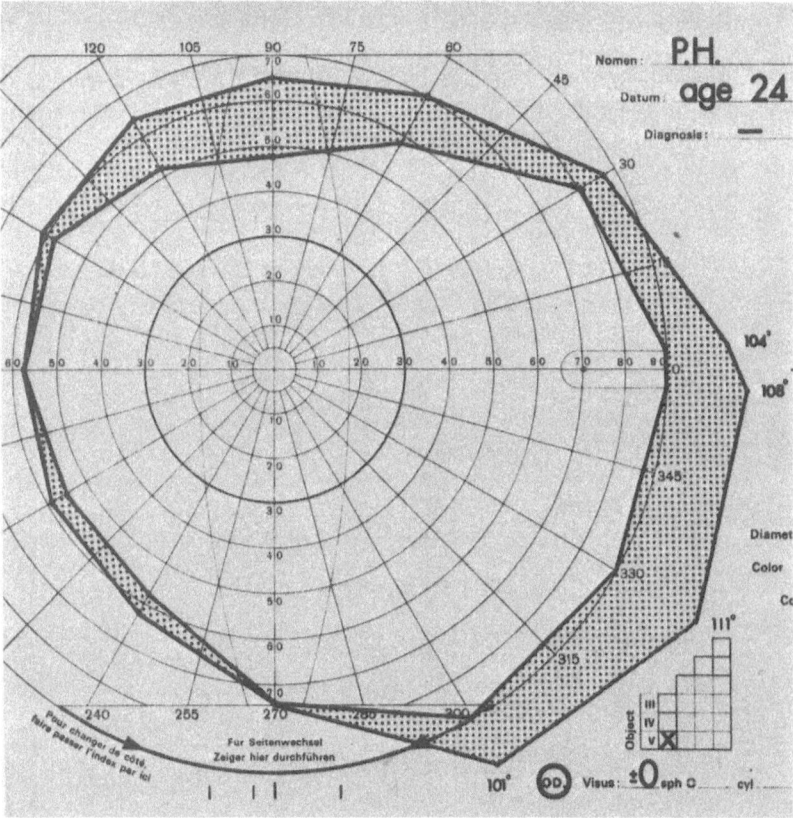

Fig. 2. Outer limits of the visual field of a normal subject (Haag-Streit perimeter, target V4). The inner curve was obtained in the conventional way, while the observations defining the outer curve were obtained with the aid of eccentric fixation marks, and retraction of the eyelids. The dotted area represents the area normally hidden from perimetric view (Frisén 1978).

cannot inform on the nature of the lesion. By analysing the distribution of the defects in the nerve fiber layer the prospects of obtaining diagnostic information become somewhat brighter. Toxic, acute demyelinating, and heredo-degenerative lesions apparently favor the papillomacular bundle in the optic nerve, with the production of a central scotoma with a more or less well conserved peripheral visual field. The papillomacular bundle is usually involved also in compressive lesions, although these lesions rarely save other bundles completely. Traumatic and vascular lesions often favour other bundles within the optic nerve, in keeping with their tendency to produce altitudinal visual field defects.

The correlation between the distribution of damage in the retinal nerve fiber layer, and the visual field defect, is generally very good in patients with substantial optic nerve lesions. Smaller lesions may be better identified by ophthalmoscopy than by routine visual field examinations (Frisén & Hoyt 1974, Hoyt, Frisén & Newman 1973, Sommer, Miller, Pollack, Maumenee & George 1977). Chronic demyelinating optic neuropathy is an example in point. This disease has a tendency, at least in the relatively early stages, to destroy quite small bundles of adjacent nerve fibers. The resulting scotomata are narrow and slit-like and they have the same orientation as the nerve fiber bundles. Such field defects are easiest to demonstrate in the arcuate

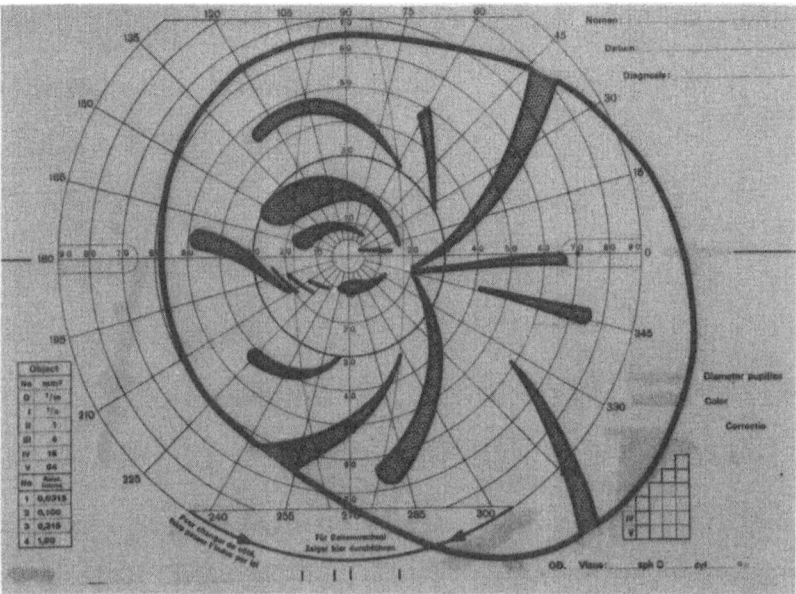

Fig. 3. Varieties of narrow, elongated scotomata expected with scattered loss of optic nerve fiber bundles, e.g. in glaucoma, drusen, and chronic demyelinating optic neuropathy. Many of these scotomata would be difficult to detect by conventional perimetry.

10

areas but they can occur also in other locations (Fig. 3). However, current perimetric procedures are not very sensitive to narrow, elongated field defects outside the arcuate areas (Frisén 1978).

Chiasmal lesions

Chiasmal lesions are regularly associated with localized wasting of retinal nerve fibers in both eyes (Lundström & Frisén 1976, 1977). Cases with extensive mid-chiasmal lesions affecting crossing nerve fibers, with complete bitemporal hemianopia, usually present very distinctive changes in the peripapillary area. The crossing nerve fibers, which have their cell bodies in the nasal hemi-retina, are then lost. This has the effect of enhancing the apparent contrast of the arcuate bundles. Sometimes there is also a horizontal band of pallor across the optic disc (Fig. 4). This picture, of course, suggests a very poor prognosis for recovery of vision upon removal of the responsible lesion. Less pronounced degrees of damage, as shown by incomplete loss of nerve fibers in nasal and papillomacular areas, and relative visual field defects, naturally indicate a better prognosis. It has been shown that there is a good correlation between the appearance of the nerve fiber layer with lesions of the chiasm due to pituitary adenoma, and the visual field defects, once the patient has reached a steady state stage after successful surgery (Lundström & Frisén 1976). Prior to surgery, many patients show field defects that are excessive in relation to the degree of atrophy (Lundström & Frisén 1977). Such excessive functional loss points to the operation of potentially reversible mechanisms for defective conduction, although the extent of recovery that is possible naturally is limited by the degree of structural damage.

Earlier stages of chiasmal disturbances, where visual impairment may be restricted to the upper temporal quadrants, are usually associated with the same distribution of nerve fiber damage as described above with hemifield visual defects (Lundström & Frisén 1976). This discrepancy is difficult to explain.

Importantly, many patients with seemingly pure temporal visual field defects also show signs of wasting of axons coming from the temporal hemi-retina. This indicates that anatomical damage in the chiasm often is more extensive than taught previously, an observation that correlates well with the usual appearance at surgery, with stretching of the whole chiasm over the tumor dome (Lundström & Frisén 1977). This affords an explanation for the sometime absence of focal visual field defects with suprasellar lesions (Möller & Hvid-Hansen 1970).

Although bitemporal hemianopia is a classical hallmark of chiasmal damage, asymmetric syndromes appear to be still more common. Again, ophthalmoscopic evaluation of the retinal nerve fiber layer improves insight into these phenomena. Take the patient with a unilateral temporal field defect and a contralateral normal field, for instance. Such a patient typically shows diffuse wasting of nerve fibers in the perimetrically normal eye. The problem of explaining a unilateral visual field defect in patients with chiasmal disorders is therefore not an anatomical problem, but an instrumental problem.

Also homonymous visual field defects are encountered now and then with suprasellar lesions. Clinical differentiation against optic tract lesion is often difficult, and the fundus changes associated with homonymous visual field defects due to anterior visual pathway lesions are better treated under a separate heading.

Optic tract and lateral geniculate lesions

Complete tract lesions, with complete homonymous hemianopia, produce distinctive changes in the ocular fundus (Hoyt & Kommerell 1973). In the eye contralateral to the lesion, the eye with the temporal field defect, the nerve fiber layer presents abnormalities that are indistinguishable from those produced by pure mid-chiasmal lesions. Abnormalities are more difficult to detect in the ipsilateral eye, the eye with the nasal hemianopia. Nasal hemianopia signifies impaired conduction from the temporal hemi-retina. This is served by fibers occupying parts of the arcuate bundles. These fibers intermingle with other fibers in the arcuate bundles, fibers that serve the *nasal* hemi-retina (Ogden 1974). Temporal hemi-retinal atrophy therefore does not produce complete loss of nerve fibers within the peripapillary area

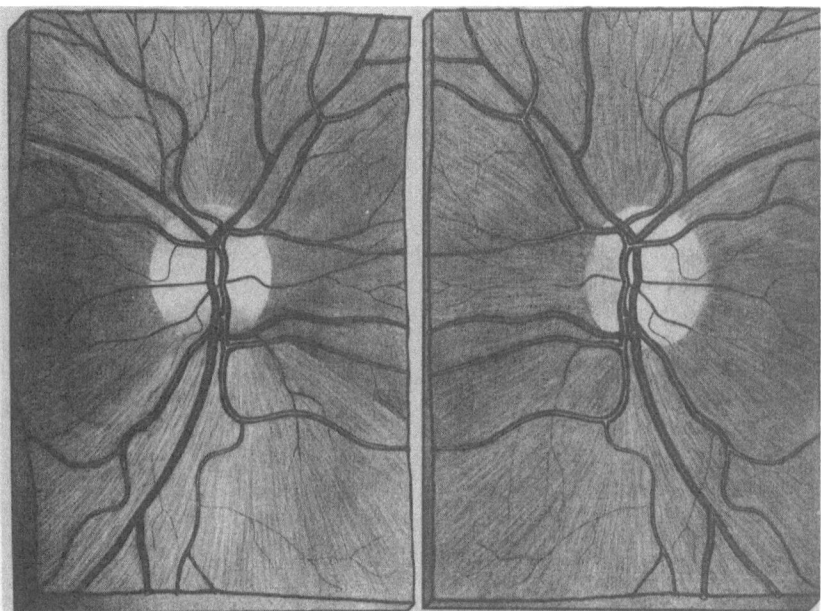

Fig. 4. Schematic representation of typical nerve fiber layer abnormalities due to a mid-chiasmal lesion, with bitemporal hemianopia.

but only thinning of the arcuate bundles (Fig. 5). Smaller degrees of damage, with relative visual field defects, are very difficult to detect ophthalmoscopically.

Tract lesions are generally impossible to distinguish from lateral geniculate lesions from the appearance of the fundus or the visual field defects (Hoyt 1975, Hoyt & Kommerell 1973). Homonymous sectorial defects, with corresponding sectorial optic atrophy, constitute an exception indicative of partial lateral geniculate damage (Frisén, Holmegaard & Rosencrantz 1978).

TIME COURSE OF OPTIC ATROPHY

A cross-sectional lesion of the optic nerve results in loss of axons about six weeks after the lesion (Lundström & Frisén 1975). Experimental studies show that degeneration does not occur step by step along the axon, but all of the axons anterior to the lesion degenerates at the same time (Anderson 1973). This observation suggests that the time course of fundus changes with anterior visual pathway lesions should be independent of the actual site of the lesion. The delay must be kept in mind when evaluating the retinal nerve fiber layer in patients with acute impairment of vision: the fiber bundles usually appear perfectly normal for several weeks following the debut of visual loss. Disc pallor is a still more protracted sign. The same

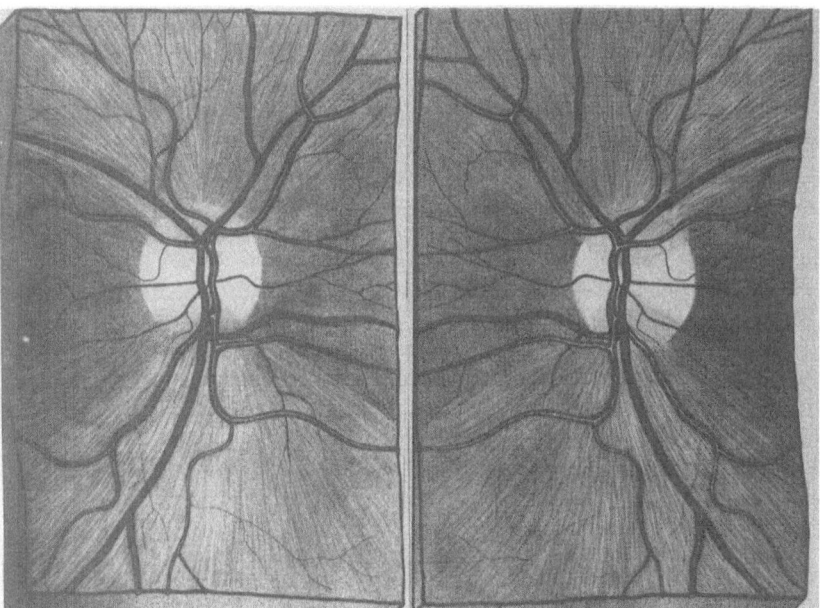

Fig. 5. Schematic representation of typical nerve fiber layer abnormalities due to a left retro-chiasmatic lesion, with right homonymous hemianopia.

delay occurs with slowly progressive lesions, so prudence needs always to be exercised when prognosticating the degree of recovery that may be possible. Further, the delayed appearance of atrophy may explain many instances of progression of optic atrophy following successful surgical treatment of the responsible lesion: the surgeon is not always to blame if atrophy progresses. Progression that occurs more than two months after surgery obviously must have another explanation, however (Lundström & Frisén 1977).

CONGENITAL VS. ACQUIRED OPTIC ATROPHY

The sequence of events outlined above is characteristic of lesions that damage the fully developed visual system. Lesions operating before complete development has occured regularly invoke compensatory mechanisms that adjust the diameters of the optic nervehead and the optic canal to the remaining mass of axons (Frisén & Holmegaard 1978). Hence lesions acquired before full development of the visual system are characterized not only by nerve fiber layer abnormalities and corollary visual field defects as described above, but also by remodelling of the optic disc. So-called hypoplasia of the optic nerve shares the characteristics of acquired optic atrophies and can be distinguished from acquired atrophy primarily by signs of disc remodelling, and lack of progression. Remodelling occurs also in de Morsier's syndrome (bitemporal visual field defects due to septo-optic dysplasia) (Davis & Shock 1975) and in early retro-chiasmal lesions (homonymous hemianopia with so-called homonymous hemioptic hypoplasia) (Hoyt, Rios-Montenegro, Behrens & Eckelhoff 1972). The size and shape of the optic disc therefore may be more important than its color in the evaluation of optic atrophy (Frisén & Holmegaard 1978).

The same type of funduscopic correlates of homonymous visual field defects that was described above is sometimes seen also in patients who have acquired *suprageniculate* lesions at an early age (Hoyt, Rios-Montenegro, Behrens & Eckelhoff 1972). This points to the possibility of trans-synaptic degeneration, at least in the immature visual system. At what age trans-synaptic degeneration no longer occurs is not yet known but there is nothing to indicate that substantial degeneration of this type occurs in adults. The oldest patient that I personally have seen with clear-cut nerve fiber layer abnormalities attributable to a suprageniculate lesion was 15 years old when she had a hemorrhage from her occipital arteriovenous malformation. This resulted in the production of a complete homonymous hemianopia. Nine years later there was a typical homonymous hemioptic atrophy with optic discs of normal size and shape. The normal disc dimensions ruled out a congenital lesion.

CONCLUSION

Evaluation of the state of the retinal nerve fiber layer in anterior visual pathway disease offers more than mere corroboration of visual field defects: it assists importantly in the development of individually appropriate perimetric strategies, it affords an objective means of identifying anatomical lesions that for various reasons may be difficult to detect by perimetry, and it allows successful prognostication of the possibilities of recovery. Under certain circumstances, it may even allow a rough timing of destructive events. Funduscopic evaluation of the peripapillary retinal nerve fiber layer is therefore a very useful complement to perimetry.

ACKNOWLEDGEMENT

Peter Hansson's assistance in producing the illustrations is gratefully acknowledged.

REFERENCES

Anderson, D.R. Ascending and descending optic atrophy produced experimentally in squirrel monkeys. *Amer. J. Ophthalmol.* 76: *693-711* (1973).

Davis, G.V. & Shock, J.P. Septo-optic dysplasia associated with see-saw nystagmus. *Arch. Ophthalmol.* 93: *137-139* (1975).

Frisén, L. The foundations of perimetric strategy. In H.S. Thompson (Ed): Topics in neuro-ophthalmology. Williams & Wilkins, in press.

Frisén, L. & Frisén, M. A simple relationship between the probability distribution of visual acuity and the density of retinal output channels. *Acta Ophthalmol.* 54: *437-444* (1976).

Frisén, L. & Hoyt, W.F. Insidious atrophy of retinal nerve fibers in multiple sclerosis. Funduscopic identification in patients with and without visual complaints. *Arch. Ophthalmol.* 92: *91-97* (1974).

Frisén, L. & Holmegaard, L. Spectrum of optic nerve hypoplasia. *Brit. J. Ophthalmol.* 62: *7-15* (1978).

Frisén, L., Holmegaard, L. & Rosencrantz, M. Sectorial optic atrophy and homonymous, horizontal sectoranopia : a lateral choroidal artery syndrome? *J. Neurol. Neurosurg. Psychiat.* 41: *374-380* (1978).

Hayreh, S.S. Optic disc edema in raised intracranial pressure. V. Pathogenesis. *Arch. Ophthalmol.* 95: *1553-1565* (1977).

Hoyt, W.F. Geniculate hemianopias: incongruous visual field defects from partial involvement of the lateral geniculate nucleus. *Proc. Austral. Assoc. Neurol.* 12: *7-16* (1975).

Hoyt, W.F. Ophthalmoscopy of the retinal nerve fiber layer in neuroophthalmologic diagnosis. *Austral. J. Ophthalmol.* 4: *13-34* (1976).

Hoyt, W.F., Frisén, L. & Newman, N.M. Funduscopy of nerve fiber layer defects in glaucoma. *Invest. Ophthalmol.* 12: *814-829* (1973).

Hoyt, W.F. & Kommerell, G. Der Fundus oculi bei homonymer Hemianopie. *Klin. Mbl. Augenheilkd.* 162: *456-464* (1973).

Hoyt, W.F., Rios-Montenegro, E.N., Behrens, M.M. & Eckelhoff, R.J. Homonymous hemioptic hypoplasia. Funduscopic features in standard and red-free illumination in three patients with congenital hemiplegia. *Brit. J. Ophthalmol.* 56: *537-545* (1972).

Ito, H., Ozawa, K., Suga, S. & Mizuno, K. Red-free light magnifying photography in neuritis and some retinal vascular lesions. *Folia Ophthalmol. Japon.* 20: *282-287* (1969).

Iwata, K., Yaoeda, H. & Sofue, K. Changes of retinal nerve fiber layer in glaucoma. Report 2. Clinical observations. *Acta Soc. Ophthalmol. Japon.* 79: *1101-1118* (1975).

15

Lundström, M. Wasting of nerve fibers in the retina. Photographic documentation. *Acta Ophthalmol.* 52: *872-880* (1974).

Lundström, M. Atrophy of optic nerve fibers in compression of the chiasm. Observer variation in assessment of atrophy. *Acta Ophthalmol.* 55: *217-226* (1977).

Lundström, M. Optic atrophy in compression of the chiasm. A funduscopic study of the human retinal nerve fiber layer. Thesis, University of Göteborg (1977). (Can be obtained from the author.)

Lundström, M. & Frisén, L. Evolution of descending optic atrophy. A case report. *Acta Ophthalmol.* 53: *738-746* (1975).

Lundström, M. & Frisén, L. Atrophy of optic nerve fibres in compression of the chiasm. Degree and distribution of ophthalmoscopic changes. *Acta Ophthalmol.* 54: *623-640* (1976).

Lundström, M. & Frisén, L. Atrophy of optic nerve fibres in compression of the chiasm. Prognostic implications. *Acta Ophthalmol.* 55: *208-216* (1977).

McLeod, D., Marshall, J., Kohner, E.M. & Bird, A.C. The role of axoplasmic transport in the pathogenesis of retinal cotton-wool spots. *Brit. J. Ophthalmol.* 61: *177-191* (1977).

Möller, P.M. & Hvid-Hansen, O. Chiasmal visual fields. *Acta Ophthalmol.* 48: *678-684* (1970).

Ogden, T.E. The nerve-fiber layer of the primate retina: an autoradiographic study. *Invest. Ophthalmol.* 13: *95-100* (1974).

Quigley, H.A. & Anderson, D.R. The histologic basis of optic disk pallor in experimental optic atrophy. *Amer. J. Ophthalmol.* 83: *709-717* (1977).

Smith, J.L., Hoyt, W.F. & Susac, J.O. Ocular fundus in acute Leber optic neuropathy. *Arch. Ophthalmol.* 90: *349-354* (1973).

Sommer, A., Miller, N.R., Pollack, I., Maumenee, A.E. & George, T. The nerve fiber layer in the diagnosis of glaucoma. *Arch. Ophthalmol.* 95: *2149-2156* (1977).

Vannas, A., Raitta, C. & Lemberg, S. Photography of the nerve fiber layer in retinal disturbances. *Acta Ophthalmol.* 55: *79-87* (1977).

Author's address:
Department of Ophthalmology
University of Göteborg
Sahlgren's Hospital
S – 413 45 Göteborg
Sweden

CORRELATIONS BETWEEN ATROPHY OF MACULOPAPILLAR BUNDLES AND VISUAL FUNCTIONS IN CASES OF OPTIC NEUROPATHIES

YUSAKU TAGAMI

(Kobe, Japan)

ABSTRACT

The various degrees of atrophy of maculopapillar bundles in 55 cases (88 eyes) of steady state optic neuropathies with central scotomas have been examined by red-free fundus photography. Furthermore, in order to facilitate the classification of the degree of the atrophy the densitometric patterns of the maculopapillar bundles were ascertained.

A close relationship was found to exist between the central field depressions in Tübinger's static perimetry and the degree of the atrophy. With developing atrophy the visual acuity decreased in a large number of cases. In some cases however an excellent visual acuity despite a marked reduction of the bundles could be observed, showing sieve-like depressions in Tübinger's perimetry. Thanks to the newly developed Quantitative Maculometry with direct fundus examination, it was possible to find an increased sensitivity at the fovea in these cases.

For the prognosis of the visual functions in optic neuropathies with central socomas it is thus recommended that accurate examinations of the central visual field as well as examination of the nerve fiber bundles should be undertaken.

INTRODUCTION

In a large number of optic neuropathy cases, central scotomas due to the involvement of maculopapillar bundles can be found thanks to kinetic or static perimetry. It is therefore important in these cases to ascertain the exact state of the maculopapillar bundles which can be done by red-free fundus photography (Behrendt & Wilson 1965, Hoyt, Schlicke & Eckelhoff 1972).

I want to present a classification of the atrophic stages of the maculopapillar bundles in their relationship with visual functions.

METHOD

55 cases (88 eyes) of optic neuropathies (retrobulbar type) with central scotomas — all admitted to the eye clinic of the Kobe University Hospital between the years 1975 and 1977 — were examined by red-free fundus photography with regard to the atrophic state of the maculopapillar bundles.

17

A Topcon TRC F3 fundus camera with a 2X magnification attachment was used for the red-free fundus photography.

A Fuji BPB53 filter was adapted to the red-free filter with a transmission peak of 530 nm (Tagami & Isayama 1975). The Kodak Tri-X Pan film was printed on Mitsubishi photographic paper Gekko V-4 and the paper prints were reproduced on Kodak Plus-X Pan film. Thanks to this double reproduction method the picture contrast could be considerably improved (Lundström & Frisén 1976).

In some cases the densitometric patterns of the maculopapillar bundles in the Kodak Plus-X films were studied with linear scanning measurements by using a dual-wavelength TLC scanner (Shimazu CS-900). These measurements allowed a more accurate establishment of the atrophic state of the nerve fiber bundles.

The visual fields were examined with Goldmann's kinetic and Tübinger's static perimetry. In some cases, Quantitative Maculometry with direct fundus examination (Isayama & Tagami 1977) was chosen in order to obtain sensitivity measurements at definit points in the retina inside the 5 degree region from the fovea. The visual functions were compared with the stage of atrophy of the maculopapillar bundles which were photographed in steadystate periods in each case at least two months following treatment.

RESULTS

A) Classification of Atrophic Stages
of Maculopapillar Bundles

In this series of optic neuropathies with central scotomas no slit-like defects (Hoyt, Frisén & Newman, 1973) in the maculopapillar bundles could be observed through red-free fundus photography. I found only diffuse and total atrophies of the maculopapillar bundles. There were various degrees of diffuse atrophy. This allowed me to classify the atrophic changes in maculopapillar bundles into four stages (Table I).

Stage 1: (normal state or only slight diffuse atrophy) Almost normal striation and nerve fiber opacity. Obvious obscuration of the vessels (crosshatching) of all sizes. No retinal mottling.

Stage 2: (moderate diffuse atrophy) Minor striation, but prominent nerve fiber opacity. Some obscuration of the vessels. No retinal mottling.

Stage 3: (severe diffuse atrophy) Hardly visible striation, but presence of nerve fiber opacity. Some obscuration of the vessels. No retinal mottling.

Stage 4: (total atrophy) No visible striation nor nerve fiber opacity. No obscuration of the vessels. Presence of retinal mottling.

The following are typical optic neuropathy cases corresponding to the four atrophic stages.

Case 1: 53-year-old male, retrobulbar optic neuritis. Atrophic stage 1. His corrected left vision was 20/20. A slight depression of the central field (minimal depression) was observed in applying Tübinger's static perimetry (Fig. 1).

Table 1. Atrophic stages of maculopapillar bundles in optic neuropathies.

	1	2	3	4
retinal striation	‖	+	±	−
nerve fibre opacity	‖	‖	+	−
crosshatching	‖	+	+	−
retinal mottling	−	−	−	‖

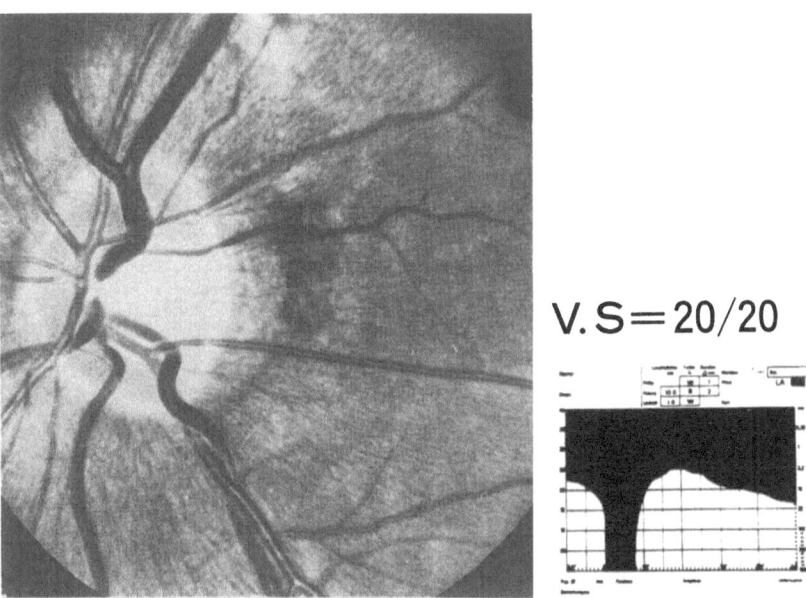

V. S = 20/20

Fig. 1. Red-free fundus photograph and Tübinger's central field (180°) in case 1 (Stage 1).

19

Case 2: 32-year-old male, retrobulbar optic neuritis. Atrophic stage 2. His corrected left vision was 20/30 and a sieve-like depression of the central field was observed in Tübinger's static perimetry (Fig. 2).

Case 3: 40-year-old male, retrobulbar optic neuritis. Atrophy stage 3. His corrected left vision was 20/60. Sieve-like depression of the central field was observed in Tübinger's static perimetry (Fig. 3).

Case 4: 28-year-old male, retrobulbar optic neuritis. Atrophic stage 4. The visual acuity in his left eye was 20/600 at the onset and it did not improve. Tübinger's perimetry revealed a complete depression of the central field (Fig. 4).

B) *Densitometric Patterns of Maculopapillar Bundles*

The densitometric patterns of the maculopapillar bundles at each atrophic stage were studied by using linear scanning of the Kodak Plus-X pan films with a 0.5 x 0,05mm blue light (wavelength 450 nm). The linear scanning was carried out vertically along 10 degrees nasal from the fovea.

Between the large peaks of the retinal vessels, small peaks of the maculopapillar bundles could be observed and their amplitude decreased with increasing atrophy. In total atrophy (Atrophic stage 4) relatively large peaks according to the retinal mottling were observed (Fig. 5).

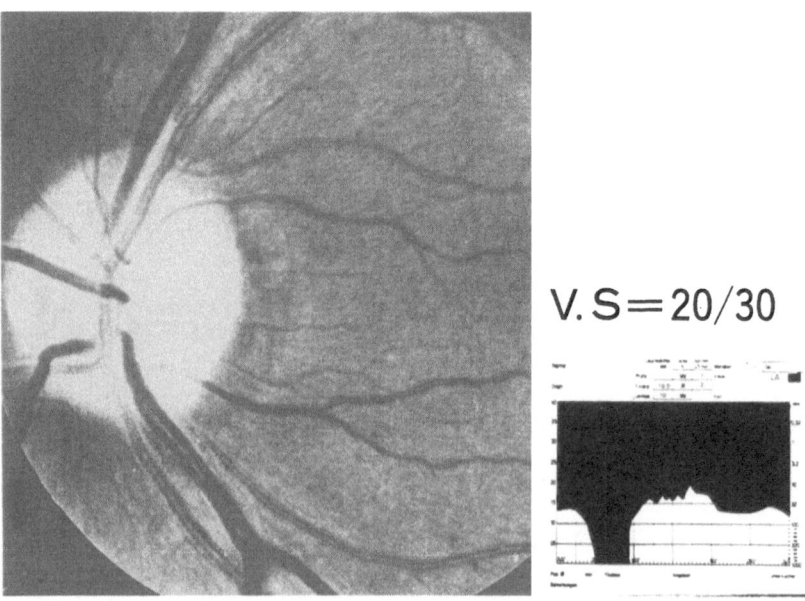

Fig. 2. Red-free fundus photograph and Tübinger's central field (180°) in case 2 (Stage 2).

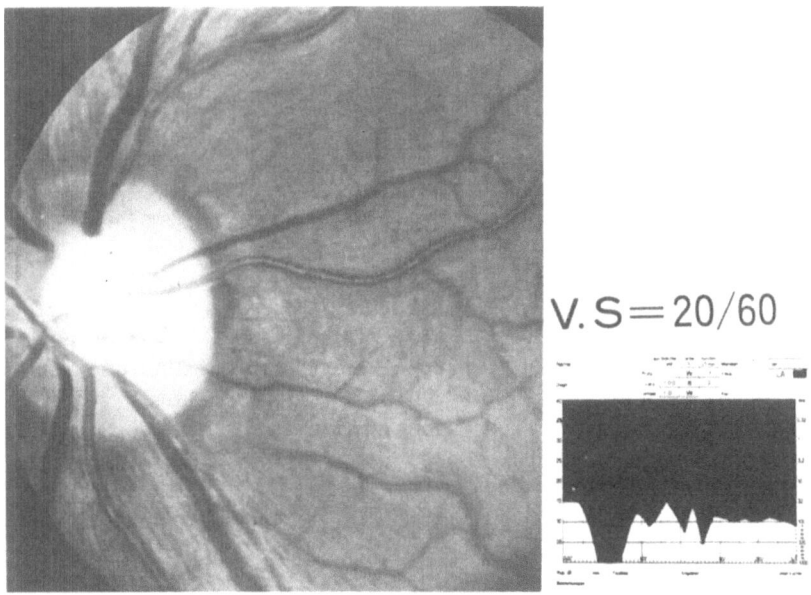

Fig. 3. Red-free fundus photograph and Tübinger's central field (180°) in case 3 (Stage 3).

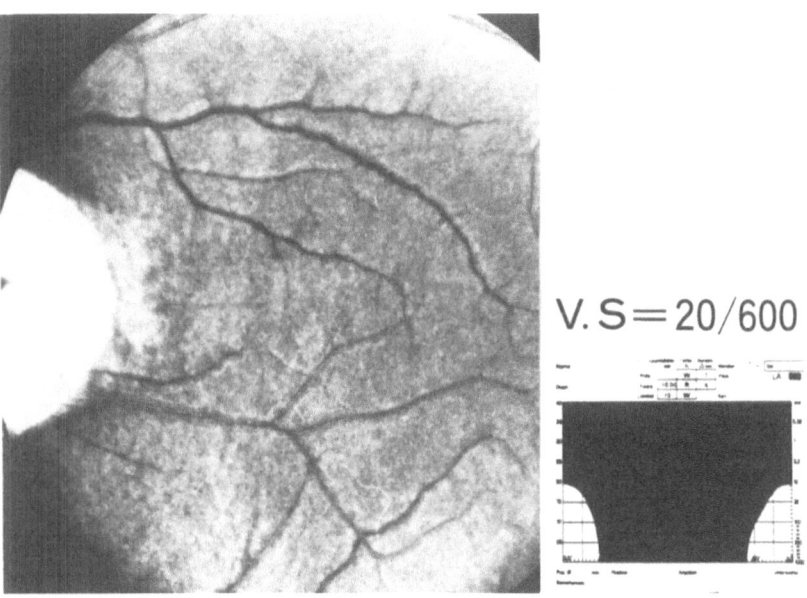

Fig. 4. Red-free fundus photograph and Tübinger's central field (180°) in case 4 (Stage 4).

C) Correlation Between Atrophic Stages
and Visual Functions

1) Visual Acuity

A rather close relationship was found to exist between the atrophic stages of the maculopapillar bundles and the decreasing of the visual acuity, except for some cases in stage 3 where the visual acuity remained excellent (Fig. 6).

2) Tübinger's Static Central
Visual Field

I devided the central visual field changes observed in cases of optic neuropathy into four types according to Tübinger's static perimetry with a 7' white stimulus on a 10 asb. white background illumination.

Type 1: minimal deficit; slight depression of the central field.

Type 2: sieve-like depression.

Type 3: Island-like fields; some small visual islands in an almost depressed central field.

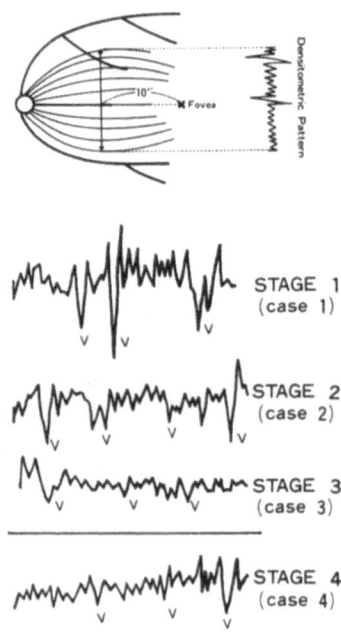

Fig. 5. Schematic drawing of the portion of which linear scanning was carried out (between arrows) and densitometric pattern of maculopapillar bundles in each atrophic stages.

V: retinal vessels.

22

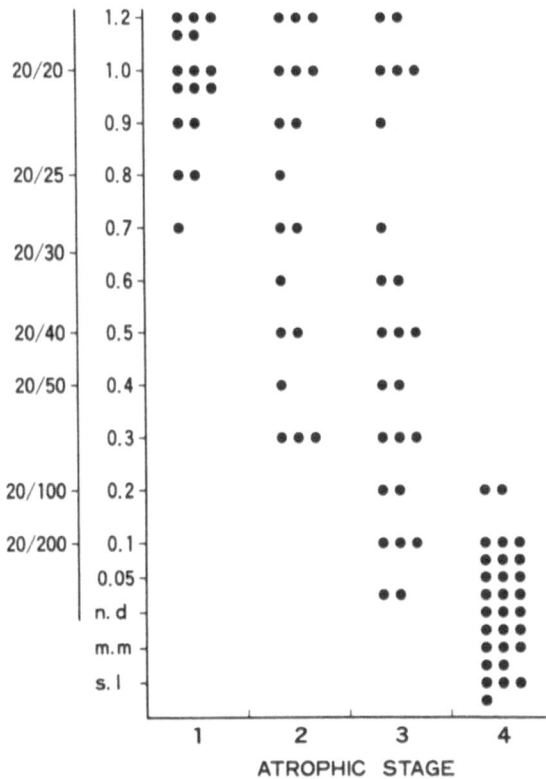

Fig. 6. Relationship between visual acuity and atrophic stages.

Table 2. Relationship between Tübinger's static central fields and atrophic stages.

	1	2	3	4
minimal deficit	16	6	0	0
general or sieve-like depression	0	12	18	0
island-like depression	0	0	6	6
complete depression	0	0	0	23

23

Type 4: complete depression.

A close relationship was found to exist between the central field depression types and the atrophic stages of the maculopapillar bundles (Table 2).

3) Quantitative Maculometry with Direct Fundus Examination

Static measurement by Quantitative Maculometry was carried out in 4 cases (6 eyes) of optic neuropathies of the atrophic stage 3 which showed excellent visual acuity of over 20/25 and presented sieve-like depression in Tübinger's static central fiedl. A 6.37' white light stimulus with a 250 asb. white background illumination was used for the measurement inside 5 degrees from the fovea. The measurement through direct fundus examination revealed increased sensitivity at the fovea in correspondance with the excellent visual acuity.

The following is a typical case of the atrophic stage 3 with excellent visual acuity of 20/20.

Case 5: 25-year-old male, retrobulbar optic neuritis. His improved vision was 20/20. A sieve-like depression in Tübinger's central field was observed. The static measurements by the Quantitative Maculometry indicated increased sensitivity at the fovea corresponding to the regained excellent visual acuity (Fig. 7).

DISCUSSION

The maculopapillar bundles are the most important retinal nerve fibers because of their close relationship with visual acuity and the central visual field. It is therefore important to examine the condition of the maculopapillary bundles when we deal with optic neuropathy cases with central scotomas.

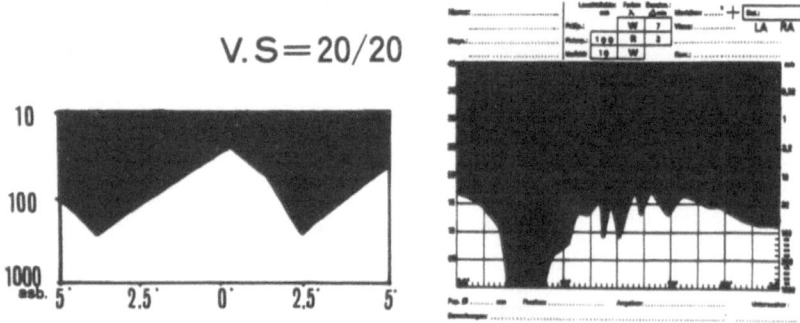

Fig. 7. Tübinger's perimetry and Quantitative Maculometry (180°) in case 5.

It could be observed, in red-free fundus photography, that the nerve fibers of squirrel monkeys disappears within 4 to 5 weeks after the severance of the optic nerve at the apex of the orbit (Anderson 1973), and Lundström & Frisén reported in 1975 the disappearance of the retinal nerve fiber layer within 4 to 8 weeks after a severe trauma of the intracranial optic nerve (Lundström & Frisén 1975).

Hoyt, Frisén & Newman (1973) described four types of atrophic changes of nerve fiber bundles, that is slit-like defects, wedge-like defects, diffuse atrophy and total atrophy. Lundström & Frisén (1976) reported a grading of ophthalmoscopic signs of diffuse atrophies in chiasmal lesions. In my series of optic neuropathy cases with central scotoma, no slit-like defects could be observed, but various degrees of diffuse atrophy and total atrophy were found.

The maculopapillar bundles are difficult to examine through ordinary ophthalmoscopes or fundus cameras, because they tend to be less compact near the optic disc than the arcuate fibers. Using a bright red-free filter such as Fuji BPB 53 (transmission peak 530 nm) enabled me to observe the minute changes of the maculopapillar bundles of the optic neuropathy cases and classify their atrophic conditions into four stages.

The densitometric patterns allow the classification of the atrophic stages of the bundles. The densitometric peaks of the maculopapillar bundles showed a reduced amplitude with developing atrophy, but a relatively high amplitude related to the retinal mottling was found in the total atrophic cases (Stage 4).

The relationship between the atrophic stages and the visual functions, was found to be close when I compared the central field depressions in Tübinger's static perimetry and the various degrees of atrophy. With developing atrophy the visual acuity decreased in a large number of cases. However in some cases at Stage 3, excellent visual acuity of over 20/25 could be observed. In these cases a sieve-like depression could be found according to Tübinger's static central field, and when I used Quantitative Maculometry with direct fundus examination, I found an increased sensitivity at the fovea.

These data suggest that the function of the nerve fiber bundles deriving from the fovea remain intact, despite a marked reduction of the function near the fovea in the cases with excellent visual acuity. In other words, there may remain normally functioning nerve fiber bundles parting from the fovea, in spite of a marked reduction of the bundles near the fovea.

There is, therefore, a great possibility of excellent visual acuity even if the atrophic stage of the maculopapillar bundles is progressing and reaches a severe degree, as could be observed through red-free fundus photography. Follow-ups and treatment over extended periods are thus advisable in cases of optic neuropathy with central scotomas even in advanced atrophic stages.

From this study it can be concluded that examination of the nerve fiber bundles through red-free photography as well as accurate measurements of the central visual field are necessary to establish the prognosis of the visual functions in optic neuropathy cases with central scotomas.

ACKNOWLEDGEMENT

I am extremely grateful to Prof. Yoshimasa Isayama for his various helpful suggestions during the course of this study.

REFERENCE

Anderson, D.R. Ascending and descending optic atrophy produced experimentally in squirrel monkeys. *Am. J. Ophthalmol.* 76: *693-711* (1973).

Behrendt, T. & Wilson, L.A. Spectral reflectance photography of the retina. *Am. J. Ophthalmol.* 59: *1079-1088* (1965).

Hoyt, W.F., Schlicke, B. & Eckelhoff, R.J. Funduscopic appearance of a nerve-fiber-bundle defect. *Br. J. Ophthalmol.* 56: *577-583* (1972).

Hoyt, W.F., Frisén, L. & Newman, N.M. Funduscopy of nerve fiber layer defects in glaucoma. *Invest. Ophthalmol.* 12: *814-829* (1973).

Isayama, Y. & Tagami, Y. Quantitative Maculometry using a new instrument in cases of optic neuropathies. *Docum. Ophthalmol. Proc. Series* 14: *237-242* (1977).

Lundström, M. & Frisén, L. Evolution of descending optic atrophy, a case report. *Acta. Ophthalmol.* 53: *738-746* (1975).

Lundström, M. & Frisén, L. Atrophy of optic nerve fibers in compression of the chiasma, degree and distribution of ophthalmoscopic changes. *Acta. Ophthalmol.* 54: *623-640* (1976).

Tagami, Y. & Isayama, Y. Funduscopic appearance of nerve fiber bundles in optic nerve disorders. *Jap. Rev. Clin. Ophthalmol.* 70: *238-242* (1976).

Author's address:
Department of Ophthalmology
School of Medicine
Kobe University
Kusunoki-cho, 7-chome, Ikuta-ku
Kobe, Japan

VISUAL FIELD DEFECTS DUE TO
TUMORS OF THE SELLAR REGION

YOSHIMASA ISAYAMA

(Kobe, Japan)

ABSTRACT

This report is based on a review of pre-operative visual field changes in 135 patients with sellar and parasellar tumors, all of them having operated either at the ophthalmological or the neurosurgical clinics of Kobe University, all in the years from 1968 to 1977.
1) Classification of 66 cases of pituitary adenoma, 31 cases of craniopharyngioma, 24 cases of meningioma and 14 cases of miscellaneous tumors.
2) Division of visual field defects into three groups: a) the symmetric type, b) the asymmetric type and c) the atypical type with detailed discussion.
3) Evaluation of various perimetric measurement methods for chiasmal tumors.
4) Discussion of central field observations including sparing macula.

INTRODUCTION

It is a wellknown fact that the ocular signs and symptomes of the chiasmal syndrome consist of a bitemporal visual field defect and pallor of the optic disc; such cardinal changes in the visual field occur only at the advanced stage of tumors. With carefully performed perimetry can be found a number of slight variations, such as scotomatous field defects and irregular depressions of the peripheral field etc. at an early stage of a chiasmal lesion. Attention to this fact has been drawn by various researchers (Adler, Austin & Grant 1948, Bakey 1950, Chamlin, Davidoff & Feiring 1955, Cushing & Walker 1915, Harms 1954, Henderson 1939, Lyle & Clover 1961, Imachi, Inoue, Kani & Umeda 1969, Walsh & Hoyt 1969).

This report is mainly based on a review of pre-operative visual field changes in 135 patients with sellar and parasellar tumors, all of them having been operated either at the ophthalmological or the neurosurgical clinics of Kobe University and the tumors having been ascertained, all in the years from 1968 to 1977.

The first table shows the list of tumors under observation: among them there are 66 cases of pituitary adenoma – of which 53 classified as chromophobe adenoma and 13 as eosinophilic adenoma – 31 cases of craniopharyngioma, 24 cases of meningioma of the tuberculum sellae (the sphenoidal ridge and the olfactory groove) and finally 14 cases of miscellaneous tumors. The main procedure of examination of the visual field defects produced by the chiasmal lesion was done kinetically with the Goldmann's perimeter.

27

As this paper will be limited to the cases of pituitary adenoma, cranio-pharyngioma and meningioma, all chiasmal lesions due to optic glioma, ectopic pinealmoma etc. are excluded.

The cases have been divided into three groups based on the type of the visual field defects observed.

The first group shows a typical progression of the defect, starting with the early loss in the upper temporal quadrant, then affecting in a clockwise movement the right field and in an anticlockwise movement the left field. Classified in the second group is the appearance of amaurosis of one eye with following field defects in the other eye. Atypical interferences of the visual field figure in the third group.

Table 1. Classification of tumors in the sellar and parasellar region.

TUMORS OF SELLAR AND PARASELLAR REGION

(1968 ~ 1977, 135 Cases)

Classification of Tumors	Number of Cases	
Pituitary Adenoma	66	
Chromophobe		53
Eosinophile		13
Craniopharyngioma	31	
Meningioma	24	
Miscellaneous	14	
Ectopic Pinealoma		4
Optic Glioma		4
Glioma of Frontal Lobe		1
Chorioepithelioma		1
Epidermoid Above the Chiasm		1
The IIIrd Ventricle Ependimona		1
Trigeminal Neurinoma		1
Chordoma		1
	Total 135	

1. FIRST GROUP: THE SYMMETRIC TYPE

The earliest changes caused by the chiasmal tumors are indicated by the central isopters. When there is a depression only in the central isopters, i.e. I-1 and I-2 with irregular loss of the peripheral field, the symbol 'a', is given; on the other hand when all isopters are affected the symbol 'b'. Contrary to the generally held opinion that the 'b' defects are more frequent than the 'a' defects in our findings the 'a' defects appear in greater number (Table 2).

In the cases of adenoma, the loss of only the central isopters dominate in the distinct loss of the temporal fields. On the contrary in craniopharyngioma 'a' and 'b' show almost identical numbers. There is less evidence of a distinct bitemporal hemianopsia in the cases of symmetric progression (13%). It has been emphasized that the quantitative analysis of the central part of a visual field is of dominant importance.

2. SECOND GROUP: THE ASYMMETRIC TYPE (TABLE 3)

The loss of the visual field may progress more rapidly in one eye than in the other and can lead to complete unilateral blindness.

It is generally said that the unilateral onset of ocular involvement is characteristic for the patients affected with meningioma of the tuberculum sellae and the cases under review here confirm indeed that there is a greater number of asymmetric existence found in patients with meningioma (54%)

Table 2. Visual field defects due to chiasmal tumors. The first group shows a typical progression of the defects.

THE FIRST GROUP

Classification of Tumors / VF Defects		Pituitary Adenoma		Cranio-pharyngioma	Meningioma
		Chromophobe	Eosinophile		
1/4 1/4	a a	1	1	1	
	a b				
	b b				
1/4 1/2	a a	4			
	b a			1	
	a b				1
	b b		1		
1/2 1/2	a a	11	2	5	2
	a b	2		1	1
	b b	9	1	6	
3/4 1/2	a a				
	a b				
	b a	1			2
	b b	2		4	
3/4 3/4	a a	1			
	a b				
	b b	1			

a   b   1/4
a   b   1/2
a   b   3/4

29

than among those with other chiasmal tumors (adenoma: 10%, craniopharyngioma: 13%).

3. THIRD GROUP: THE ATYPICAL
VISUAL FIELD DEFECTS (TABLE 4)

Under this heading are classified scotomas of various sizes and types, irregular defects of either the central or the peripheral isopters and altitudinal defects. 35 cases, accounting for 29% of the total 121 cases, can be considered as atypical with regard to the visual field changes they produced. Such changes, particularly those of scotomatous nature, have been considered as the earliest manifestation of a pressure exercised by a tumor. In various cases however the operation finding of the location of the tumor does not explain the particular kind of visual field defects. It can be assumed that various other factors than the contact of the visual pathway with the tumor, cause such atypical field defects. The visual field defects of these 3 groups have been summarized (Fig. 1). In the meningioma cases a different tendency was found when compared with the other two tumor groups. The correlation between the surgical findings and the visual field defects and suggested explanations for the possible cause of the atypical defects are presented in the following cases. (Isayama & Takahashi et al. 1975, Takahashi, Nakamura & Isayama 1976).
Case 1: Temporal hemianoptic scotoma in one eye (Fig. 2). The peripheral visual field of both eyes was normal. Only a right hemianoptic scotoma

Table 3. Visual field defects due to chiasmal tumors. The second group: Ammaurosis of one eye appears with following field defects in the other eye.

SECOND GROUP

Classification of Tumors VF Defects		Pituitary Adenoma		Cranio-pharyngioma	Meningioma
		Chromophobe	Eosinophile		
0, Normal					1
0, Central Scotoma		1			1
0, 1/4	a				
	b				
0, 1/2	a				2
	b	2	1	3	7
0, 3/4	a				
	b	3		1	1
0, 0					1

Table 4. Visual field defects due to chiasmal tumors. In the third group the atypical field defects such as scotomas of various sizes and types, irregular defects, defects of altitude are classified.

THE THIRD GROUP

Classification Tumors / VF Defects	Pituitary Adenoma		Cranio-pharyingioma	Meningioma
	Chromophobe	Eosinophile		
Normal, Normal		7		
Normal, Irregular			1	
Normal, 1/4	2			
Normal, 1/2	2		1	
Normal, Altitudinal				1
Normal, C.S.	1			1 Hemi-anoptic
C.C., C.S.				1
C.S., C.S.			1	
1/2, C.S.	1		1, Para 1	
Irregular, Irregular	1			
Irregular, 1/2	1		1	
Irregular, 3/4	1			
Altitudinal, Altitudinal				1
1/2, Altitudinal	1		1	
C.C., 1/2	2		1	
C.C., 3/4	1			
Homonymous	2		1	
Total	15	7	9	4

C.C. = Concentric Concentration

C.S. = Central Scotoma

could be observed. Verification of the tumor revealed a meningioma of the tuberculum sellae. The right optic nerve was distended and rather thin and looked as being compressed laterally. The left optic nerve however was found to be in an almost normal position. The extention of the tumor below the chiasm was slight. It is difficult to explain the cause of the central visual defect.

Case 2: Central and paracentral scotoma due to a homonymous defect (Fig. 3a, b). Temporal paracentral scotoma on the right side and central scotoma and upper-nasal quadrantpsia on the left side. The operation revealed that the chiasm was prefixed. A cystic chromophobe adenoma extended in a left nasal direction to the interpreduncular cistern. The chiasm, both optic nerves and the left optic tract were humped over by the tumor and the nerves were thin. The short optic nerves of either side were pushed against the bone at the entrance of the optic canal. Prefixation may have been the cause of the involvement of the left optic tract, producing an atypical homonymous defect and the optic nerve compression may have caused the central scotoma.

Case 3: Notching by the anterior cerebral artery (Fig. 14a, b). Perimetric patterns indicated irregular lower field defects in some of the central isopters. Operation findings revealed an upward extention of the chromophobe adenoma. The atrophic thin chiasm was humped over by the tumor. Above the

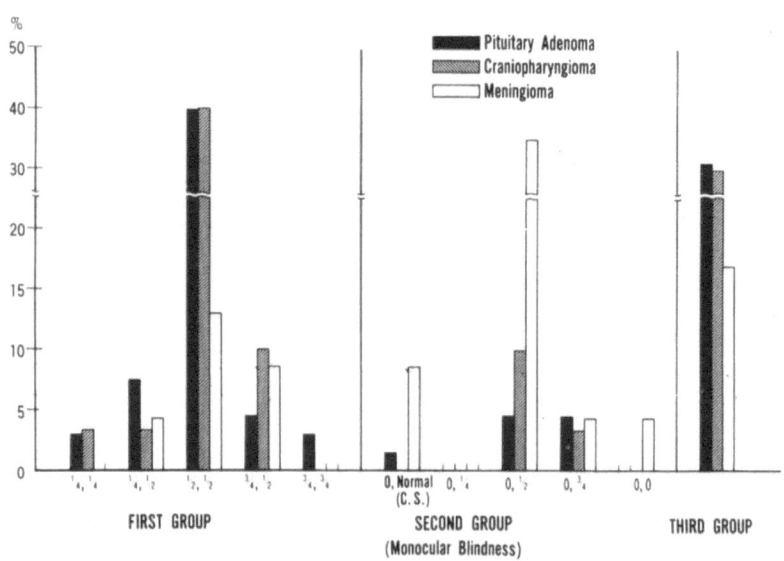

Fig. 1. Summarization of the visual field defects of the 3 groups.

chiasm and above either of the optic nerves however no tumor was found. The anterior cerebral artery was notched into the chiasm. The defect of the lower field may have derived from the notching of the anterior cerebral artery.

Case 4: Temporal hemianopsia on one side (Fig. 5). The visual field showed a temporal hemianopsia only in the central isopters of the right eye and normal findings in the left. Tumor verification indicated craniopharyngioma. The cystic tumor had enclosed the right optic nerve and the internal carotide artery, and extended to the anterior fossa. The right optic nerve was slightly pushed upward. After puncture of the cyst, the tumor

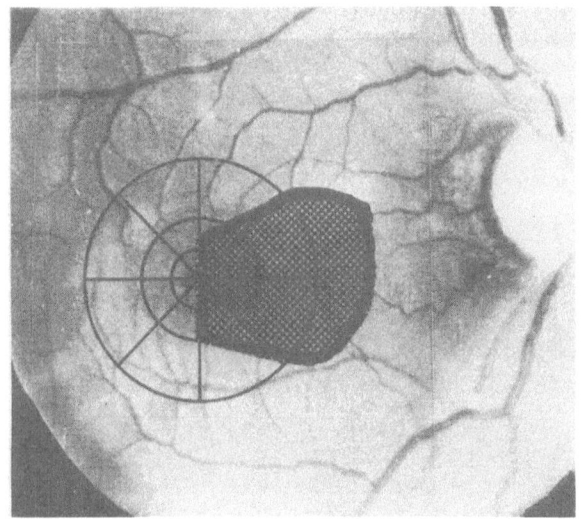

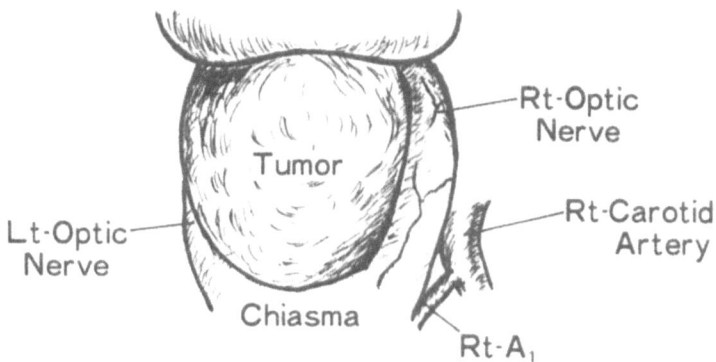

Fig. 2. Case 1 Upper: A hemianoptic central scotoma in the right eye observed by our Fundus Maculometry. Lower: The operation findings.

33

around the right optic nerve could be removed without difficulty. It is puzzling that the slight visual field variation had appeared only in the right side.

Case 5: Central scotoma prior to bitemporal defects. A 39 year-old-woman complained on Nov. 10, 1969 of the sudden loss of vision in her left eye. She had consulted an other ophthalmologist. Examination showed a visual acuity of 20/20 in the right and 20/200 in the left eye. Except for the visual field the ocular examination showed nothing abnormal, neither in the appearance of the optic disc. There was a central scotoma with a normal peripheral field. Retrobulbar optic neuritis could be considered as an explanation. However the visual acuity showed progressive impairment in both eyes until it reached on Jan. 12, 1970, 20/600 for the right eye and finger counting for the left eye. The woman being pregnant no definite treatment could be undertaken. Post parturtum, her visual acuity improved to 20/20

CASE 2   49y.o. Female, Chromophobe Adenoma

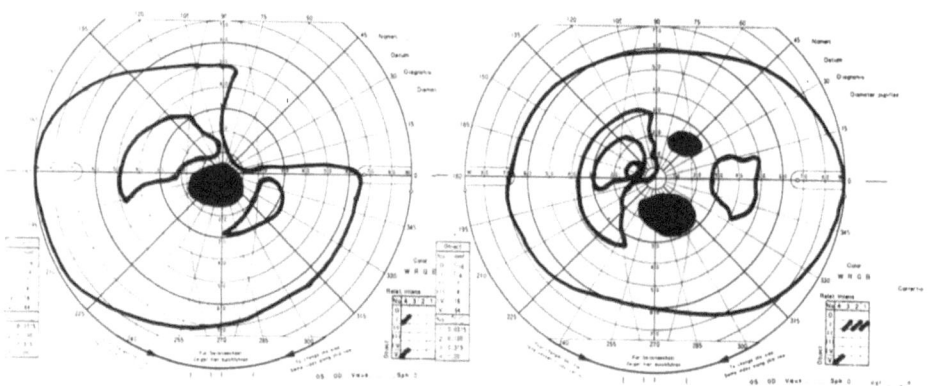

Fig. 3a. Case 2: An atypical homonymous hemianopsia with central scotoma and paracentral scotoma.

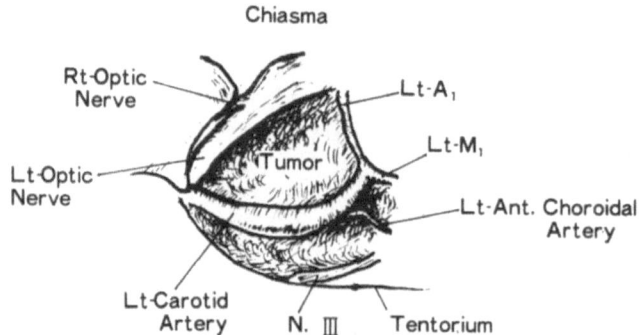

Fig. 3b. Case 2: Operation findings to Fig. 3a.

34

and 20/40 for the respective eyes thanks to steroid therapy. A new loss of the visual field developed however after long term recovery of one and a half years. Perimetric findings indicated a tendency for bitemporal hemianopsia. Verified tumor revealed meningioma of the tuberculum sellae.

Case 6: Central scotoma and irregular defects without bitemporal hemianopsia leading to blindness (Fig. 6). A 35 year-old-woman had been followed up after being diagnosed as suffering from retrobulbar optic neuritis. During the growth of a tumor she developed central scotoma with irregular peripheral defects and concentration. No bitemporal defects however could be detected through measurements. Verified tumor revealed meningioma of the tuberculum sellae.

It is uncertain whether a mechanical distortion is in fact responsible for certain visual field defects (Huber 1976). There is no distinct resistance such as a bone above the chiasm and this allows the nerve fibers to move freely upward, without being harmed. Bergland & Rey (1969) have come to the conclusion that the chiasm receives its arterial supply from the superior vessels, derived from the anterior cerebral arteries and from the inferior group of vessels, derived from the internal carotide arteries, the posterior cerebral arteries and the posterior communicating artery. The decussing fibers of the central chiasm receive their arterial supply only from the inferior group. The above mentioned authors therefore conclude that bitemporal defects caused by intrasellar tumors are the results of ischemia rather than of neural compression. At an early stage a rough irregular depression of the peripheral field may be explained by the partial damage of the supplying arteries, in other words, some capillaries derived from the same artery may disturb the blood flow while others maintain some blood flow and thus maintain a limited function of the nerve fibers.

Various factors may be involved in the nerve function mentioned above.

CASE 3 54y.o. Male, Chromophobe Adenoma, Notching by the anterior cerebral artery

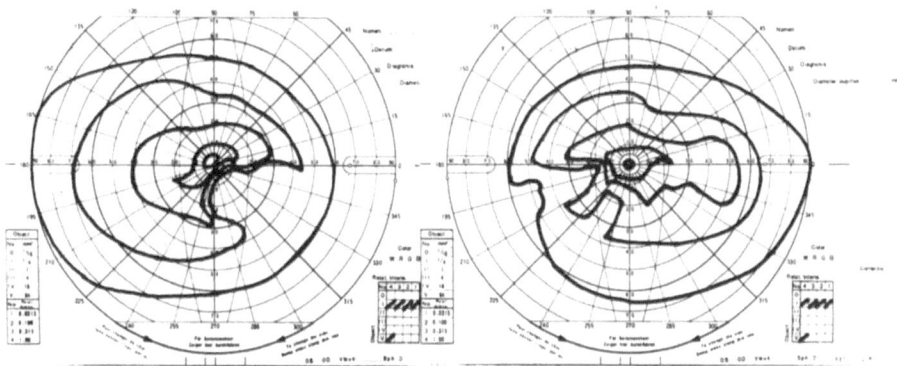

Fig. 4a. Case 3: Irregular lower field defects.

35

In Case 3 notching by the anterior cerebral artery could have been the cause of the lower field defects. Of great importance seems to be the presence of central (non hemianoptic) scotoma. They seem to be due to the impairement of the optic nerve, produced by the associated arachnoiditis or the pressure toward the bone. Some cases illustrated above cannot be explained by the operation findings.

A further exact examination of the capillary distribution inside the nerve fasciculus should prove important for a satisfactory explanation.

Evaluation of the various perimetric methods applied in neuro-ophthalmology

As a general rule the kinetic methods was used in order to measure the visual field defects due to chiasmal lesions. There are however possibe

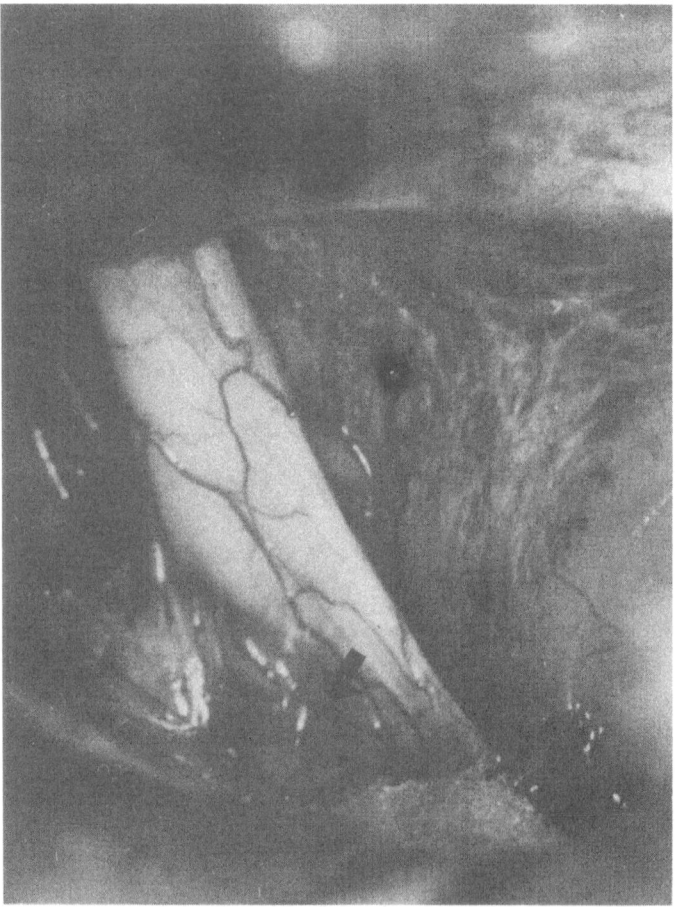

Fig. 4b. Anterior cerebral artery (arrow) was notched into chiasm.

advantages of applying other perimetric methods. Thus the multiple stimulus static perimetry may be of value for the observation of the visual field defects caused by a chiasmal lesion and it can be expected that it would produce more accurate information about central field defects inside the 25 degree radius. It must be remarked that it will hardly contribute to the earliest diagnosis of chiasmal tumors although it reveals more accurate visual field defects unless they are bitemporal. As for the Friedmann's visual field analyzer and the Goldmann's perimeter it could be noticed that the findings of the two methods were almost identical and that even when using the 1.2 log. unit filters as stimulus luminance for screening, the result did

CASE 4 7y.o. Female, Craniopharyngioma

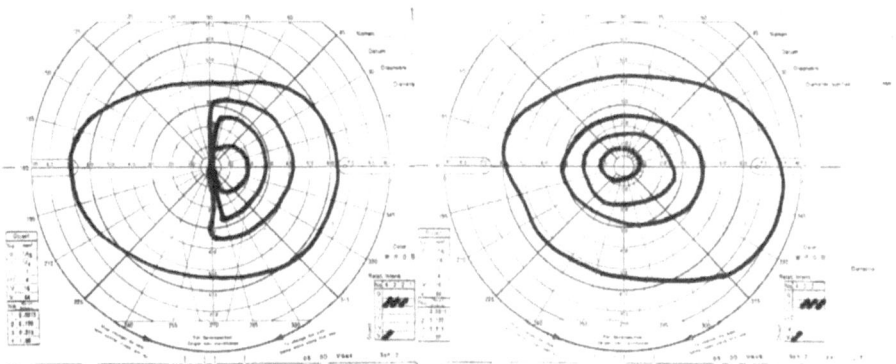

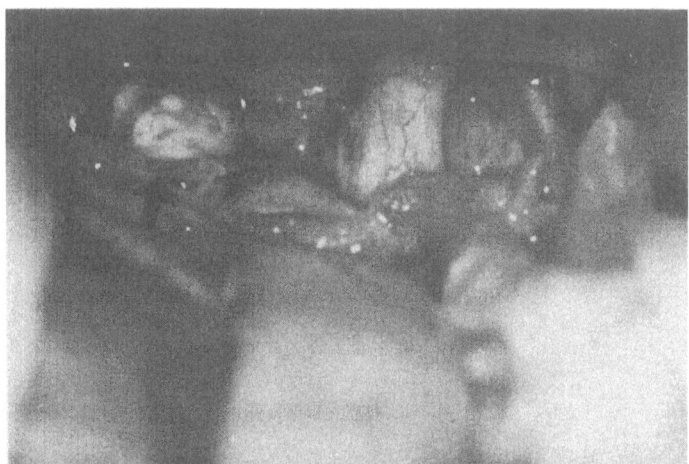

Fig. 5. Case 4 Upper: A temporal hemianopsia on one side. Lower: The surgical findings. Arrow shows the tumor enclosed the right optic nerve.

37

not fall positive. In our opinion the Tübinger's perimetry should be employed in the cases of dubious hemianoptic defects detected by the kinetic perimetry in the central isopters.

Central vision – A problem of macular sparing

The visual acuity of chiasmal tumor patients varies considerably in the cases where there is splitting hemianopsia. Generally, patients with good vision are those having a sparing field near the fovea. The cases of complete hemianopsia can be divided into two groups. In the first there is a genuine reservation of the macular fibers while in the second there is a pseudo-macular sparing. Cases of the first group can easily be detected by means of routine kinetic perimetry and they show a sparing over 3 degree radius from the fovea attributed in 7 of our cases to pituitary adenoma, in 1 case to craniopharyngioma, while there was no case of meningioma. Cases of the second

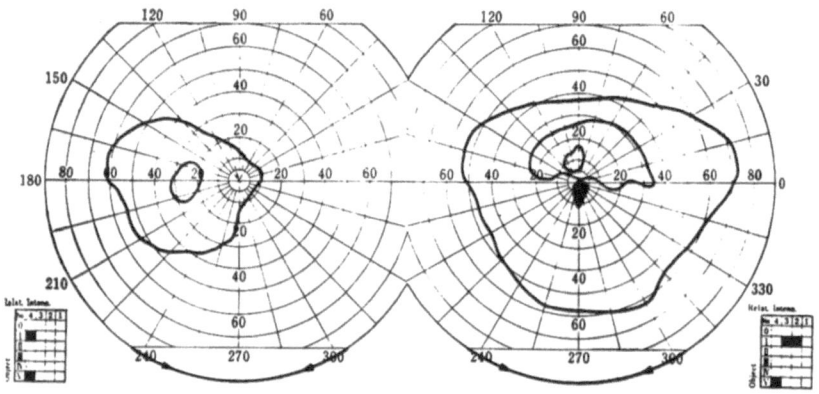

CASE 6 35y.o. Female, Meningioma of tuberculum sellae

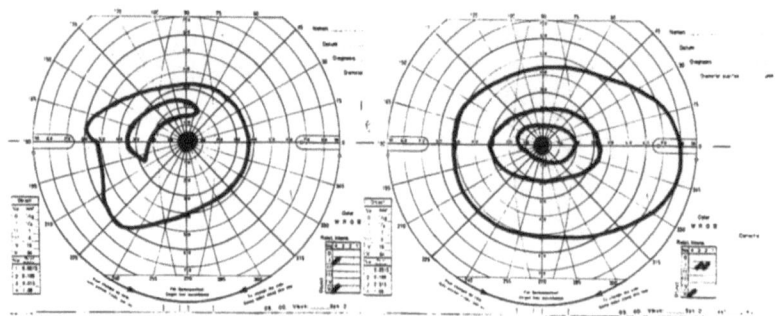

Fig. 6. Case 5. Central scotoma and irregular defects without bitemporal hemianopsia leading to blindness.

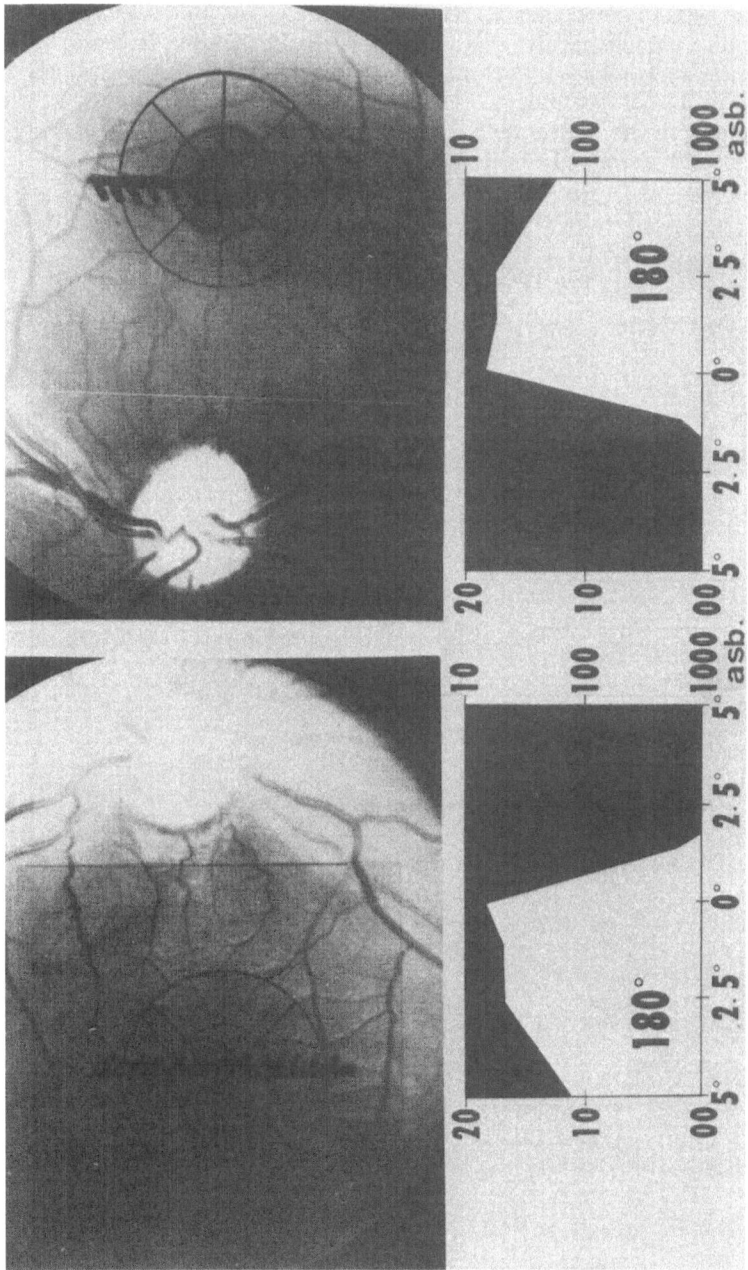

Fig. 7. The pseud-macular sparing: Results obtained by our own Fundus Maculometry. In left figure sparing is observed at about 2 degrees from the fovea with kinetic
method. Right: using the static method in a 180 dagrees radius.

group were found thanks to our own apparatus for fundus maculometry. Here the pseudo-macular sparing appears inside the 2 to 3 degree radius from the fovea (Fig. 7). The cause seems to be a shift of fixation toward the blind field and according to Harrington (1976) this fixation shift is more noticeable in the central field. It has been supposed that an overshoot field developes a characteristic displacement of the vertical border of the field

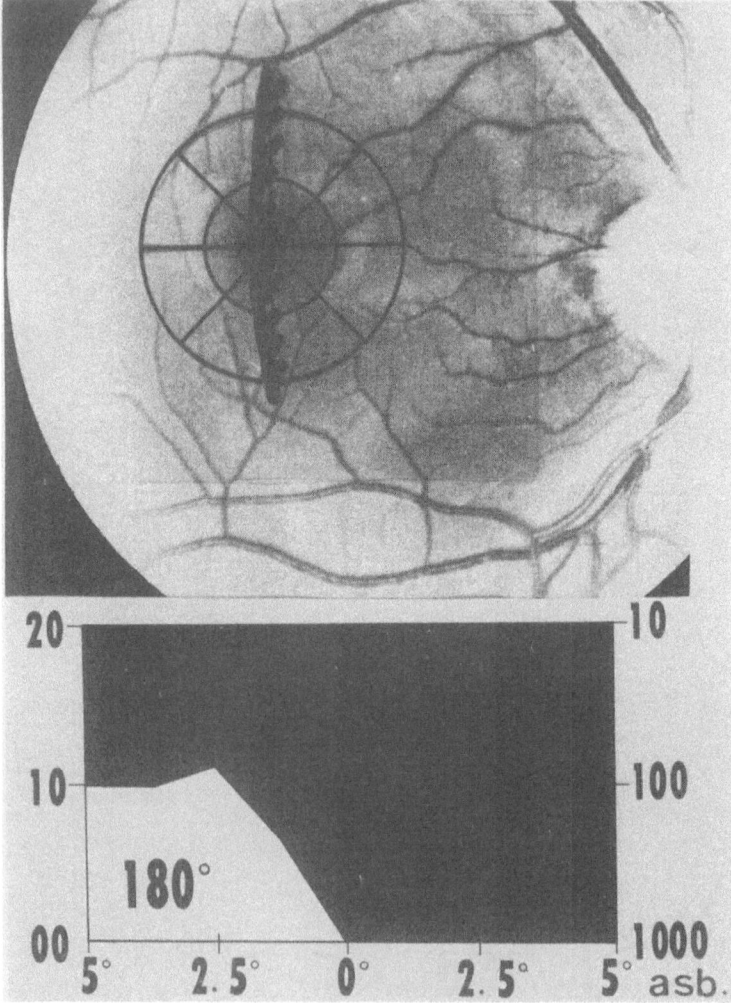

Fig. 8. Central field defect on a splitting macula case using our own Fundus Maculometry. The upper picture shows kinetic measurement while the lower shows static measurement at a radius of 180 degrees. This photograph illustrates how it is possible to detect very small and low density scotomas thanks to our Fundus Maculometry where conventional perimetry does not yield any results.

defect due to central integration or the retinal ganglion supply to the blind field (Bunt & Minckler). In the cases of defective visual acuity on a splitting macula hemianoptic scotomas of various kinds and of various densities and sizes can be found. Denser scotomas can easily be detected by routine campimetry. If however profile perimetry or our own new method for fundus maculometry is used, 4 types of central defects, i.e. the complete depression type, the island-like depression type, the sieve-like depression type and the general depression type similar to central scotoma in optic neuropathies, can be distinguished. Therefore the visual acuity in these cases will be in direct relation with the sort of depression. A case of this kind which have been measured with our own apparatus is presented (Fig. 8). Attention should be paid to the investigation of the macular threshold because of its importance with regard to the prognosis of the visual acuity of the patients and also with regard to the origin of the defect.

REFERENCE

Adler, F.H., Austin, G. & Grant, F.C. Localizing value of visual fields with early chiasmal lesions. *Arch. Ophthalmol.* 40: *579* (1948).

Bakey, L. The results of 300 petuitary adenoma operations. *J. neurosurg.* 7: *240* (1950).

Bergland, R. & Ray, B.S. The arterial supply of the human optic chiasm. *J. neurosurg.* 31: *327* (1969).

Bunt, A.H. & Minckler, D.S. Foveal sparing. A new anatomical evidence for bilateral representation of the central retina. *Arch. Ophthalmol.* 95: *1445* (1977).

Chamlin, M., Davidoff, L.M. & Feiring, E.H. Ophthalmologic changes produced by pituitary tumors. *Am. J. Ophthalmol.* 40: *353* (1955).

Cushing, H. & Walker, C.B. Chismal lesions with special reference to bitemporal hemianopsia, *Brain* 37: *341* (1951).

Harms, H. Quantitative perimetrie bei sellanahen Tumoren. *Ophthalmologica* 127: *255* (1954).

Harrington, D.O. The visual fields. A textbook and atlas of clinical perimetry. 4th ed., The C.V. Mosby. St. Louis (1976).

Henderson, W.R. The pituitary adenomas. *Br. J. Surg.* 26: *811* (1939).

Lyle, T.K. & Clover, P. Ocular symptoms and signs in pituitary tumours. *Proc. Roy. Soc. Med.* 54: *611* (1961).

Huber, A. Eye signs and symptoms in brain tumors. 3rd., The C.S. Mosby. St. Louis (1976).

Imachi, J., Inoue, K., Kani, K. & Umeda, M. Clinico-statiscal evaluation in cases of tumors of chiasmal region. *Jap. J. Clin. Ophthalmol.* 23: *283* (1969).

Isayama, Y., Takahashi, T., et al. Prechiasmal syndrome. *Jap. J. Clin. Ophthalmol.* 29: *463* (1975).

Takahashi, T., Nakamura, A. & Isayama, Y. Analysis of the visual fields in tumors of the chiasmal region. *Jap. J. Clin. Ophthalmol.* 30: *543* (1976).

Walsh, F.B. & Hoyt, W.F. Clinical neuro-ophthalmology Vol. 3. The Williams, Wilkins. Co. (1969).

Note: A report 'on atypical chiasmal visual field defects' by E.L. Greve and M.A.C. Rakkman has been published in Documenta Ophthalmologica Proceedings Series vol 14: *315-326* (1977).
(Second Int. Visual Field Symposium, Tübingen 1976).
A paper by F. Dannheim related to this subject is published in this volume.

Author's address:
Department of Ophthalmology
School of Medicine,
Kobe University
Kusunoki-cho, 7-chome, Ikuta-ku
Kobe, Japan

Docum. Ophthal. Proc. Series, Vol. 19

VISUAL FIELDS BEFORE AND AFTER TRANSNASAL REMOVAL OF A PITUITARY TUMOR

Correlation of topographical features with
sensorial disturbance for liminal and
supraliminal stimuli

F. DANNHEIM, D. LUEDECKE & D. KUEHNE

(Hamburg, GFR)

ABSTRACT

In 111 patients with pituitary tumors, central visual fields were obtained preoperatively, in halve of them postoperatively as well. Kinetic perimetry as well as supraliminal stimuli have been applied. The correlation of the radiologically (skull x-ray, PEG, CT) and surgically evaluated extent of tumor and visual fields is good. Deviations occur only towards more functional damage than to be expected. 11 patients showed sensorial alterations with intrasellar tumors, some of them as changes of sensation, but normal kinetic fields. Those findings – never observed in normal subjects – seem to represent the first functional damage produced by a 'compressing' lesion, and they are the last to disappear after decompression. Recovery of visual function may show a rapid and a slow phase, complete recovery from even those minimal changes is not frequent. An affection of the nasal field is more frequent than generally accepted, sometimes following a nerve fibre pattern. Classical nerve fibre defects are observed with large tumors. Binasal or homonymous changes of sensation – however – occur especially with small tumors.

INTRODUCTION

Conventional perimetry is based on perception of light by means of threshold measurements as in kinetic and static perimetry. The application of supraliminal stimuli for an assessment of sensation proved valuable especially in chiasmal syndromes with discrete functional damage (Chamlin 1949, Frisén 1973, Dannheim 1977, 1978). This study was made to find out the accuracy and limitations of this second method by correlating it's results with patho-anatomical features of pituitary tumors and by observing the characteristics of visual recovery following removal of the compressing lesion.

MATERIAL AND METHOD

111 patients of 15 - 75 years of age suffering from a pituitary tumor have been evaluated before transnasal removal both ophthalmologically and radiologically within the last 2 years. The central visual fields were performed with a Tuebinger or a modified Rodenstock perimeter using a background

43

luminance of 3.2 cd/m², a target of 10' and multiple isopters. An attempt was made for a randomized direction of presentation of the stimulus. (Heijl & Krakau 1977). Static perimetry was not performed routinely since it did not offer additional information (Dannheim 1977).

The visual sensation was tested with a supraliminal white target of 10ʳ, 3-6/10 log units above threshold, and with the largest red target of maximal luminance. These targets have been presented alternating 5° nasal and temporal of the fixation spot while observing the eye being tested. The targets were then presented just nasal and temporal of the vertical meridian about 5° above and below the centre. Finally the targets were moved circularly with 5 and 8° excentricity. The patient was asked to keep steady fixation and simultaneously watch for differences or alterations of the subjective appearance of the target in brightness, contour, and saturation of colour. 100 normal subjects served as a control group (Dannheim 1978).

The cooperation of some patients especially with very large tumors was not sufficient as to warrant consistent responses – they were excluded from this study. In one half of the patients perimetry was repeated about 1 to 2 weeks following surgery. Some patients were re-tested up to more than 1 year later.

Small steps in the paracentral isopters of about 5° extent at the upper vertical meridian were judged as discrete changes of perception, since they are the typical early perimetric changes (Chamlin 1949, Dannheim 1977). They are often missed when only peripheral kinetic fields are traced. Severe changes of perception were divided in those of the temporal hemifield only and those crossing the midline and affecting the nasal field as well.

Radiological examination included skull x-rays, sella-tomography, computer tomography and in most cases pneumencephalography (PEG) – especially in tumors with questionable and definite suprasellar extent. In every case with significant suprasellar extension PEG was intraoperatively carried out to make sure that the chiasm was completely decompressed. Carotide arteriography was applied only exceptionally. Only the upward extent of the pituitary tumor was evaluated for this report, classified as intra- or suprasellar.

The amount of suprasellar expansion was judged as discrete, if the cisterna suprachiasmatica was slightly impressed. The growth of the tumor was moderate or extensive suprasellar, if the 3rd ventricle showed slight or severe impression. All tumors had been verified histologically.

RESULTS

I. Case reports

2 examples might demonstrate the different type of sensorial damage.
1. H. F., record-no. 96 916, 43 year old lady, extensively suprasellar growing prolactinoma. The intraoperative findings, including PEG, verified the decompression of the chiasm.

In the preoperative fields of this patient (Fig. 1, top) severe bitemporal disturbance of perception is visible as deformations of the isopters. The absolute scotoma is larger in the left eye, a relative scotoma crosses the midline centrally and below fixation resulting in a reduced visual acuity of 0.4. A disturbance of sensation in the right eye has hemiopic distribution temporally, with a sector-shaped accentuation near the upper vertical merid-

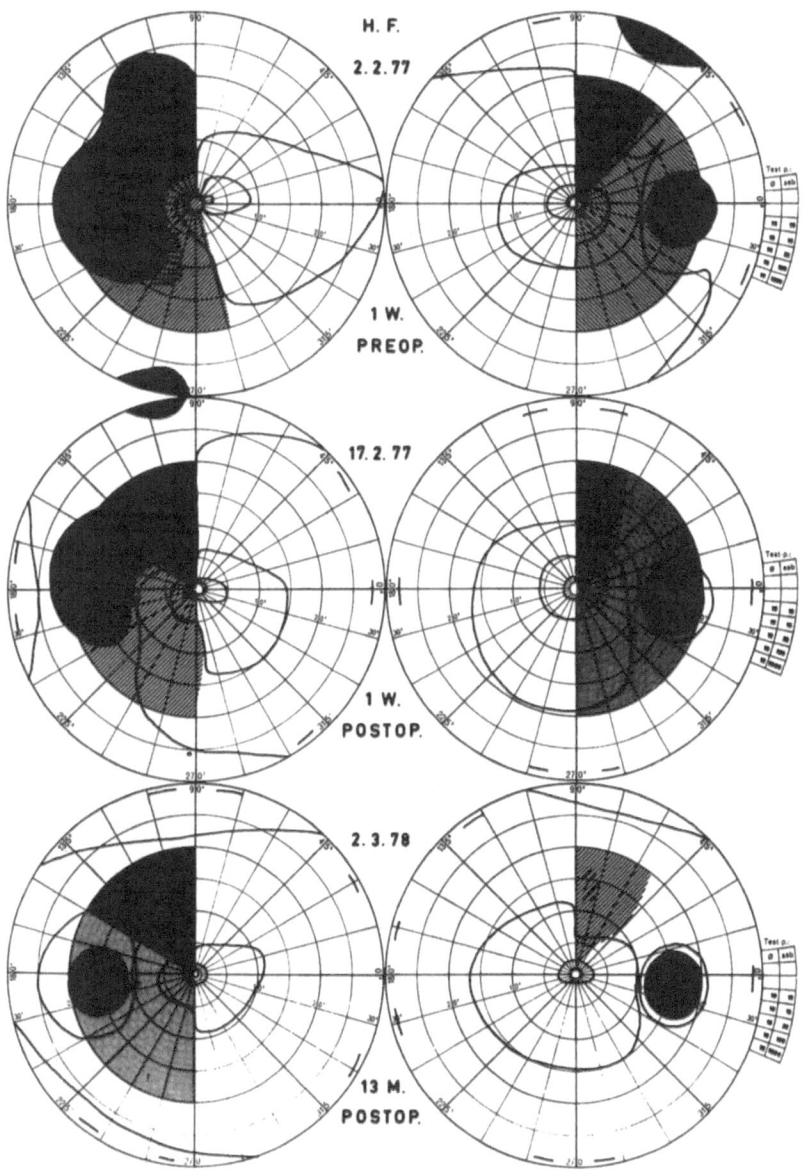

Fig. 1. (Description in the text).

45

ian. In the left eye the disturbance of sensation is crossing the midline as to be expected by the deformation of isopters.

1 week postoperatively (Fig. 1, middle) the right eye shows only discrete changes of perception, visible as small steps at the upper vertical meridian. In the left eye the absolute scotoma is significantly smaller and the central field has recovered resulting in a normal visual acuity. The nasal field is practically unaffected now.

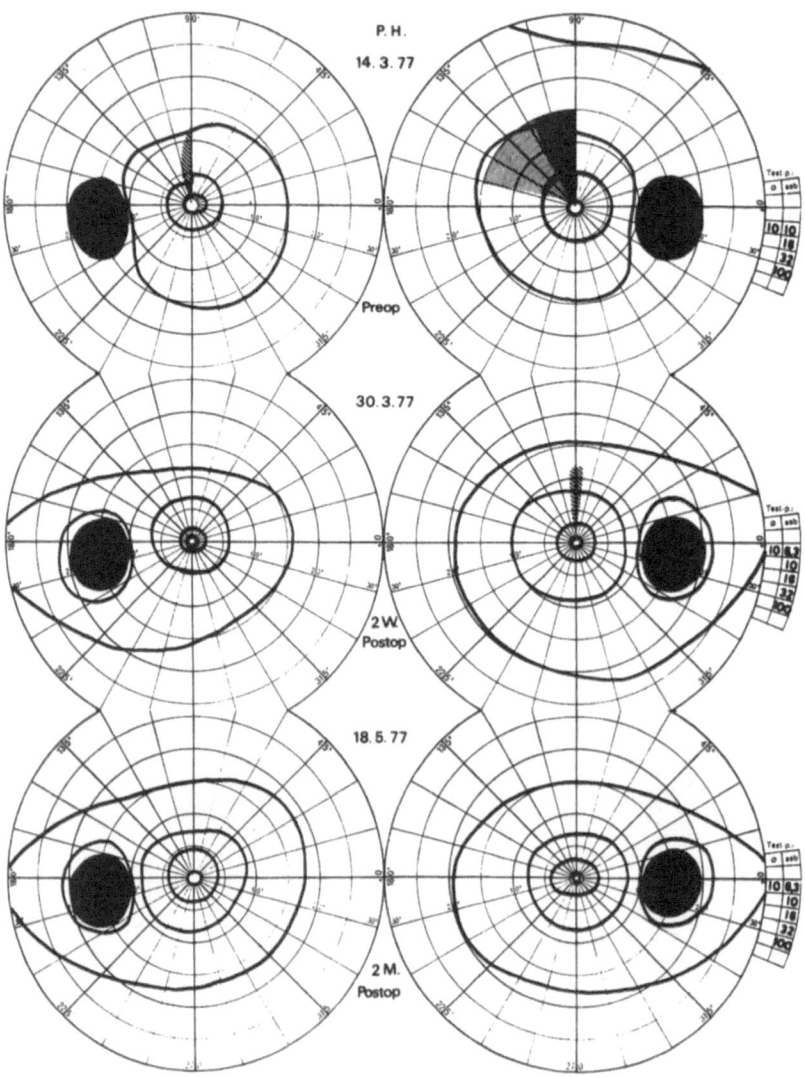

Fig. 2. (Description in the text).

Supraliminal stimuli still show a bitemporal hemiopic disturbance, just more pronounced in the left eye, and again a sector-shaped accentuation in the upper temporal field. There is only a circumscript affection of the nasal field paracentrally below fixation, adjacent to the vertical meridian.

13 months postoperatively (Fig. 1, bottom) the changes of isopters of the left eye have improved so far as to reach the same level of disturbance as the right eye, which shows constant findings. The extent of changes of sensation is contracted to a sector in the upper temporal field of the right eye. The left eye still presents a hemiopic distribution but no crossing of the midline.

2. P. H., record-no. 97 767, 39 year old acromegalic male with an intrasellar adenoma.

The isopters show preoperatively (Fig. 2, top) for the right eye small steps nasally, for the left eye minimal steps temporally only $5°$ above fixation. Changes of sensation are present in sectors, more pronounced for the right eye. 2 weeks postoperatively the isopters are normal, whereas the right eye has still an alteration of sensation in a tiny area above fixation. 2 months postoperatively even those minimal sensorial changes have disappeared.

II. Correlation of visual fields with extent of tumor

The correlation between preoperative visual fields and the extent of the tumor is given in table 1 for all 111 patients.

1. It is self evident that the higher a tumor extends into the suprasellar space, the more severely visual fields are affected (Bynke & Cronqvist 1964, Gauvin & Bourgnon 1976). No deviation from a linear relationship occured towards less functional damage than to be expected (Lloyd & Grant 1924, Møller & Hvid-Hansen 1970): None of the patients with moderate or extensive suprasellar spread of tumor had normal fields or even minimal changes. All patients with extensive tumors showed severe field damage. In only 4 patients with discrete suprasellar findings fields were 'normal'. Yet 2 of them had some concentric contraction (marked as stars) without any alterations of vertical orientation. A deviation from linearity towards more functional affection than expected was frequent, however:

2. 2 patients had discrete suprasellar findings only but severely affected fields. The individual topographic relation between the chiasm and the direction of growth of tumor must be responsible for such a discrepancy (Bynke & Cronqvist 1964, Walsh & Hoyt 1969).

3. 11 patients presented discrete sensorial alterations − as typically found in well-established chiasmal syndromes − but without radiological or surgical evidence of a suprasellar expansion. All these 11 patients had changes of sensation, half of them changes in isopters in addition. There is no explanation for this discrepancy. A similar observation was recently reported (Riss 1976), even though not confirmed by others (Bynke & Cronqvist 1964). Changes of sensation have been found in normal subjects only as a physiolo-

gical effect in the upper and lower periphery wedge-shaped at the vertical meridian (Dannheim 1978). In 10% such an effect could be traced as far as 5° toward the centre.

4. There is a high frequency of fields with discrete changes in isopter perimetry and a high frequency in the group with severe changes of isopters already with affection of the nasal field. A definite affection of both temporal hemifields is a relatively rare condition even though being the 'classical' type of defect (Chamlin, Davidoff & Feiring 1955, Bynke & Cronqvist 1964, Huber 1977).

5. The crossing of the midline occurs often paracentral above or below fixation in an arcuate way resembling the nerve fibre arrangement. In 3 of our patients with large tumors, growing asymmetrically and producing very severe affection of one eye, the visual field was restored greatly after surgery, leaving a typical nerve fibre defect as the dominating feature (Adler, Austin & Grant 1948, Rucker & Kernohan 1954, Kearns & Rucker 1958, Møller & Hvid-Hansen 1970, Harrington 1971, O'Connell 1973, O'Connell & Du Boulay 1973, Schmidt 1975, Sugita, Sato, Hirota, Tsugane & Kageyama 1975). All 3 patients had been misdiagnosed originally as retrobulbar neuritis (Knight, Hoyt & Wilson 1972, Greve & Raakman 1977).

6. Binasal changes of the fields were observed in 2 patients of this group with intrasellar tumors, present as symmetrical zones of changes of sensa-

Table 1. Correlation of preoperative visual fields with the extend of a pituitary tumor in 111 patients.

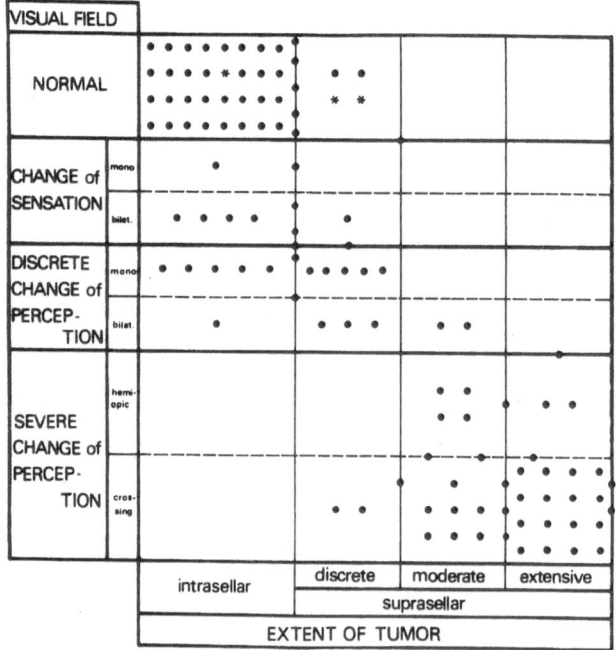

48

tion (Dannheim 1977, 1978). These findings are different from those severe binasal nerve fibre scotomata, which had been attributed to compression of the displaced chiasm by the adjacent structures.

7. Homonymous alterations were present in 4 patients, 3 times as discrete changes with an intrasellar tumor (Dannheim 1978) and once with severe damage by a very large tumor (Bynke & Cronqvist 1964, Walsh & Hoyt 1969, & Harrington 1971).

III. Regression of field changes after removal of tumor

45 of the patients, in whom perimetry was also postoperatively performed, had field changes prior to surgery. Their findings are given in table 2. The scale for the time interval between the operation and the repetition of perimetry favours the time immediately after surgery since the phase is biologically more significant.

1. Cases with severe field damage do not differ from those with discrete changes in their reversibility of sensorial damage.

2. The marked interindividual variation in reversibility of field changes must be due to the different degree of optic atrophy depending, for example, on the time lag between the first sensorial affection and the removal of the tumor, and on the characteristics of the growth of tumor (Nover 1962, Sugita, Sato, Hirota, Tsugane & Kageyama 1975). These factors have not been included in this report.

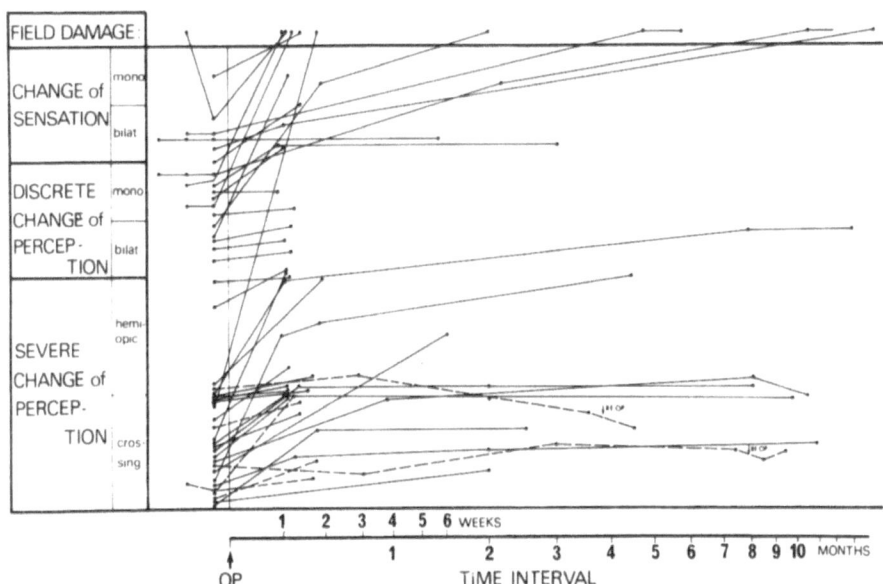

Table 2. Regression of visual field changes after removal of a pituitary tumor in 45 patients.

49

3. In quite a number of cases the maximal amount of recovery was not yet obtained 1 to 2 weeks after surgery (Fig. 1 and 2). The final level was reached in most cases about 1 to 2 months postoperatively. This finding corresponds with a differentiation of a rapid and a slow phase of recovery (Nover 1962, Kayan & Earl 1975, Frisén, Sjostrand, Norrsell & Lindgren 1976). This fact calls for a close postoperative follow-up to document the full amount of recovery. Only in this way the degree of deterioration necessary as a signal of recurrence of the tumor is minimal.

4. In 6 patients the tumor could only partially be removed (broken line). After a slight postoperative improvement 2 of these presented a progression of defects later on. They were re-operated trans-cranially (arrows), however, with no substantial benefit for the visual field.

5. In table 2 the relatively low frequency of fields with definite, but only hemiopic damage is visible as in table 1.

6. Changes of sensation persisted longer than those in isopter perimetry. 15 of all 45 patients regained normal fields according to isopter perimetry after surgery. But only 9 of them recovered with completely normal fields without changes of sensation, even though many had only discrete preoperative functional damage. In 1 patient the preoperative follow-up revealed a progression from a normal field to typical sector-shaped changes of sensation only within 4 months. These alterations disappeared following surgery.

REFERENCES

Adler, F.H., Austin, G. & Grant, F.C. Localizing value of visual fields in patients with early chiasmal lesions. *Arch. Ophthal.* 40: *579-600* (1948).

Bynke, H.G. & Cronqvist, S. Relationship between visual field defects and encephalographic changes in 48 cases of pituitary chromophobe adenoma. *Acta Ophthal.* (Kbh) 42: *465-482* (1964).

Chamlin, M. Minimal defects in visual field studies. *Arch. Ophthal.* 42: *126-139* (1949).

Chamlin, M., Davidoff, L.M. & Feiring, E.H. Ophthalmologic changes produced by pituitary tumors. *Amer. J. Ophthal.* 40: *353-368* (1955).

Dannheim, F. Perimetrie beim Chiasmasyndrom, schwellennahe und überschwellige Reize. *Klin. Mbl. Augenheilk.* 171: *468-477* (1977).

Dannheim, F. Early sensorial disorders in chiasmal lesions. Docum. Ophthal. Proc. Series 17: *239-246* (1978).

Frisén, L. A versatile color confrontation test for the central visual field. A comparison with quantitative perimetry. *Arch. Ophthal.* 89: *3-9* (1973).

Frisén, L., Sjöstrand, J., Norrsell, K. & Lindgren, S. Cyclic compression of the intracranial optic nerve: patterns of visual failure and recovery. *J. Neurol., Neurosurg. Psychiat.* 39: *1109-1113* (1976).

Gauvin, P. & Bourgon, P. Étude de la récupération visuelle après exérèse transphénoidale de tumeur hypophysaire. *Un. Med. Canada* 105: *1551-1554* (1976).

Greve, E.L. & Raakman, M.A.C. On atypical chiasmal visual field defects. *Docum. Ophthal. Proc. Series* 14: *315-325* (1977).

Harrington, D.O. The visual fields. pp 251-298, Mosby, St. Louis (1971).

Heijl, A. & Krakau, C.E.T. A note on fixation during perimetry. *Acta Ophthal.* (Kbh) 55: *854-861* (1977).

Huber, A. Chiasmasyndrome – Klinik. *Klin. Mbl. Augenheilk.* 170: *266-278* (1977).

Kayan, A. & Earl, C.J. Compressive lesions of the optic nerves and chiasm. Pattern of recovery of vision following surgical treatment. *Brain* 98: *13-28* (1975).

Kearns, T.P. & Rucker, C.W. Arcuate defects in the visual fields due to chromophobe adenoma of the pituitary gland. *Amer. J. Ophthal.* 45: *505-507* (1958).

Knight, C.L., Hoyt, W.F. & Wilson, C.B. Syndrome of incipient prechiasmal optic nerve compression. Progress toward early diagnosis and surgical management. *Arch. Ophthal.* 87: *1-11* (1972).

Lloyd, J.H. & Grant, F.C. Tumor of the Hypophysis. Report of a case. *Arch. Neurol. Psychiat.* (Chic.) 12: *277-287* (1924).

Møller, P.M. & Hvid-Hansen, O. Chiasmal visual fields. *Acta Ophthal.* (Kbh) 48: *678-684* (1970).

Nover, A. Über das Verhalten des Optikus nach längerdauernder Kompression. *Fortschr. Neurol., Psychiat., Grenzgeb.* 30: *228-233* (1962).

O'Connell, J.E.A. The anatomy of the optic chiasma and heteronymous hemianopia. *J. Neurol., Neurosurg., Psychiat.* 36: *710-723* (1973).

O'Connell, J.E.A. & Du Boulay, E.P.G.H. Binasal hemianopia. *J. Neurol., Neurosurg., Psychiat.* 36: *697-709* (1973).

Riss, M. Discussion at 2nd Symp. Internat. Perimetr. Soc., Tübingen 1976 (not printed).

Rucker, C.W. & Kernohan, J.W. Notching of the optic chiasm by overlying arteries in pituitary tumors. *Arch. Ophthal.* 51: *161-170* (1954).

Schmidt, D. Zur Differentialdiagnose bitemporaler parazentraler Gesichtsfeldausfälle bei 'Glaukom ohne Hochdruck' und chiasmanahen Tumoren. *Klin. Mbl. Augenheilk.* 166: *483-488* (1975).

Sugita, K., Sato, O., Hirota, T., Tsugane, R. & Kageyama, N. Scotomatous defects in the central visual field in pituitary adenomas. *Neurochirurgica* 18: *155-162* (1975).

Walsh, F.G. & Hoyt, W.F. Clinical Neuro-Ophthalmology. 3rd ed., Vol.I., Williams & Wilkins, Baltimore 1969.

Authors' address:
Universitaets-Augenklinik
Martinistrasse 52
2000 Hamburg 20
GFR

Docum. Ophthal. Proc. Series, Vol. 19

VISUAL FIELD DEFECTS IN ANTERIOR ISCHEMIC OPTIC NEUROPATHY

S.S. HAYREH & P. PODHAJSKY

(Iowa City, Iowa U.S.A.)

ABSTRACT

In 120 patients (168 eyes) with anterior ischemic optic neuropathy (AION), the pattern of visual field defects, and their relationship to the optic disc changes and visual acuity, were evaluated, both at the start of the disease and after a follow-up period; the various factors which influence the progress of visual field defects were also investigated. Visual field defects were seen much more frequently than defects in the visual acuity in AION. The field defects were present in 100% and 97% of the eyes with AION associated with temporal arteritis (Group I) and without temporal arteritis (Group II) respectively. The pattern of field defects, although complex and diverse, could be classified as optic-disc-related. In Group II, the commonest defects were inferior nasal segmental defect, inferior altitudinal hemianopic defect and central scotoma. In Group I, there was usually massive visual loss so that either no fields were obtained or only a small island field was seen, and in the rest the pattern was otherwise similar to that seen in Group II. In Group II, a marked potential for visual recovery was seen after systemic corticosteroid therapy, as compared to untreated cases (p<0.0005), especially when they were treated soon after the onset of AION while the optic disc still showed a fair amount of edema.

Anterior ischemic optic neuropathy (AION) is one of the commonest severely blinding disorders in old age. Its apparent rarity is due to frequent misdiagnosis and a lack of awareness on the part of physicians. AION results from acute ischemia of the anterior part of the optic nerve (the part supplied by the posterior ciliary artery circulation), including the optic nerve head, and is caused by circulatory occlusive disorders of the posterior ciliary arteries and/or the peripapillary choroid (Hayreh 1975). Most commonly it involves a segment of the nerve, and only occasionally the entire thickness of the nerve; the latter happens most frequently in temporal arteritis. In this disease, there is sudden onset of visual disturbance, although rarely a person may not be aware of it if the central vision is preserved. Ophthalmic examination during the acute stage reveals optic disc edema associated with optic-disc-related visual field defects, and, frequently, poor visual acuity. The optic disc becomes atrophic, usually within 2 months, but the visual loss persists. There is a high incidence of involvement of the fellow eye which further confuses physicians not fully aware of this entity. This sometimes

* This study was supported by Public Health Service Grant EY-001151.

Table 1. Incidence of age, sex and cause of AION

AION associated with	Age (years) and sex distribution																		Total # of patients
	0-10		11-20		21-30		31-40		41-50		51-60		61-70		71-80		81-90		
	M	F	M	F	M	F	M	F	M	F	M	F	M	F	M	F	M	F	
Temporal arteritis	–	–	–	–	–	–	–	–	–	–	–	–	–	5	3	10	1	4	23
Diabetes mellitus	–	–	2	–	–	2	1	–	2	–	3	6	3	–	2	2	–	–	23
Others	–	–	–	–	2	2	1	–	4	3	9	4	24	15	4	5	1	2	74
Total # of patients	–	–	2	–	4	–	2	–	6	3	12	10	27	20	9	17	2	6	120

54

results in unnecessary and hazardous neurosurgical investigation, yielding no positive findings other than the optic disc and visual field changes, with or without disturbance of the visual acuity. Our experience has shown that the most important single investigation in AION, apart from optic disc examination, is the meticulous recording of the visual fields.

We conducted the present study to evaluate fully the pattern of visual field defects in AION and their relationship to the optic disc changes and visual acuity, and also to investigate the various factors which influence the progress of the visual field defects. Apart from a casual reference, no detailed account is available on the subject in the literature.

MATERIAL AND METHODS

This investigation was carried out in 120 patients (168 eyes) with AION. All patients initially had the visual fields (in 97 patients by a Goldmann perimeter and in 23 patients by a tangent screen) and visual acuity recorded. Usually Targets I-2e, I-4e and V-4e were used in the Goldmann perimeter. All patients were investigated to find out the cause of the AION, particularly to rule out temporal arteritis (by erythrocyte sedimentation rate, by Westergren method and whenever indicated by temporal artery biopsy); this was so that corticosteroid therzpy could be started immediately in case of temporal arteritis, to prevent any further loss of vision. A number of the patients without temporal arteritis were treated with systemic corticosteroids if they were first seen with an appreciable amount of optic disc edema, to determine the role of steroids in reversing or arresting the visual loss. 114 patients (162 eyes) were followed up for variable lengths of time, the maximum being 7 years. The initial visual acuity and visual fields were compared with those at the end of follow-up to evaluate progress. The data was subjected to statistical analysis.

OBSERVATIONS

Age and sex

There were 60 males and 60 females between the ages of 15 and 88 years of age. The data are summarized in Table I.

Table 2. Laterality and cause of AION in 120 patients

Cause of AION	Laterality			Total # of	
	Right eye	Left eye	Both eyes	Patients	Eyes
Temporal arteritis	30.4%	17.4%	52.2%	23	35
Diabetes mellitus	26.1%	30.4%	43.5%	23	33
Others	32.4%	32.4%	35.1%	74	100

Table 3. Time interval between the onset of AION in the two eyes in patients with bilateral disease.

Cause of AION	Simultaneous	≤ One month	2 months	4-5 months	7-8 months	12 months	2 years	3-5 years	6-10 years	15-18 years	? years	Total of patients
Temporal arteritis	7	1	2	–	1	–	–	1	–	–	–	12
Diabetes mellitus	2	2	–	1	1	1	–	1	2	–	–	10
Others	3	3	2	3	1	–	1	4	5	3	1	26

Although the disease started in one eye, it involved both eyes in many patients, the proportion depending upon the length of follow-up. Table 2 summarizes the findings.

Time interval between the onset of AION
in the two eyes in patients with bilateral
disease:

The two eyes were involved in 48 patients (Table 3). The time interval varied from almost simultaneous onset of AION in the two eyes, of 12 patients, to 18 years, and the findings are summarized in Table 3.

Causes of AION:

Following were the known or probable causes in this series (Table 4). The group labelled as 'others' consisted essentially of individuals with arteriosclerosis, atherosclerosis, hypertension and other cardiovascular disorders, or with no other apparent abnormality.

Erythrocyte sedimentation rate (ESR)
and temporal artery (T.A.) Biopsy:

ESR was investigated whenever indicated, and always in patients aged 50 years or older; if it was over 20 mm/hour, T.A. biopsy was performed to

Table 4. Causes of AION

Cause	Number of patients	Number of eyes
Temporal arteritis	23	35
Diabetes mellitus	23	33
Post-cataract extraction	6	8
Raised intraocular pressure	5	7
Post-hemorrhagic amaurosis	2	4
Carotid stenosis	1	2
Chronic lymphocytic leukemia	1	2
Others	59	77
Total	120	168

Table 5. Initial and final visual acuities and their progress in AION with temporal arteritis (Group I).

Visual Acuity	6/6	6/9	6/12	6/15	6/18	6/24	C.F.	H.M.	P.L.	N.P.L.	Total # of eyes
Initial Visual Acuity	14.2%	2.8%	8.6%	8.6%	2.8%	2.8%	14.3%	11.4%	5.7%	28.6%	35
Final Visual Acuity	20 %	2.8%	5.7%	5.7%	2.8%	–	20 %	5.7%	5.7%	31.4%	35
Progress ↑	8.5%	–	–	–	2.8%	–	5.7%	2.8%	2.8%	–	8
↓	–	–	2.8%	–	–	–	–	–	2.8%	8.5%	5
0	11.4%	2.8%	2.8%	5.7%	–	–	14.3%	2.8%	–	22.9%	22

↑ = Improved, ↓ = Deteriorated, 0 = No change

Table 6. Initial and final visual acuities and their progress in AION without temporal arteritis (Group II).

Visual Acuity	6/6	6/9	6/12	6/15	6/18	6/21	6/24	6/30	6/60	6/120	C.F.	H.M.	P.L.	N.P.L.	Total # of eyes
Initial Visual Acuity	26.3%	6.8%	7.5%	5.3%	5.0%	3%	0.7%	8.3%	8.3%	3.8%	17.3%	5.0%	1.5%	2.2%	133*
Final Visual Acuity	38.6%	7.9%	6.3%	6.3%	1.6%	0.8%	1.6%	6.3%	11.0%	3.1%	11.8%	3.9%	–	0.8%	127
Progress ↑	11.8%	2.4%	3.1%	2.3%	1.6%	0.8%	1.6%	2.4%	3.1%	1.6%	1.6%	1.6%	–	–	42
0	26.8%	4.7%	2.4%	3.1%	0.8%	–	–	3.1%	4.7%	0.8%	7.9%	1.6%	–	–	72
↓	–	0.8%	0.8%	0.8%	–	–	–	0.8%	3.1%	0.8%	2.4%	0.8%	–	–	13

* 6 eyes were seen only once and their visual acuity was L.P., C.F., 6/120, 6/21, 6/6.
↑ = Improved, ↓ = Deteriorated, 0 = No change

rule out temporal arteritis. In patients with temporal arteritis, confirmed by T.A. biopsy, the ESR ranged from 21 to 135 (87.6 ± 27.9)mm, while in those without temporal arteritis it was 1 to 133 (34.5 ± 33.0) mm/hour.

CLASSIFICATION:

The eyes were divided into two main classes − Group I having AION with temporal arteritis, and Group II having AION without temporal arteritis.

Visual Acuity (V.A.):

'Improvement' or 'deterioration' were defined as a change of 2 or more lines on Snellen's test type. The various lines on the chart, each representing one line, were 6/6, 6/9, 6/12, 6/15, 6/18, 6/21, 6/24, 6/30, 6/60, 6/90 and 6/120. If the vision was less than 6/120, each of the steps from 'counting fingers (C.F.)' to 'hand motion (H.M.)', from H.M. to 'light perception (L.P.)', and from L.P. to 'no light perception (NPL)', were considered equal to 2 lines.

A) GROUP I − The initial and final visual acuity varied from 6/6 to no perception of light (NPL) in these patients (Table 15). It improved in 8 eyes, deteriorated in 5 and did not change in 22. The optic disc at the initial visit was edematous in 26 eyes and atrophic in 9 eyes; in 8 eyes with optic atrophy there was no change in vision and in one it improved (Table 15).

B) GROUP II − The initial and final visual acuity varied from 6/6 to NLP in these patients also (Table 6). It improved in 42 eyes, deteriorated in 13 and showed no change in 72 eyes (Table 6). The state of the optic disc at the initial visit and its relationship to the change in visual acuity is shown in Table 7.

VISUAL FIELD DEFECTS:

These were analysed under three categories because of their complexity and diversity. These three categories were:
1) Generalized peripheral visual field contraction.
2) Localized peripheral visual field defect.
3) Localized scotoma, showing no peripheral breakthrough.

In each category these were further analysed, subdivided according to whether temporal arteritis was present or not (i.e., Group I or II) and also as seen at the first visit ('initial') and at the end of follow-up ('final').

In Group II, no visual field defect could be recorded initially in 4 eyes (except for an enlarged blind spot in one). On follow-up the visual fields remained normal in all 4 eyes; 15 other eyes also recovered normal vision. All 19 eyes had optic disc edema at the first visit. In the remaining eyes the following field defects were recorded:

1. Generalized peripheral visual field contraction: The detailed incidence is given in Table 8. There was no contraction initially in 37.1% and 76.7% of eyes of Group I and II respectively, and on follow-up at the final visit it

Table 7. State of the optic disc at the initial visit and its relationship to progress in visual acuity in Group II.

Progress	State of optic disc	FINAL VISUAL ACUITY														Total # of eyes
		6/6	6/9	6/12	6/15	6/18	6/21	6/24	6/30	6/60	6/120	C.F.	H.M.	P.L.	N.P.L.	
Improved	ODE	11.8%	2.4%	3.1%	0.8%	0.8%	0.8%	1.6%	2.4%	2.4%	0.8%	1.6%	1.6%	–	–	38
	OA	–	–	–	1.6%	–	–	–	–	0.8%	0.8%	–	–	–	–	4
No change	ODE	17.3%	1.6%	0.8%	0.8%	–	–	–	2.4%	0.8%	0.8%	3.1%	–	–	–	35
	OA	9.5%	3.1%	1.6%	2.4%	0.8%	–	–	0.8%	3.9%	–	4.7%	1.6%	–	0.8%	37
Deterio-rated	ODE	–	0.8%	0.8%	–	–	–	–	–	1.6%	–	2.4%	0.8%	–	–	8
	OA	–	–	–	0.8%	–	–	–	0.8%	1.6%	0.8%	–	–	–	–	5

ODE = Optic disc edema
OA = Optic atrophy

was absent in 31.4% and 74.8% respectively (Table 8).

2. *Localized peripheral visual field defects:* In Group II, the most common peripheral field defects were the inferior altitudinal and inferior nasal — frequently the former was a relative defect and the latter an absolute defect in the same eye. In Group I, the commonest defect was the inability to plot any visual fields because of either complete blindness or extremely poor visual acuity (Table 9). The various types of localized peripheral visual field defects at first visit and at the end of follow-up are shown in Table 9. Some of the eyes had more than one localized peripheral visual field defect.

3. *Localized scotomata:* In AION the commonest form of scotoma was the central scotoma. Some of the eyes had more than one scotoma. The various types of scotomata and their incidence in both Groups is shown in Table 10.

RESPONSE TO TREATMENT WITH SYSTEMIC CORTICOSTEROIDS:

GROUP I: Every patient with temporal arteritis was treated with large doses of systemic corticosteroids to prevent further loss of vision. The response of these eyes to the treatment is given in Tables 5, 8, 9 and 10.
GROUP II: Some of the patients of Group II, if seen with an appreciable optic disc edema at first visit, were treated with systemic corticosteroids. The effects on visual acuity and visual field defects were evaluated to find out if systemic corticosteroids in adequate doses have a beneficial effect on the visual loss.
Visual acuity: The results are shown in Table 11. In the treated group, a chi-square test established that a significant number of eyes showed improvement in visual acuity, ($p = 0.004$). (Table 11)

Table 8. Incidence of generalized peipheral contraction of visual fields in Groups I and II at the first and final visits.

Type of defect	AION without temporal arteritis		AION with temporal arteritis	
	Initially	Finally	Initially	Finally
Contraction Absent	76.7%	74.8%	37.1%	31.4%
Contraction Present	10.5%	16.5%	8.6%	14.3%
No fileds obtained	7.5%	3.9%	42.9%	42.9%
Peripheral Island field only	5.2%	4.7%	11.4%	11.4%
Totaal # Eyes	133	127	35	35

Visual field defects: Table 12 summarizes the results. A chi-square test established that a significant number of eyes on treatment showed improvement in visual field defects ($p < 0.0005$). The effect of the treatment was further analysed in the three types of visual field defects separately and showed the following results:

1) *On generalized peripheral visual field contraction:* The results are shown in Table 13. A chi-square test showed the *p* value to be between 0.1 and 0.05 level, which is not conclusive but could be considered to show an appreciable improvement in the treated group as compared to the other groups.

2) *On localized peripheral visual field defects:* The results are shown in Table 14. The treated group showed a significant improvement on chi-square test ($p < 0.025$) as compared to the rest.

Table 9. Localized peripheral field defects in AION in Groups I and II at the first and final visits.

Type of field defect	AION without temporal arteritis		AION with temporal arteritis	
	Initially	Finally	Initially	Finally
i. No peripheral defect	16.5%	25.5%	5.7%	8.6%
ii. Inferior nasal	29.3%	29.9%	11.4%	8.6%
iii. Inferior altitudinal	28.6%	27.6%	5.7%	14.3%
iv. Superior altitudinal	7.5%	5.5%	5.7%	–
v. Superior nasal	6.8%	7.1%	14.3%	8.6%
vi. Superior temporal	2.3%	3.2%	5.7%	2.9%
vii. Inferior temporal	3.8%	3.1%	2.9%	2.9%
viii. Nasal vertical hemianopia	5.3%	3.9%	–	2.9%
ix. Temporal vertical hemianopia	2.3%	1.6%	–	–
x. Superior arcuate	1.5%	–	–	–
xi. Inferior arcuate	0.7%	0.8%	–	–
xii. Peripheral island field only	5.3%	4.7%	11.4%	11.4%
xiii. No fields obtained	7.5%	3.9%	42.9%	42.9%
Total # of defects	156	148	37	36
Total # of eyes	133	127	35	35

3) *On scotomata:* Table 15 summarizes the results. A statistical analysis (chi-square test) of these showed no significant correlation between treatment and the number of scotomata present at the end of follow-up; however, relative size of scotoma was not measured because of the obvious difficulties.

Table 10. Incidence of localized Scotomata in Groups I and II at the first and final visits.

Type of scotoma	AION without temporal arteritis		AION with temporal arteritis	
	Initially	Finally	Initially	Finally
1. No scotoma	39.8%	52.8%	28.6%	25.7%
2. Central scotoma	32.3%	26.0%	8.6%	11.4%
3. Centrocecal scotoma	5.3%	3.1%	2.9%	2.9%
4. Inferior central	2.3%	0.8%	–	–
5. Paracentral	5.3%	6.3%	2.9%	2.9%
6. Peripheral	3.8%	4.7%	2.9%	2.9%
7. Arcuate	1.5%	–	–	–
8. Enlarged blind spot	4.5%	–	–	–
9. Peripheral island field only	5.3%	4.7%	11.4%	11.4%
10. No fields obtained	7.5%	3.9%	42.9%	42.9%
Total # of scotoma	143	130	35	35
Total # of eyes	133	127	35	35

Table 11. Effect of systemic corticosteroid treatment on visual acuity in Group II

Progress	With optic disc edema				With optic atrophy	
	Treated group		Non-treated group			
	Incidence	Lines of Snellen chart	Incidence	Lines of Snellen chart	Incidence	Lines of Snellen chart
Improved	65.9%	2-13 (5.5 ± 3.4)	50 %	3-5 (4 ± 0.8)	15.1%	2-4 (3.4 ± 0.9)
Deteriorated	9.8%	4-12 (8.2 ± 3.9)	12.5%	2	21.2%	2-8 (3.6 ± 2.1)
No change*	24.4%	–	37.5%	–	63.6%	–
Total # of eyes		41		8		33

* In addition to these eyes with no change, in 19, 4 and 13 eyes in groups with treatment, without treatment and optic atrophy respectively the initial and final visual acuity was normal. These eyes were excluded from the analysis.

Effect of the time lag between the onset of AION and start of the therapy: This was also analysed. It revealed that in eyes which improved it was 0.55 ± 0.42 months, in those which showed no change it was 0.94 ± 0.93 months, and in the ones with deterioration the treatment was started 1 ± 0.52 months after the onset of AION. A statistical analysis (student's t test) revealed that this time lag made a significant difference to the outcome of treatment at a confidence level of $p < 0.05$ between those who improved and those who showed no change, and at a level of $p < 0.0125$ between those who improved and those who deteriorated. The follow-up period from first examination in these eyes was for $\leqslant 3$ months in 21 eyes, for 3-12 months in 37 eyes and 12-84 (27 ± 15) months in 55 eyes, and the time from onset to the end of follow-up was $\leqslant 3$ months in 10, 3-12 months in 37 and 12-240 (52 ± 52) months in 66 eyes.

Effect of treatment on visual field defects and/or visual acuity: The effect of the treatment on visual acuity and/or visual fields was evaluated in each

Table 12. Effect of systemic corticosteroid treatment on visual field defects in Group II

Progress	With optic disc edema		With optic atrophy
	Treated group	Non-treated group	
Improved	70.0%	45.5%	10.9%
No change	15.0%	45.5%	56.5%
Deteriorated	15.0%	9.0%	32.6%
# of eyes	60	11	46

Table 13. Effect of systemic corticosteroid treatment on generalized peipheral contraction of fields in Group II

Type of field defect	With optic disc edema				Optic atrophy	
	Treated group		Non-treated-group			
	Initially	Finally	Initially	Finally	Initially	Finally
Contraction Absent	81.7%	81.7%	90.9%	100%	69.6%	58.7%
Contraction Present	8.3%	11.7%	–	–	19.6%	28.3%
No fields obtained	6.7%	5.0%	9.1%	–	4.3%	4.3%
Island field only	3.3%	1.7%	–	–	6.5%	8.7%
Total # eyes	60	60	11	11	46	46

eye, to find out if either or both of them showed any improvement on treatment. The results are shown in Table 16. A statistical analysis of these results showed a highly significant improvement in the treated group as compared to the others ($p < 0.0005$).

DISCUSSION

It is well-established that AION due to temporal arteritis is a serious condition and if not treated promptly tends to involve both eyes and produce

Table 14. Effect of systemic corticosteroid treatment on localized peripheral field defects in Group II

| | | With optic disc edema | | | | Optic atrophy | |
| | | Treated group | | Non-treated group | | | |
Type of field defect		Initially	Finally	Initially	Finally	Initially	Finally
i.	No peripheral defect	20.0%	36.7%	36.4%	27.3%	8.7%	13.0%
ii.	Inferior nasal	18.3%	21.7%	27.3%	36.4%	39.1%	34.8%
iii.	Inferior altitudinal	28.3%	21.7%	27.3%	27.3%	28.3%	28.3%
iv.	Superior altitudinal	8.3%	5.0%	–	–	8.7%	4.3%
v.	Superior nasal	5.0%	8.3%	–	9.1%	8.7%	6.5%
vi.	Superior temporal	3.3%	3.3%	9.1%	9.1%	–	–
vii.	Inferior temporal	6.7%	5.0%	–	–	2.2%	2.2%
viii.	Nasal vertical hemianopia	6.7%	3.3%	–	–	6.5%	6.5%
ix.	Temporal vertical hemianopia	3.3%	1.7%	–	–	2.2%	2.2%
x.	Superior arcuate	3.3%	–	–	–	–	–
xi.	Inferior arcuate	1.7%	1.7%	–	–	–	–
xii.	Island peripheral field	5.0%	1.7%	–	–	13.0%	19.6%
xiii.	No fields obtained	6.7%	5.0%	–	9.1%	4.3%	2.2%
Total # of defects		70	69	11	13	56	55
Total # of eyes		60	60	11	11	46	46

Table 15. Effect of systemic corticosteroid treatment on localized scotomata in Group II

| Type of scotoma | With optic disc edema | | | | Optic atrophy | |
| | Treated group | | Non-treated group | | | |
	Initially	Finally	Initially	Finally	Initially	Finally
1. No scotoma	31.7%	56.7%	54.5%	63.6%	43.5%	39.1%
2. Central scotoma	40.0%	23.3%	27.3%	27.3%	28.3%	32.6%
3. Centrocecal scotoma	33.3%	5.0%	–	–	6.5%	2.2%
4. Inf. central	1.7%	–	–	–	2.2%	–
5. Paracentral	5.0%	8.3%	–	–	6.5%	8.7%
6. Peripheral	6.7%	5.0%	9.1%	9.1%	–	2.2%
7. Arcuate	1.7%	–	–	–	2.2%	–
8. Enlarged blind spot	10 %	–	–	–	–	–
9. Island fields only	33.3%	1.7%	–	–	8.7%	10.9%
10. No fields obtained	8.3%	5.0%	9.1%	–	4.3%	4.3%
Total # of scotomata	67	63	11	11	47	46
Total # of eyes	60	60	11	11	46	46

Table 16. Effect of treatment on visual acuity and/or visual field defects (VFD) in Group II

| Progress | With optic disc edema | | With optic atrophy |
	Treated group	Non-treated group	
VA and/or VFD improved	77.6%	36.4%	19.6%
VA and VFD no change	13.8%	45.4%	47.8%
VA and/or VFD deteriorated	8.6%	18.2%	32.6%
Total # of eyes	58	11	46

serious visual impairment However, the fact that AION due to causes other than temporal arteritis, particularly in diabetics and elderly individuals, also tends to become a bilateral disease over a period of weeks, months or years, producing serious visual loss, has not been duly appreciated. In the present study 43.5% of the diabetic group and 35.1% of the others developed bilateral AION, as compared to 52.2% in those with temporal arteritis.

In the diagnosis of temporal arteritis, estimation of ESR is usually considered to be the main investigation. In the present study although the mean ESR in temporal arteritis (Group I) was much higher (87.6 mm/hour) than in those without temporal arteritis (Group II) (34.5 mm/hour), *a low ESR does not rule out temporal arteritis* (Bethlenfalvay, Nusynowitz 1964, Cullen 1963, Eagling, Sanders & Miller 1974, Hayreh 1978, Kansu, Corbett, Savino & Schatz 1977, Permin, Juhl, Wiik & Balsløv 1977). For example, an ESR of 21 mm/hour was seen in temporal arteritis and 133 mm/hour without any temporal arteritis. In view of this, *it is essential to carry out temporal artery biopsy* in eyes with AION *if there is an ESR of more than 20 mm/hour, a massive visual loss and fluorescein angiography* shortly after the onset of visual loss *shows a marked non-filling of the choroid*. There is still the possibility of biopsy revealing no evidence of temporal arteritis, due to 'skip areas' in rare cases (Albert, Ruchman & Keltner 1976, Klein, Campbell, Hunder & Carney 1976) although we have not come across one so far.

In the diagnosis of AION, the visual acuity may be perfectly normal and reliance on this parameter may be misleading. The visual acuity was 6/9 or better in 1/3 of patients in Group II (Table 6) and in 17% of those in Group I (Table 15). Thus *a normal visual acuity does not rule out AION* – a fact not realized by most of the ophthalmic profession. The most important investigation in the diagnosis and management of AION is a painstaking and critical plotting and evaluation of the visual fields. None of the Group I eyes showed normal visual fields. In Group II AION no visual field defect was detected in 3% of the eyes and the diagnosis was based on other evidence of AION. The various types of visual field defects seen in AION are obviously optic-disc-related. A massive visual field loss was seen in more than half of the eyes of Group I, and far less commonly in Group II. A generalized peripheral visual field contraction was seen in some of the eyes of both Groups (Table 8). The commonest type of visual field defect was a localized peripheral defect (Table 9): in Group II it is consisted most commonly of an inferior altitudinal and/or inferior nasal defect, with the former frequently being a relative and the latter an absolute defect in the same eye. A central scotoma was the most frequent type of localized scotoma, particularly in Group II (Table 10).

Patients with AION due to temporal arteritis (Group I) have to be treated as an emergency with large doses of systemic corticosteroids, primarily to prevent involvement of the second eye. The involved eye showed some improvement in visual acuity in about a quarter of the eyes – the improvement being only of a small degree (e.g., from NPL to PL or HM, or from PL to HM or CF in an island) and, surprisingly, taking months to show up in some cases.

67

In contrast to Group I, usually no treatment is considered beneficial in Group II. Following earlier reports suggesting a beneficial effect of large doses of systemic corticosteroids during the early stages of AION with a significant optic disc edema (Foulds 1969, Georgiades, Stangos & Iliadelis 1976, Hayreh 1974, 1975), we treated a number of patients with optic disc edema by this therapy. The results on statistical analysis showed a highly significant improvement of both the visual acuity and visual field defects in the treated group and the results were very highly significant when improvement in visual acuity and/or visual field defects was considered. The study further indicated that the chances of recovery were much greater if the treatment was started within 2 weeks after the onset of AION than if treatment was started any later. Once the optic disc became atrophic (i.e., in about 2 months after the onset of AION), no appreciable improvement was seen, and 1/3 of the eyes showed some further deterioration on follow-up. 70% of the eyes with optic disc edema treated with steroids showed improvement of visual fields (Table 12). In a number of patients of Group II, with bilateral disease with one eye having optic atrophy (due to old AION) and the fellow eye with optic disc edema (due to fresh AION), the eye with optic atrophy usually showed no appreciable improvement when these

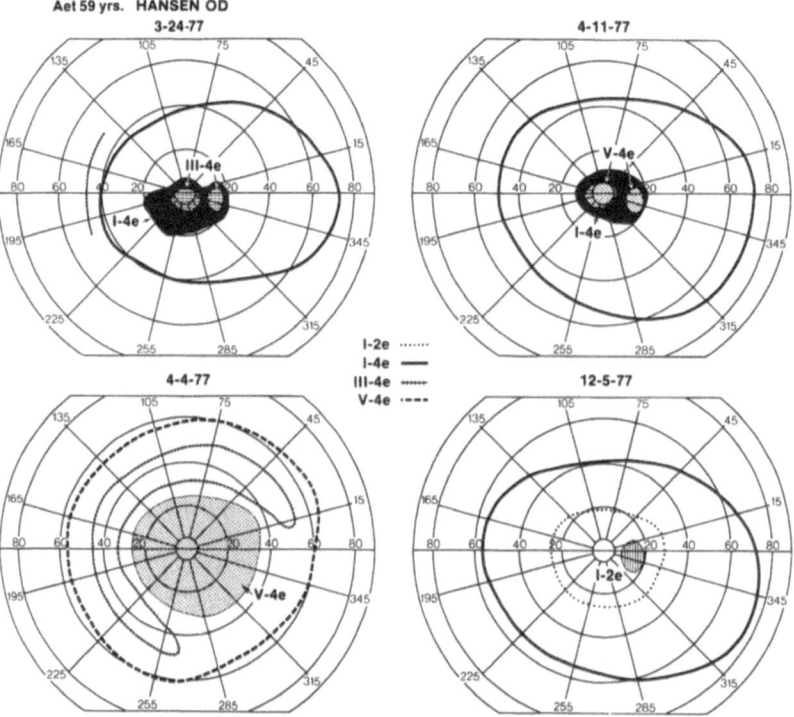

Fig. 1. (See text).

patients were treated with systemic corticosteroids. This suggests that during the early stages of the disease when the disc is still swollen, a number of the optic nerve fibers are still viable although not functioning, and are capable of recovering a normal function. In Group I, a few of the eyes suddenly recovered some function months after the onset of the disease; however, this recovery was only of a minor degree. The fact that the nerve fibers have such surprising powers of recovery, before the process has passed 'the point of no return' (i.e., when edema of the disc changes to optic atrophy) makes it absolutely essential for the physician to institute adequate treatment at the earliest possible moment where recovery is still possible, if he is to obtain any recovery at all; and, conversely, makes it pointless to use corticosteroids in cases where atrophy is already present. The degree of recovery must depend upon the amount of ischemic damage already inflicted (much more massive in Group I than II), as well as the time lag between onset of AION and start of treatment, so that by no means all cases will show improvement even if treatment is started promptly and vigorously. In Group II there is no indication when the patient is first examined whether and what degree of improvement will take place after treatment, which makes the evaluation of the therapy very difficult in small

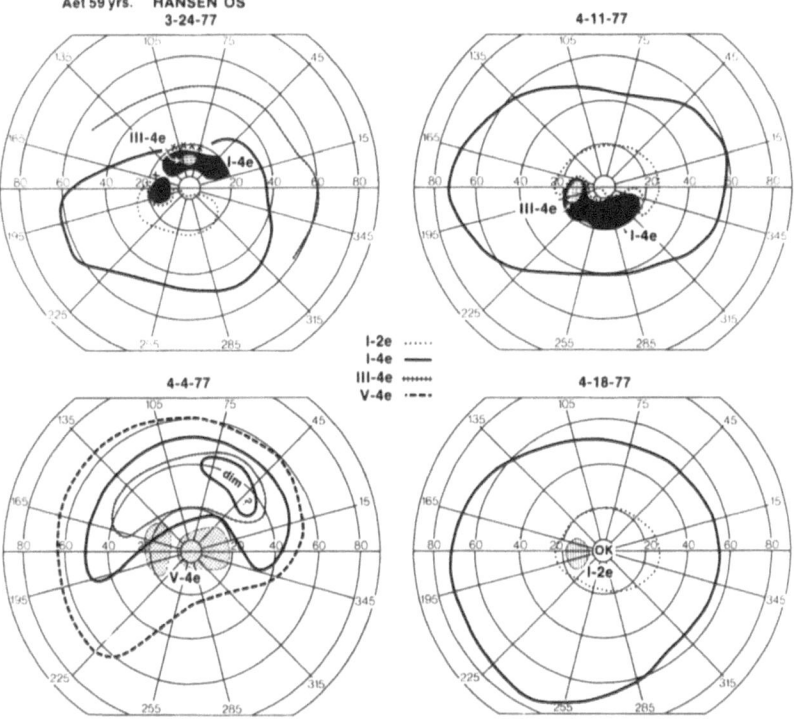

Fig. 2. (See text).

series. The following case vividly illustrates the tremendous potential for visual recovery after ischemia.

A 59-year-old woman was first seen in our clinic on March 24, 1977 with a history that she had developed blurred vision on about March 7, 1977 and had experienced deterioration of the vision in the right eye for one week prior to attending the clinic. Her visual acuity at the first visit was 6/60 and 6/15-2 in the right and left eye respectively and she had bilateral mild optic disc edema. ESR was 13 mm/hour. She was again seen in the clinic on April 4 with visual acuity of C.F. and 6/30 in the right and left eye respectively and more marked optic disc edema in both eyes, and the following day the acuity was C.F. and 6/60 respectively. Temporal artery biopsy showed no evidence of temporal arteritis. She was put on systemic prednisone, starting with 100 mg. daily orally. The prednisone was maintained at that dose for 12 days and then gradually tapered off over the following 6 weeks. Evolution of the visual fields is shown in Fig. 1 (right eye) and 2 (left eye). On April 18 the visual acuity was 6/7.5-3 and 6/6-3 in right and left eye respectively and on August 2, 1977 it was 6/7.5-1 and 6/6-2, with mild pallor of the optic disc in both eyes — right more than the left. On follow-up she has maintained the same visual acuity and normal visual fields.

The functional recovery is usually well maintained; however, the presence of chronic ischemia following the acute episode in some eyes could be responsible for a gradual deterioration after the initial recovery.

ACKNOWLEDGEMENTS

We are grateful to Ms. Miriam Leinen and Ms. Ginny Colston for their expert and painstaking perimetry in these patients, to Dr. R.F. Woolson for the biostatistical help, and to Miss Jane Duwa for the secretarial help. We are also grateful for the co-operation of Dr. H.S. Thompson.

REFERENCES

Albert, D.M., Ruchman, M.C. & Keltner, J.L. Skip areas in temporal arteritis. *Arch. Ophthal.* (Chicago) 94: *2072-2077* (1976).

Bethlenfalvay, N.C. & Nusynowitz, M.L. Temporal arteritis, A rarity in the young adult. *Arch. Inter. Med.* 114: *487-489* (1964).

Cullen, J.F. Occult temporal arteritis. *Trans. Ophthal. Soc. U.K.* 83: *725-736* (1963).

Eagling, E.M., Sanders, M.D. & Miller, S.J.H. Ischaemic papillopathy. *Brit. J. Ophthal.* 58: *990-1008* (1974).

Foulds, W.S. Visual disturbances in systemic disorders — optic neuropathy and systemic disease. *Trans. Ophthal. Soc. U.K.* 89: *125-146* (1969).

Georgiades, G., Stangos, N. & Iliadelis, E. The anterior ischemic opticopathy or vascular pseudothilitis. *Ophthal. Chron.* (Athens) 13: *32-56* (1976).

Hayreh, S.S. Anterior ischaemic optic neuropathy-III. Treatment, prophylaxis, and differential diagnosis. *Brit. J. Ophthal.* 58: *981-989* (1974).

Hayreh, S.S. Anterior ischemic optic neuropathy. Springer Verlag, New York (1975).

Hayreh, S.S. Ischemic optic neuropathy. *Internation. Ophthal.* 1: *9-18* (1978).

Kansu, T., Corbett, J., Savino, P. & Schatz, N. Giant cell arteritis with normal sedimentation rate. *Arch. Neurol.* (Chicago) 34: *624-625* (1977).

Klein, R.G., Campbell, R.J., Hunder, G.G. & Carney, J.A. Skip lesions in temporal arteritis. *Mayo Clin. Proc.* 51: *504-510* (1976).

Permin, H., Juhl, F., Wiik, A. & Balsløv, J. Immunoglobulin deposits in the dermo-epidermal junction zones in patients with systemic lupus erythematosus. Rheumatoid arthritis and temporal arteritis compared by serological testing including a_2 – macroglobulin. *Scand. J. Rheum.* 6: *105-110* (1977).

Authors' address:
Department of Ophthalmology
University of Iowa
Iowa City, Iowa – 52242
USA

Docum. Ophthal. Proc. Series, Vol. 19

COMPARISON OF VISUAL FIELD DEFECTS IN GLAUCOMA AND IN ACUTE ANTERIOR ISCHEMIC OPTIC NEUROPATHY

E. AULHORN & M. TANZIL

(Tübingen, B.R.D.)

ABSTRACT

The location, size and shape of field defects in over 60 cases of anterior ischemic optic neuropathy are described. The frequency distribution of the location of these defects in the visual field is determined and compared with the frequency distribution of early defects in glaucoma.

INTRODUCTION

With all visual field defects, where the form corresponds to the nerve fibre pathway in the retina, the underlying damage is to be looked for in the area of the optic disc. Here the defect area can lie in the papillar tissue itself as well as in the immediate vicinity of the optic disc. Apart from optic disc anomalies the causes of damage that come into consideration are above all juxta-papillary inflammatory foci, glaucoma, and ischemic optic neuropathy. From the location of the scotoma in the visual field, the area of damage in the region of the optic disc can always be deduced. An example of this is the typical sector-like defect in a juxta-papillary chorioretinitis. Similar considerations applie to early glaucomatous visual field defects. The five stages of the development of glancomatous visual field defects are illustrated in fig. 1.

The spot-like or arcuate defects of the second or third stages appear superior and inferior in the visual field with approximately the same frequency. They lie, however, at different positions in the superior and inferior halves of the visual field, as can be seen from the frequency distribution of the location of the defects (Fig. 2). If one deduces from this location the area of disturbance in the optic disc, then different disturbance areas result in the superior and inferior halves: superior closer to the vertical axis of the optic disc, and inferior somewhat further away from it, more temporally displaced than in the superior part.

To gain information concerning the areas in the optic disc favoured by the defects in anterior ischemic optic neuropathy (AION) we have now determined the visual field defects in this disease systematically as well. Our visual field study is based on 61 eyes with typical AION. Cases of ischemic optic neuropathy caused by temporal arteriitis with a total loss of sight or with an almost total visual field defect were not included in our study as

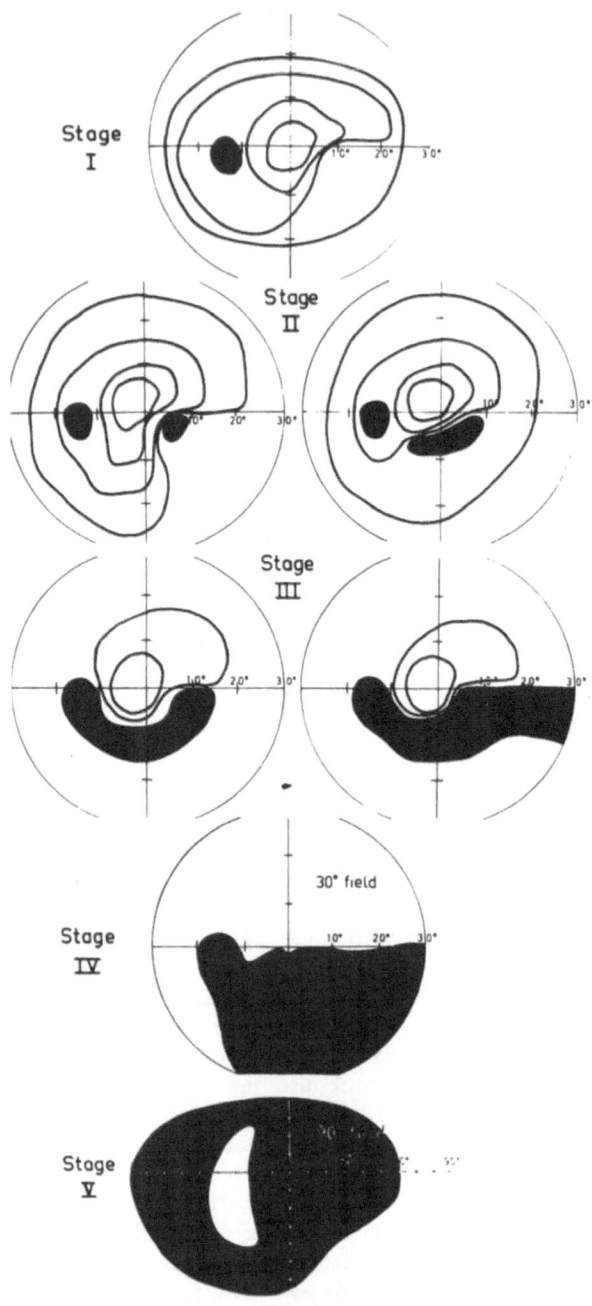

Fig. 1. 5 stages of glaucomatous field defects.

well as cases due to Diabetes. As criteria for the disease we have taken the following six points:

1. Sudden appearance of the visual field defect.
2. Sector-like or general edema of the papillary tissue, frequently with small hemorrhages in the area of the optic disc.
3. Form of visual field defects corresponding to the nerve fibre pathway in the retina. All our cases belong to the group 'localised scotomata' of Hayreh (see this Proceedings).
4. Visual field defect irreversible.
5. Sector-like or general optic disc atrophy in check-up examinations.
6. Typical sparing of the capillary filling in fluorescence angiography.

Points 1 to 3 of these criteria were given with all 61 eyes. Points 4 and 5 could not be proved present in all cases, since not all of the patients came to the check-up required. Point 6 was not always found in cases, which had already become diseased some years earlier, because we had at that time not carried out fluorescence angiography in AION regularly. Where fluorescence angiography was carried out, however, the result was not always typical either.

On examining these 61 visual field defects, their similarity to the glaucoma-induced defects of stages 2 and 3 is at once obvious (Fig. 3), whereas we have never observed defects resembling the sector-like defects in chorioretinitis juxta-papillaris.

There are, however, typical differences to glaucoma as well, affecting

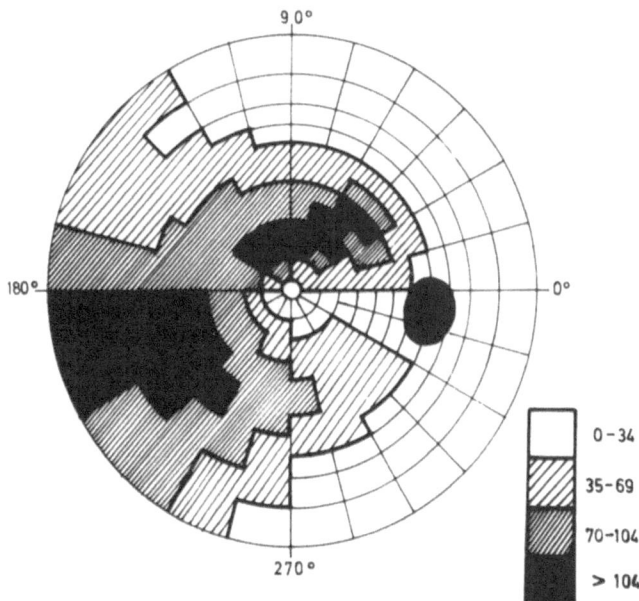

Fig. 2. Frequency distribution of the location of the glaucoma defects in stage 2 within 400 cases.

75

above all the preference for the superior or inferior halves of the visual field. Whilst in terms of figures there is a strikingly even distribution of the defects in the superior and inferior halves in glaucoma, the inferior half is clearly favoured in AION (table I).

With regard to the characteristics of the superior and inferior defects, the defects in glaucoma and in AION are astonishingly similar: the superior defects are usually smaller and they lie nearer the centre, mostly directly above it and close to the vertical axis of the visual field (Fig. 4). This is true

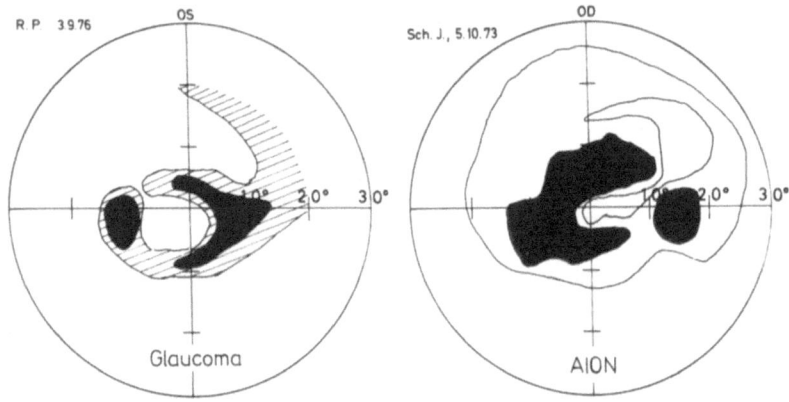

Fig. 3. Example of the similarity of VF defects in glaucoma and AION; arcuate scotoma above and below still without combination to the blind spot.

Table 1. Distribution of VF defects in the superior and inferior half of the VF in AION and glaucoma.

Ischemic optic neurop. Defects in 61 vis.f.		Glaucoma, stage II Defects in 100 vis.f.
4 (6%)	superior only	40 (40%)
48 (79%)	inferior only	44 (44%)
9 (15%)	sup. and inferior	16 (16%)
13 (19%)	superior	56 (48%)
57 (81%)	inferior	60 (52%)

76

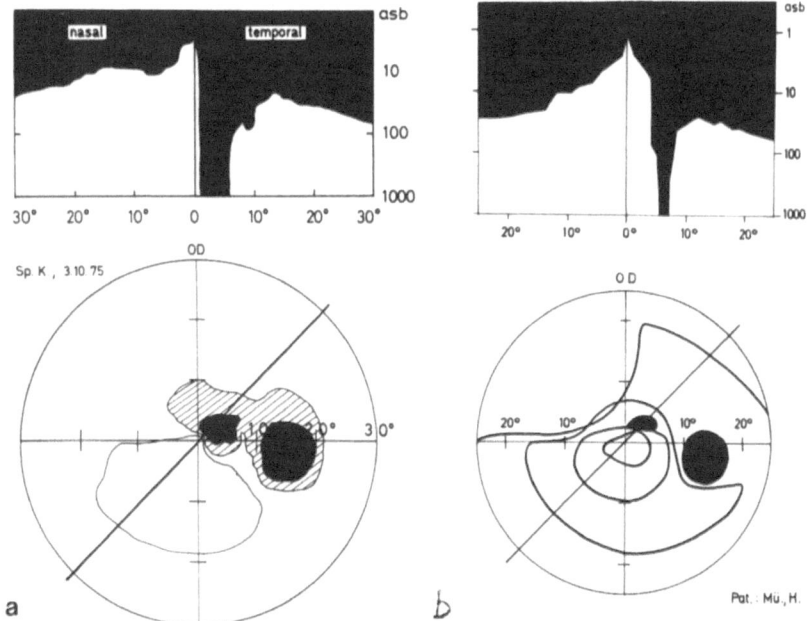

Fig. 4. Typical defects of the superior part in both diseases
   a) AION
   b) glaucoma

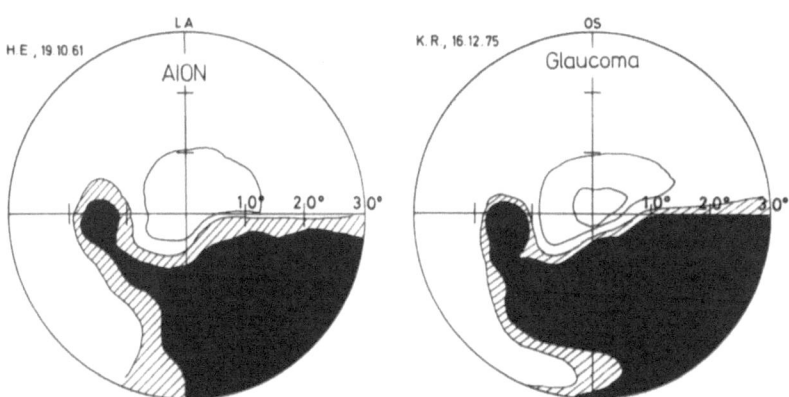

Fig. 5. Typical defects of the inferior part in AION and glaucoma.

77

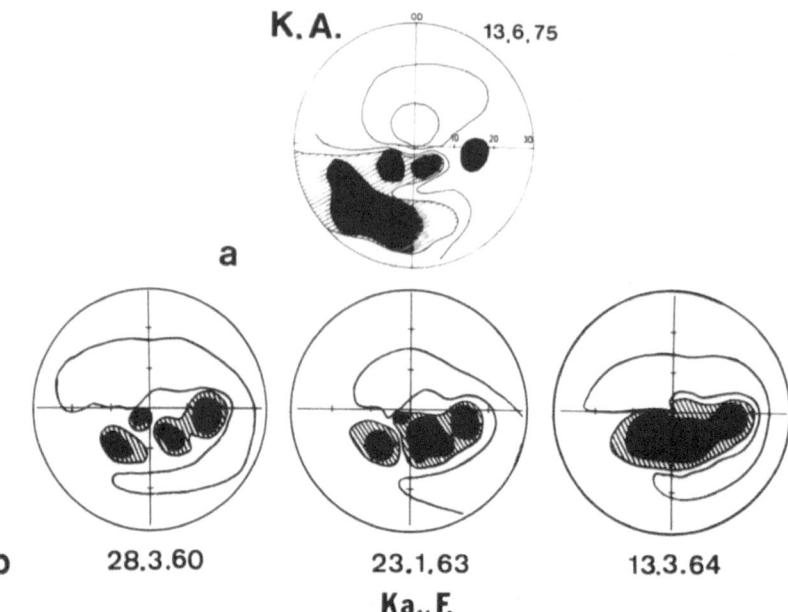

Fig. 6. No direct contact to the blind spot in spite of large defects.
a) AION
b) glaucoma

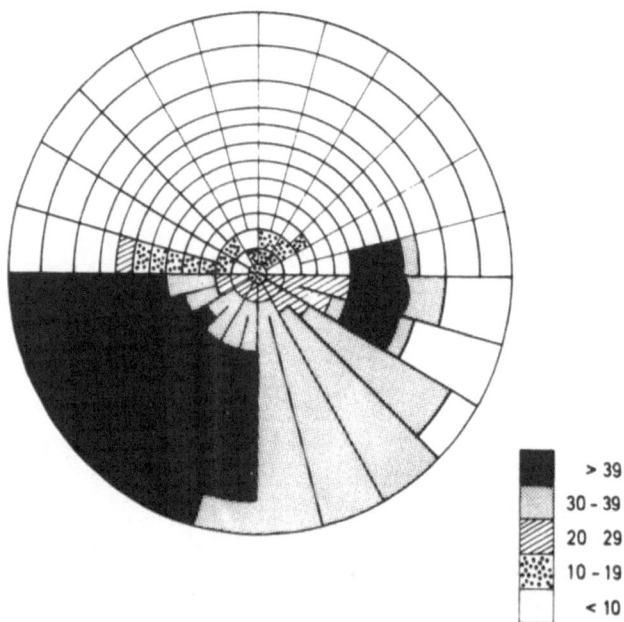

> 39
30 - 39
20 29
10 - 19
< 10

Fig. 7. Frequency distribution of the location of localized scotomas in 61 cases with
AION.

of both diseases, just as the inferior defects are usually very much larger than the superior ones in both diseases (Fig. 5). If we disregard the defects in AION, which affect the whole of the inferior half, then the inferior defects lie, as in glaucoma further from the centre than the superior ones and predominantly nasal to the vertical axis.

A further point, in which the defects in AION resemble those in glaucoma, is the spatial relation of the defects to the blind spot (Fig. 6). In as far as the defects in AION do not affect the whole inferior half of the visual field, the remaining 38 inferior defects very often – that is in 24 cases – have no connection as yet to the blind spot, just the same as the defects of stage 2 in glaucoma. The superior defects in AION have even more often no contact with the blind spot (in 9 out of 13 cases). This, too, is true of early glaucomatous defects.

In summary it follows that the defects in AION are, in so far as they are not very large, very similar in shape, size, and location to the defects, which we have determined in stages 2 and 3 of glaucomatous defects (Fig. 7). The large defects closely resemble those of stage 4. The differences in the large defects in both diseases lie not only in the higher frequency of defects in AION in the inferior part of the field, but also that in AION the field centre is sometimes included in the defect. This normally appears in glaucoma only in the final stage (Stage V of Fig. 1).

As we have seen, the defects in AION correspond partly to the defects of stage 2 and partly to those of stage 3 and 4 of glaucomatous defects. Whilst in the glaucoma these stages develop one after the other in the course of deterioration as the defects gradually become bigger, the defect in AION emerges suddenly. It corresponds then from the start in size, shape, and location to any one stage of development of glaucomatous defects and remains irreversibly in this stage. In AION we have before us as it were 'snapshots' in the course of glaucomatous damage – nevertheless always with the difference, that the inferior half of the visual field is more affected than the superior half. However, in the 21% of cases, in which a superior defect emerged, it had all the criteria shown also by early glaucomatous defects lying superior. The ischemic infarct of the papillary tissue, at the root of the visual defects in AION, must as a result be similar to glaucoma, as regards position and extent of the probable ischemic damage in the papillary tissue.

Our comparative study can give no information concerning the patho genesis of the damage in both diseases, but I believe that the observation made above can on its own represent an interesting contribution to the problem of glaucoma development.

REFERENCES

Hayreh. S.S. & Podhajsky, P. Visual fields defects in anterior ischemic optic neuropathy. Documenta Ophthalmologica Proceedings Series, 19: *53-71* (1979).

Authors' address:
Eberhard-Karls-Universität Tübingen
Universitäts-Augenklinik
7400 Tübingen
B.R.D.

VISUAL FIELD DEFECTS DUE TO HYPOPLASIA
OF THE OPTIC NERVE

LARS FRISÉN

(Göteborg, Sweden)

ABSTRACT

Any visual field defect associated with hypoplasia of the optic nerve is a reflection of the distribution and severity of axonal deficit. Patients with a uniformly distributed, low-degree lack of nerve fibers cannot be expected to produce clearcut perimetric defects. Patients with an advanced, diffuse deficit of neurons have more or less concentric contractions of the visual field, and subnormal visual acuity. Finally, patients with focal lack of nerve fibers may display any type of focal visual field defect. Visual acuity is often normal in these latter cases. Diagnostic hallmarks are a stationary visual deficit, and ophthalmoscopic signs of adaption of the optic disc to the remaining mass of nerve fibers. A subnormal diameter of the disc is not obligatory in minor hypoplasia. It is argued that optic nerve hypoplasia should be regarded as the unspecific result of visual pathway damage sustained some time before full development of the visual system.

Hypoplasia of the optic nerve is classically defined as a congenital condition characterized by a stationary deficit of vision, and an optic disc that is smaller than one half of normal size. More than one hundred cases of this type are on record and their visual deficits [primarily poor central vision and concentric or altitudinal contractions of the visual field (Gardner & Irvine 1972, Hittner, Desmond & Montgomery 1976, McKinna•1966, Petersen & Walton 1977, Seeley & Smith 1972] have been described well in the past. However, the classical definition of optic nerve hypoplasia (ONH) is inadequate in at least two regards. Firstly, there are no reasons to believe that hypoplasia always must be severe enough to reduce the disc diameter to one half of normal, or less. It is much more likely that ONH has a wide spectrum, abutting on optic nerve aplasia at the one end, and overlapping with the normal state at the other (Frisén & Holmegaard 1978). Secondly, the classical definition is inconsistent with the known fact that there is a two-fold range in dimensions among normal optic discs (Bengtsson 1976, Franceschetti & Bock 1950, Frisén & Holmegaard 1978). These arguments carry enough weight to call for a more comprehensive definition of OHN. Such a definition should be centered on the histopathologic hallmark, the reduction in number of optic nerve axons (Whinery & Blodi 1963), in combination with evidence of a prenatal or perinatal origin. Such an origin can be deduced from signs of compensatory adjustment of the diameter of the optic nervehead to the remaining mass of neurons. Diagnostic hallmarks of *minor* ONH therefore include a defective retinal nerve fiber layer, compensatory adjustment of the optic disc borders, and a corollary and stationary visual defect. The funduscopic abnormalities characteristic of minor ONH have recently been analysed elsewhere: here it may suffice to note that the disc abnormalities usually consist in foreshortening and remodelling of the disc border in areas adjacent to defects in the retinal nerve fiber layer. Disc remodelling usually involves the production of incomplete peripapillary rings. An outer, lighter ring is often separated from the true disc border by a narrow, pigmented ring (Frisén & Holmegaard 1978). The corollary visual field defects will be exemplified in the following.

It is likely that the clinical picture of ONH may be produced by a variety of mechanisms, not only a primary failure of development of retinal ganglion cells (Davis & Shock 1975, Hittner, Desmond & Montgomery 1976, McKinna 1966, Petersen & Walton 1977). Similar defects occur in patients with retrochiasmal visual pathway lesions acquired in the prenatal or perinatal periods: in these cases the abnormalities are bilateral (Hoyt, Rios-Montenegro, Behrens & Eckelhoff 1972). ONH can therefore be regarded as the unspecific result of a visual pathway lesion acquired some time before full development of the visual system (Frisén & Holmegaard 1978). It is practical to classify ONH in topical terms, whenever this is possible.

UNILATERAL OPTIC NERVE HYPOPLASIA

The spectrum of visual field defects in unilateral ONH ranges from minimal over severe contraction to complete blindness. The more severe varieties require no comment here. The same is the case with the upper temporal depressions associated with 'tilted' discs (Dorrell 1978). This latter syndrome can be regarded as the most common variant of ONH. Other variants may be more difficult to diagnose. In my experience, they usually take the form of a localized contraction and depression of the visual field (Figs. 1 and 2). Visual acuity is commonly within normal limits in these cases (Frisén & Holmegaard 1978, Gardner & Irvine 1972). An afferent pupillary defect is rarely observed when the central visual field is spared. Diagnosis is facilitated by juxta-positioning well focused fundus photographs and comparing the appearance of the peripapillary retinal nerve fiber layers, and the sizes and configurations of the optic discs.

BILATERAL OPTIC NERVE HYPOPLASIA

Bilateral ONH may be due to bilateral optic nerve lesions, chiasmal lesions, or retrochiasmal lesions, Bilateral prechiasmal lesions usually share the characteristics of unilateral lesions as described above, although binasal visual field defects seem to be more common in this latter group (Fig. 3).

Chiasmal lesions

A chiasmal localization of the responsible lesion appears likely whenever visual field defects are explicable in terms of the known arrangement of nerve fibers in the chiasm, and when the defects are combined with corresponding abnormalities of the retinal nerve fiber layer and the optic discs. A typical example is septo-optic dysplasia, where congenital bitemporal hemianopia is combined with absence of the septum pellucidum. In these cases, there is bilateral nasal foreshortening of the optic discs, and absence of the retinal nerve fiber layer within nasal and papillomacular sectors (Davis & Shock 1975). Less pronounced abnormalities may be more difficult to refer to a chiasmal origin with a similar degree of confidence (Fig. 4). The syndrome of bilaterally tilted optic discs is an important differential diagnosis (Dorrell 1978).

Retrochiasmal lesions

The picture of homonymous hemi-optic hypoplasia with complete homonymous hemianopia due to a congenital retrochiasmal lesion has been well described previously (Hoyt, Rios-Montenegro, Behrens & Eckelhoff 1972). These patients often have other signs of neurological abnormalities, i.e. cerebral palsy. The optic discs are smaller than average normal discs. The defects in the retinal nerve fiber layer are not the same on both sides. The eye contralateral to the lesion, the eye with the temporal hemianopia, shows a picture indistinguishable from that described above in the septo-optic dysplasia syndrome. The ipsilateral eye, the eye with a nasal hemianopia, shows a reduced prominence of the arcuate bundles of the retinal nerve fiber layer. This is due to the fact that nerve fibers coming from the temporal hemiretina are concentrated primarily to the arcuate bundles. Although

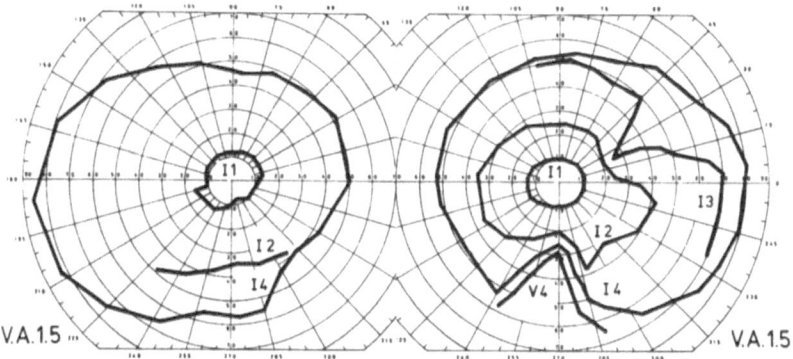

Fig. 1. Visual field defect due to right optic nerve hypoplasia. Fundus photographs showed faint peripapillary rings bilaterally. The right ring was twice as broad as the left on its nasal side; the vascularized area of the right disc was foreshortened similarly. Both discs were within normal limits in size but the horizontal diameter of the right disc was only 85 per cent of that on the left. The patient was a 26-year-old female laboratory assistant, who was referred for evaluation because of chronic headaches. No other abnormalities were disclosed.

83

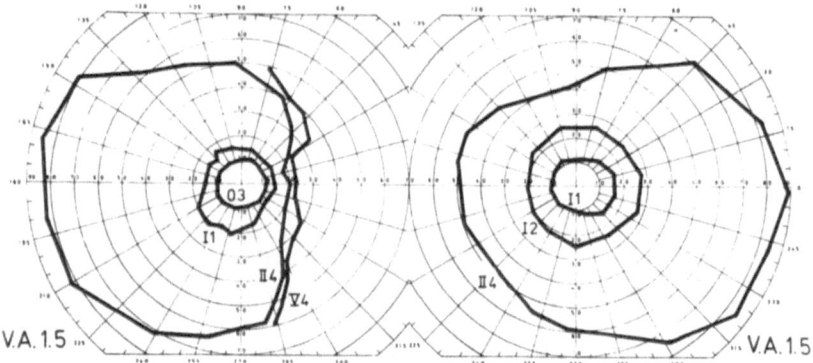

Fig. 2. Visual field defect due to left nerve hypoplasia. Fundus photographs showed faint peripapillary rings bilaterally. The two discs had the same width. The height of the left disc was only 79 per cent of that on the right, and there was corresponding thinning of the arcuate bundles. The patient was a 23-year-old with secondary amenorrhea. There were no signs of a pituitary tumor.

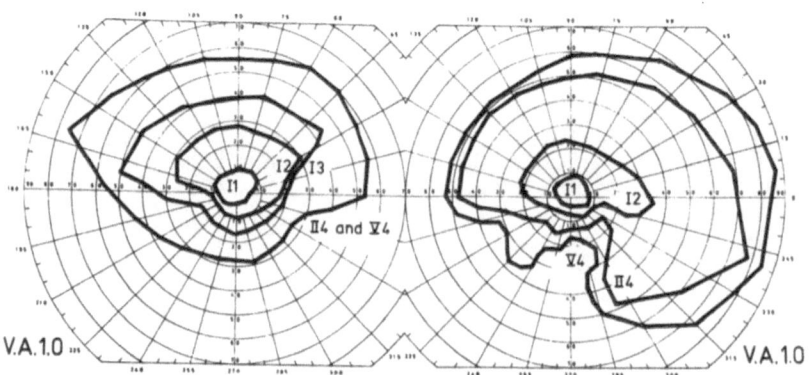

Fig. 3. Visual field defects due to bilateral optic nerve hypoplasia. Measurements on fundus photographs showed that both optic discs were just below the normal range in size. There were no peripapillary rings but the discs showed signs of remodelling superiorly, corresponding to the defects in the retinal nerve fiber layer. The patient was a 22-year-old female examined because of chronic headaches. No other abnormalities were disclosed.

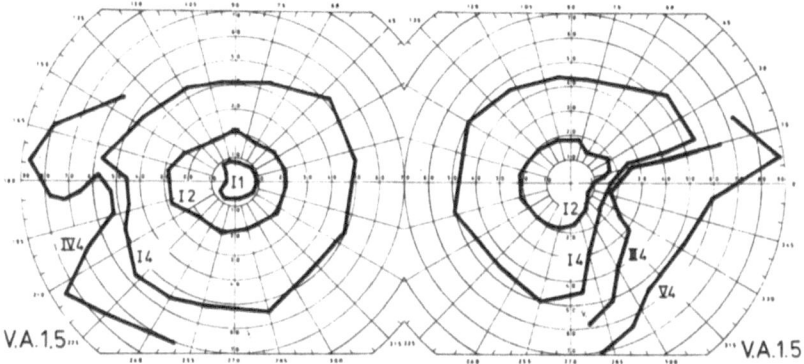

Fig. 4. Bilateral optic nerve hypoplasia, possibly due to a congenital chiasmal lesion. Measurements on fundus photographs showed that the optic discs had heights within the normal range, but the horizontal diameters were subnormal. There were no peripapillary rings. There was pronounced thinning of the retinal nerve fiber layer within horizontal sectors of the fundus. The patient was a 38-year-old epileptic female. The visual field defects had been stationary for at least 10 years.

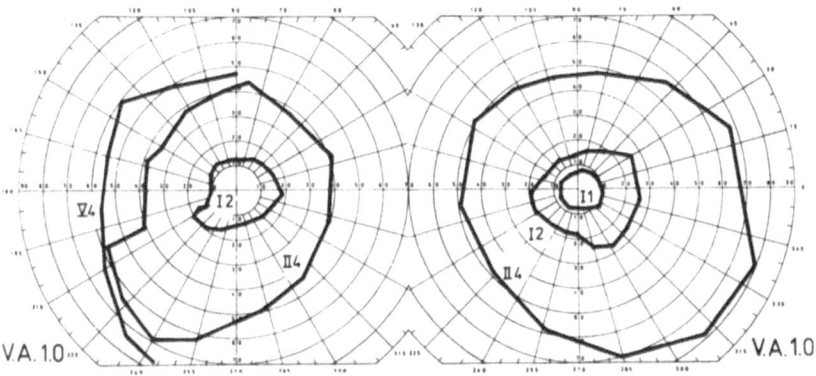

Fig. 5. Unilateral optic nerve hypoplasia mimicking loss of the temporal crescent due to a retrochiasmal lesion. The optic discs had the same height but the horizontal diameter was 20 per cent less on the left. There were no peripapillary rings but there was contraction of the left disc corresponding to the thinned horizontal sectors of the retinal nerve fiber layer. The patient was a 44 year old female referred in connection with a work-up for possible neurological disease. The subsequent examinations disclosed nothing abnormal.

85

less complete lesions certainly are conceivable, and their funduscopic characteristics can be predicted from present knowledge, such lesions have not yet been reported. The case presented in Fig. 5 mimics one variety of a suprageniculate lesion, namely loss of the temporal crescent in the contralateral eye. In this particular instance, truly unilateral hypoplasia was a more likely diagnosis as a retrochiasmal lesion producing a temporal defect of this magnitude would be expected to produce a congruent cut in the nasal field of the other eye.

REFERENCES

Bengtsson, B. The variation and covariation of cup and disc diameters. *Acta Ophthalmol.* 54: *804-818* (1976).

Davis, G.V. & Shock, J.P. Septo-optic dysplasia associated with see-saw nystagmus. Arch. Ophthalmol. 93: *137-139* (1975).

Dorrell, D. The tilted disc. *Br. J. Ophthalmol.* 62: *16-20* (1978).

Franceschetti, A. & Bock, R.H. Megalopapilla: a new congenital anomaly. *Am. J. Ophthalmol.* 33: *227-235* (1950).

Frisén, L. & Holmegaard, L. Spectrum of optic nerve hypoplasia. *Br. J. Ophthalmol.* 62: *7-15* (1978).

Gardner, H.B. & Irvine, A.R. Optic nerve hypoplasia with good visual acuity. *Arch. Ophthalmol.* 88: *255-258* (1972).

Hittner, H.M., Desmond, M.M. & Montgomery, J.R. Optic nerve manifestations of human congenital cytomegalovirus infection. *Am. J. Ophthalmol.* 81: *661-665* (1976).

Hoyt, W.F., Rios-Montenegro, E.N., Behrens, M.M. & Eckelhoff, R.J. Homonymous hemioptic hypoplasia. Funduscopic features in standard and red-free illumination in three patients with congenital hemiplegia. *Br. J. Ophthalmol.* 56: *537-545* (1972).

McKinna, A.L. Quinine induced hypoplasia of the optic nerve. *Canad. J. Ophthalmol.* 1: *261-266* (1966).

Petersen, R.A. & Walton, D.S. Optic nerve hypoplasia with good visual acuity and visual field defects. *Arch. Ophthalmol.* 95: *254-258* (1977).

Seeley, R.L. & Smith, J.L. Visual field defects in optic hypoplasia *Am. J. Ophthalmol.* 73: *882-889* (1972).

Whinery, R.D. & Blodi, F.C. Hypoplasia of the optic nerve: a clinical and histopathologic correlation. *Trans. Am. Acad. Ophthalmol. Otolaryngol.* 67: *733-738* (1963).

Author's address:
Department of Ophthalmology
University of Göteborg
Sahlgren's Hospital
S-413 45 Göteborg
Sweden

Docum. Ophthal. Proc. Series, Vol. 19

VISUAL FIELD DEFECTS IN
CONGENITAL HYDROCEPHALUS

H. BYNKE & L. VESTERGREN-BRENNER

(Lund, Sweden)

ABSTRACT

Various kinds of visual field defects were found in 15 patients with congenital hydrocephalus and optic atrophy. Paracentral defects and caecocentral scotomata were most frequent and occurred in 8 patients. These defects were ascribed to direct or indirect compression of the chiasma and the optic nerves by a distended third ventricle during attacks of intracranial hypertension. Although the pale optic discs had abnormally sharp borders, transient papilloedema had occurred in the majority of these cases. Concentric contraction and optic atrophy with blurred discs after papilloedema were found in 2 patients and dense central scotomata due to macular changes in 3. The remaining 2 patients had homonymous hemianopic defects, i.e. lesions of the post-chiasmatic visual pathway.

INTRODUCTION

The mechanisms behind the optic atrophy in congenital hydrocephalus are not fully understood, largely since this disease has made the patients uncooperative during perimetry. However, it is wellknown that in aqueduct stenosis the distended third ventricle may act as a tumour and compress the chiasma with resulting bitemporal hemianopia. Hughes (1946) demonstrated that paracentral scotomata may precede the development of this bitemporal hemianopia. Lassman et al. (1960) described a child with aqueduct stenosis and a unilateral upper quadrantanopia, which was ascribed to damage to the optic nerve by the enormously dilated third ventricle. Hughes (1946) and Lassman et al. (1960) also presented excellent reviews of the previous literature on this topic. Smith et al. (1966) mentioned that optic atrophy may also be due to papilloedema, associated developmental anomalies, and other mechanisms, and reported five cases of congenital hydrocephalus with cortical blindness after shunt-operations.

Thanks to modern shunt-operations, many patients with congenital hydrocephalus can now cooperate during perimetry. This report deals with such patients.

MATERIAL

The material consists of 15 patients, 9 male and 6 female, aged between 10 and 43 years (Table 1). It comprises a selection of cases with congenital and

87

probably congenital hydrocephalus with concomitant optic atrophy. These patients had previously been treated in the Department of Neurosurgery in Lund.

In 9 patients the initial signs of disease, e.g. delayed development, tense fontanels and abnormally rapid growth of head, had appeared at birth or during the first months of life. In 6 patients the initial symptoms, e.g. headache, vomiting, or visual deterioration, had occurred after the age of 6 years.

Aqueduct stenosis was found in 10 cases. There was communication between the third and fourth ventricles in 5 cases. The hydrocephalus was associated with other congenital malformations in 7 patients.

Repeated eye examinations had been performed at the Department of Neuro-Ophthalmology. Transient papilloedema of a low or moderate degree had been observed in 8 patients. Except in cases 2 and 9 the optic atrophy was not present at the first examination but developed insidiously, often after attacks or intracranial hypertension, whether papilloedema had been found or not.

Single or repeated shunt-operations had been performed in 12 patients. The subdural hygromas of case 1 had been evacuated and the arteriovenous malformation (AVM) in Sylvian fossa of case 7 extirpated. The myelomeningoceles of cases 6, 10 and 11 had been treated operatively at an early stage. At the time of the present study the patients' general condition was good.

Table 1. Material. AS = aqueduct stenosis.

Case	Sex years	Age at initial symptoms	Observed papill- oedema	Other findings	Shunt- operation(s)
1	m 13	4 mos.	–	Subdural hygromas	–
2	m 26	24 yrs.	–	AS + Arnold-Chiari malform.	+
3	m 10	7 yrs.	+	AS	+
4	m 22	9 yrs.	+	AS	+
5	m 19	6 mos.	+	AS	+
6	m 10	0	+	AS + myelomeningocele	+
7	m 14	0	–	AVM in Sylvian fossa	–
8	f 16	8 yrs.	+	AS + deformed skull bones (Mb. Recklinghausen)	+
9	f 23	18 yrs.	–	–	+
10	f 14	0	+	AS + myelomeningocele	+
11	f 11	0	+	AS + myelomeningocele	+
12	f 13	0	–	AS. Congen. toxoplasmosis	+
13	m 13	0	–	AS. Congen. toxoplasmosis	+
14	m 15	0	–	–	+
15	f 43	6 yrs.	+	–	–

METHODS

The patients were re-examined by the authors in 1977.

Goldmann's kinetic perimeter was used in all cases. Because of mental defects 6 patients did not cooperate perfectly and were examined once more after some months. Additional methods were automatic computerized perimetry (Heijl & Krakau 1975, Bynke & Heijl 1978, Bynke, Heijl & Holmin 1978), which was performed in 9 patients, and Friedmann's Visual Field Analyser, which was used in 5 patients.

The colour vision was tested with Ishihara's and Boström-Kugelberg's pseudo-isochromatic charts.

The fundi were examined with ophthalmoscopy and photography. We used a Carl Zeiss Fundus Camera with its 2X magnification attachment. Black and white negative film (Kodak Tri-X Pan) was exposed through a built-in Kodak Wratten gelatine filter no. 40. The negatives were developed in Kodak Microdol 1:3 and printed on Ilfospeed paper 3. Colour diapositives (Kodak Ektachrome 64) were also obtained.

The ocular findings were taken into account in a revaluation of the roentgenograms.

RESULTS

The three perimetric methods gave approximately the same results.

Cases 1 - 8 had paracentral defects and caecocental scotomata, reduced visual acuity and defective colour vision in one or both eyes (Table 2).

In visual fields the paracentral defects were small, partly scotomatous and located in the temporal hemi-fields (Fig. 1). In 3 fields the paracentral nasal

Table 2. Results.

Case	Visual acuity RE	LE	Visual field RE	Visual field LE
1	0.9	0.7	paracent. def.	normal?
2	0.5	1.0	caecocent. scot.	normal?
3	0.9	1.0	paracent. def.	paracent. def.
4	0.9	0.8	caecocent. scot.	normal?
5	0.9	1.0	caecocent. scot.	paracent. def.
6	0.7	0.9	paracent. def.	paracent. def.
7	0.4	1.0	paracent. def.	paracent. def.
8	1.0	0.9	paracent. def.	caecocent. scot.
9	0.4	0.06	concent. contr.	concent. contr.
10	0.5	0.2	concent. contr.	concent. contr.
11	0.04	1.0	cent. scot.	normal
12	0.1	0.04	cent. scot.	cent. scot.
13	0.2	0.2	cent. scot.	cent. scot.
14	0.7	0.2	lt. quadrantanopia	lt. quadrantanopia
15	0.7	0.4	rt. hemianopia	rt. hemianopia

area was involved as well. In 4 fields (cases 2, 4, 5 and 8) the temporal paracentral scotomata were connected with a central scotoma, thus forming a caecocentral scotoma (Fig. 2). Two patients had small paracentral defects in one visual field and a caecocentral scotoma in the other one. In 3 fields no significant defect was found despite the occurrence of slight optic atrophy. In 2 of these eyes there was defective colour vision.

The optic discs of these 8 patients were pale and had abnormally sharp borders. The defects of the retinal nerve fibre layer were either diffuse or focal and corresponded to the field defects (Fig. 3).

Cases 9 - 15 had other kinds of field defects. Their visual acuity was generally lower than in the first group of cases.

In 4 visual fields (cases 9 and 10) there was concentric contraction of the isopters. These eyes were the only ones in this series with blurred disc borders and diffuse retinal nerve fibre degeneration.

Five eyes (cases 11, 12 and 13) had dense central scotomata, pronounced macular changes and temporal optic atrophy. In case 11, whose left fundus was normal, there was a cystic degeneration of the right macula. Cases 12 and 13 had heavily pigmented macular scars typical of congenital toxoplasmosis.

In case 14, there was a homonymous left inferior quadrantanopia and a diffuse retinal nerve fibre degeneration. Several shunt-operations had been made in this patient, who had also had a post-operative, transient left hemi-

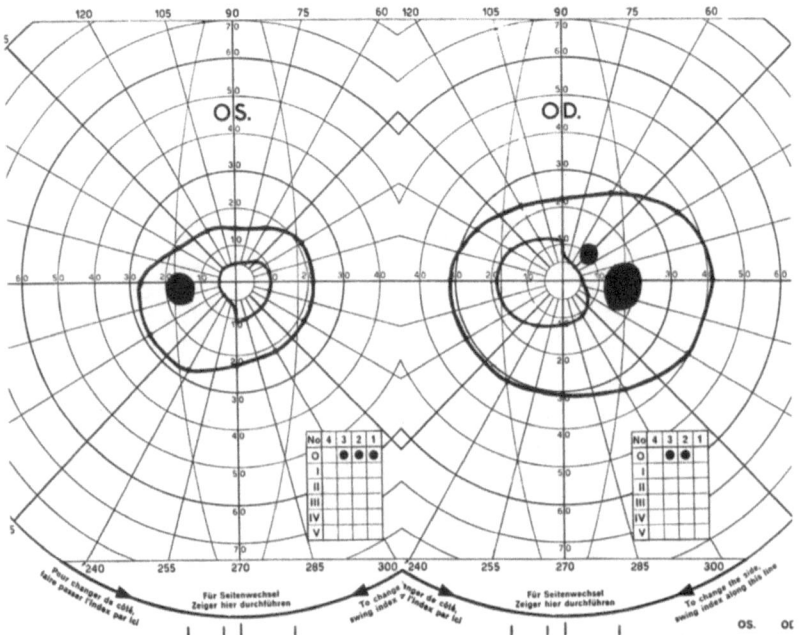

Fig. 1. Visual fields in case 7. Paracentral defects in both fields.

paresis. Case 15 had a subtotal right homonymous hemianopia and a homonymous hemioptic nerve fibre degeneration with normal-sized optic discs.

Other findings in *both groups* of cases were amblyopic pupillary response, jerky or pendular nystagmus, and heterotropia. In some eyes the latter seemed responsible for the reduced visual acuity.

The third ventricle was enormously dilated and extended into the partly empty sella in cases 2, 4, 8 and 9. It was moderately dilated and did not extend into the sella in cases 1, 3, 7, 12, 14 and 15. In the latter case the lateral ventricles were very wide. The third ventricle could not be evaluated on the roentgenograms of cases 5, 6, 10, 11 and 13.

DISCUSSION

The caecocentral scotomata and the paracentral visual field defects of *cases 1 - 8* indicated that the lesion was situated in the optic nerves or in the

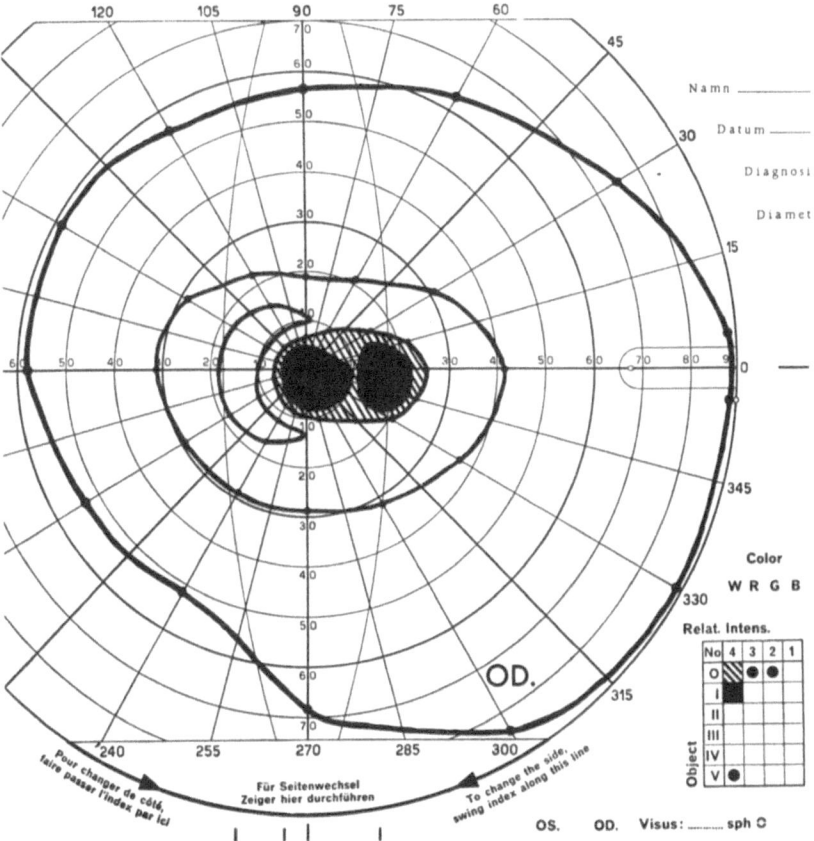

Fig. 2. Right visual field in case 2. Caecocentral scotoma. No field defect was found in the left eye, but the colour vision was defective.

91

chiasma. Although transient papilloedema had been found in 5 of these patients, the pale discs had abnormally sharp borders.

In at least 3 out of the 4 cases with caecocentral scotomata, the third ventricle was enormously dilated and extended into the sella. We suggest that during attacks of intracranial hypertension, the distended third ventricle had compressed the optic nerves or pushed and pressed them against bone or other structures. The course of case 2 supports this hypothesis, since the caecocentral scotoma decreased and the visual acuity increased from 0.1 to 0.5 after shunt-operation.

It seems reasonable to assume that the paracentral defects were the result of a similar mechanism. As mentioned, Hughes (1946) demonstrated that paracentral scotomata may precede the development of a bitemporal hemianopia. In agreement with this, the field defects of case 7 may be interpreted as an intermediate stage between paracentral scotomata and bitemporal hemianopia (Fig. 1).

In *cases 9 - 15* the mechanisms were easier to explain. The concentric contraction of the fields in cases 9 and 10 was evidently secondary to

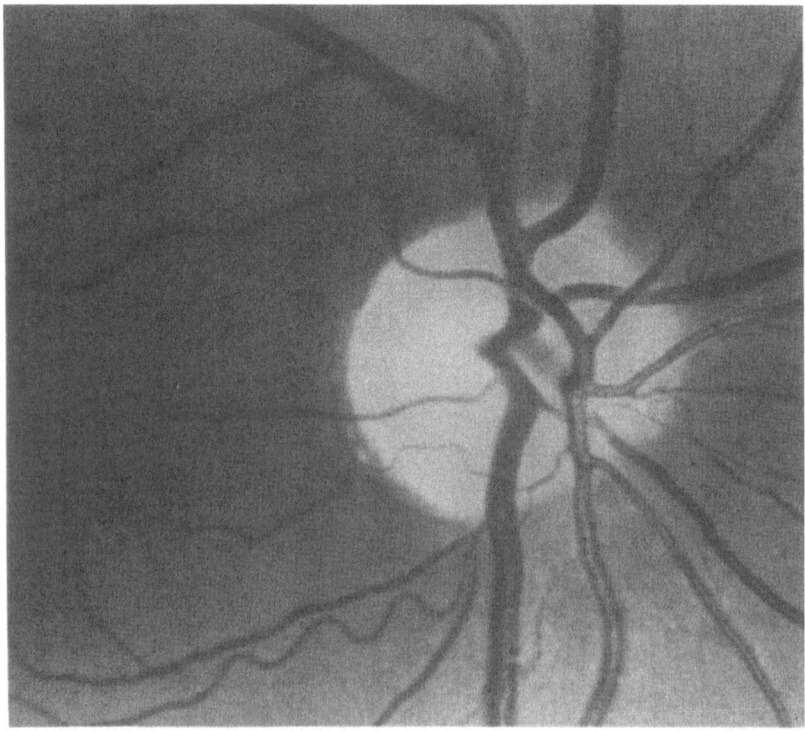

Fig. 3a. Right (a) and left fundus (b) in case 2. The right optic disc is pale with an abnormally sharp temporal border. The degeneration of the retinal nerve fibre layer is most marked in the papillomacular area. The left fundus has similar but less pronounced changes.

papilloedema. The dense central scotomata in cases 11, 12 and 13 were caused by macular changes. The homonymous inferior quadrantanopia of case 14 seemed to be due to surgical injury to the optic radiation. This complication has also been described by Smith et al. (1966). In case 15 with homonymous hemioptic nerve fibre degeneration and very wide lateral ventricles, the homonymous hemianopia was caused by a lesion to the optic tract or an early lesion to the optic radiation (Hoyt et al. 1973).

To sum up, the commonest cause of optic atrophy in this material seemed to be direct or indirect compression of the anterior visual pathway by a distended third ventricle. Other causes were papilloedema, macular changes, and lesions to the post-chiasmatic visual pathway.

ACKNOWLEDGEMENTS

The authors' thanks are due to S. Cronquist, M.D., Dept. of Neuroradiology, for revaluation of the roentgenograms, and to Å. Kjällquist, M.D., Dept. of Neurosurgery, for valuable advice.

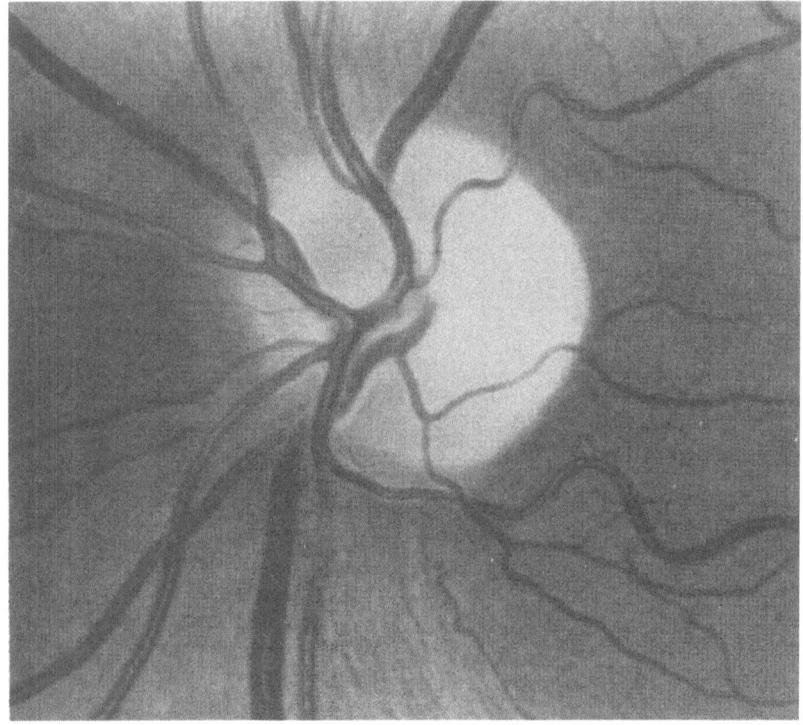

Fig. 3b.

REFERENCES

Bynke, H. & Heijl, A. Automatic computerized perimetry in the detection of neurological visual field defects. A pilot study. *Graefes Arch. Ophthal.* (1978).

Bynke, H., Heijl, A. & Holmin, C. Automatic computerized perimetry in neuro-ophthalmology. *Docum. Ophthal. Proc. Series* (1978).

Heijl, A. & Krakau, C.E.T. An automatic perimeter for glaucoma visual field screening and control. Construction and clinical cases. *Graefes Arch. Ophthal.* 197: *13-23* (1975).

Hoyt, W.F. & Kommerell, G. Der Fundus oculi bei homonymer Hemianopie. *Klin. Monatsbl. f. Augenheilk.* 162: *456-464* (1973).

Hughes, E.B.C. Some observations on the visual fields in hydrocephalus. *J. Neurol., Neurosurg. & Psychiat.* 9: *30-39* (1946).

Lassman, L.P., Cullen, J.F. & Howat, J.M.L. Stenosis of the aqueduct of Sylvius. *Am. J. Ophthal.* 49: *261-266* (1960).

Smith, J.L., Walsh, T.J. & Shipley, T. Cortical blindness in congenital hydrocephalus. *Am. J. Ophthal.* 62: *251-257* (1966).

Authors' address:
University Eye Clinic
S-221 85 Lund
Sweden

Docum. Ophthal. Proc. Series, Vol. 19

CENTRAL CRITICAL FUSION FREQUENCY IN NEURO-OPHTHALMOLOGICAL PRACTICE

TOSHIFUMI OTORI, TAKASHI HOHKI
& YUZO NAKAO

(Osaka, Japan)

ABSTRACT

Clinical usefulness of determining central CFF in the diagnosis of optic nerve diseases was studied on over 10.000 cases using a flicker apparatus developed by the authors. Dissociation of central vision and CFF was so remarkable that 'flicker test' can be used as the most important and reliable test in the diagnosis of optic nerve diseases in neuro-ophthalmological practice.

INTRODUCTION

Critical fusion frequency (CFF) and flicker fields have been studied by many investigators in an attempt to apply them to the examination of ophthalmological diseases. However, neither of them have been established as one of the routine examinations.

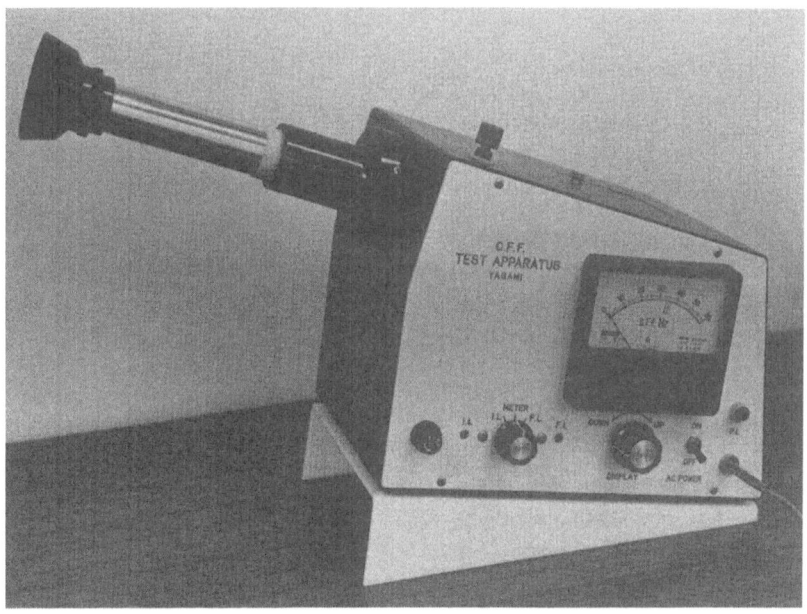

Fig. 1. Photograph of flicker test apparatus.

95

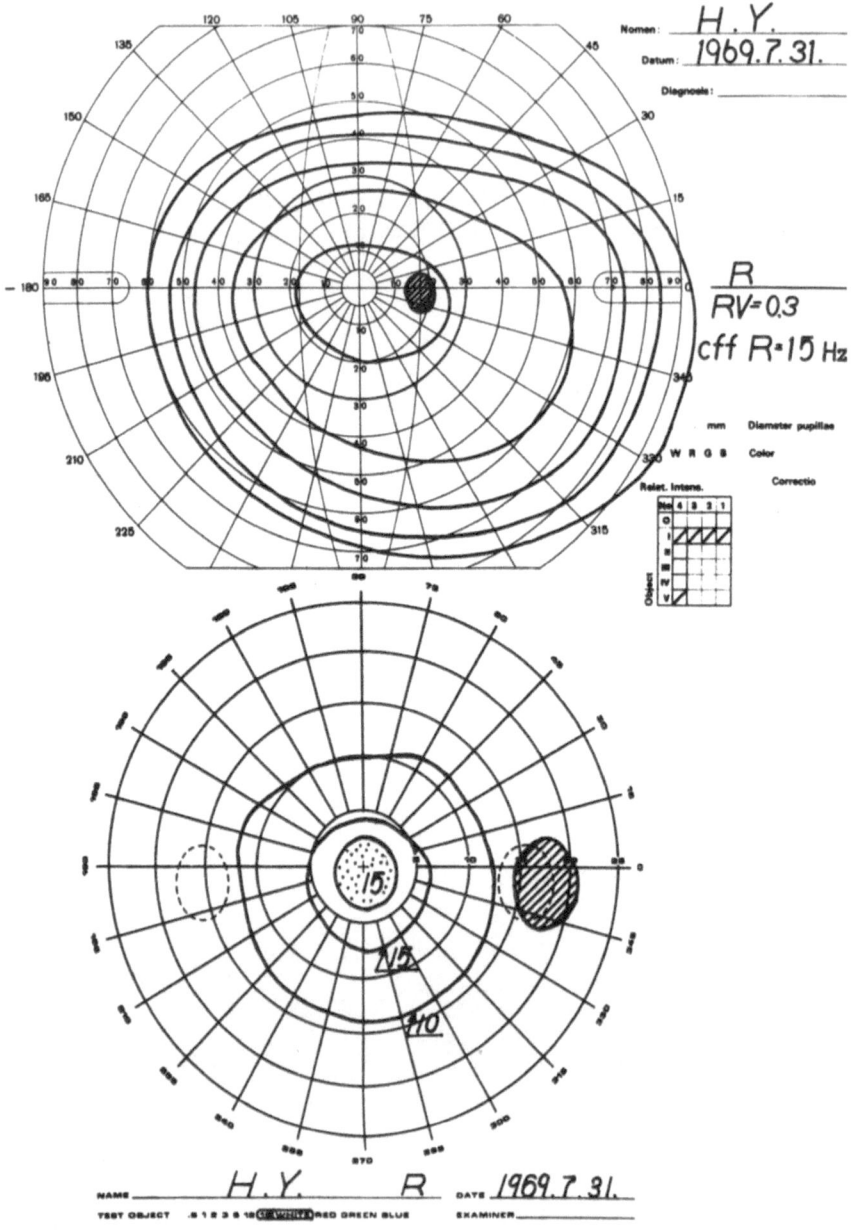

Fig. 2. Comparison of visual fields in a case of optic neuritis using goldmann perimeter and modified flicker Autoplot Tangent Screen.

We have been interested in flicker perimetry and campimetry since 20 years ago and we have made a few reports on these subjects (Mizukawa, Nakabayashi, Manabe, Otori & Kosaki 1960). For the last 8 years, we have studied the clinical usefulness of determining central CFF in neuro-ophthalmological practice.

It is the purpose of this study to demonstrate that measurement of central CFF ('flicker test') is the most important and reliable method of examination for the diagnosis and follow-up of optic nerve diseases.

MATERIALS AND METHODS

We have developed an apparatus for the measurement of central CFF as shown in figure 1. Servo- or control circuit was employed to assure smooth stabilized frequency of the flickering target whose diameter was 10 mm. The target subtended 2 degrees at a 300 mm test distance. Luminosity of the background was set at approximately 4 asb and that of the flickering target was equal to 1,000 asb when the disc was kept motionless.

We also used a modified flicker tangent screen for the studies of central

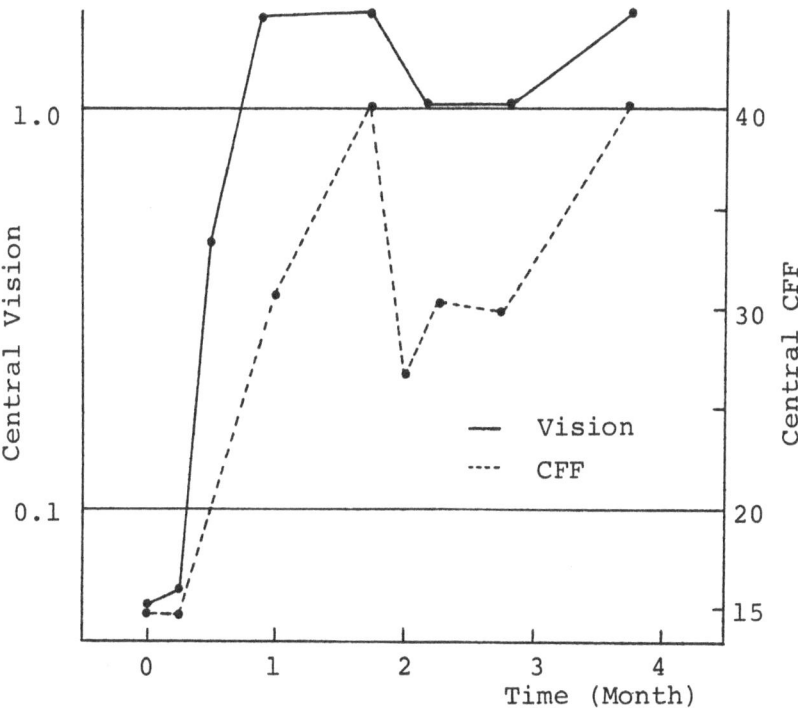

Fig. 3. A typical course of recovery of vision and CFF in optic neuritis (with recurrence).

97

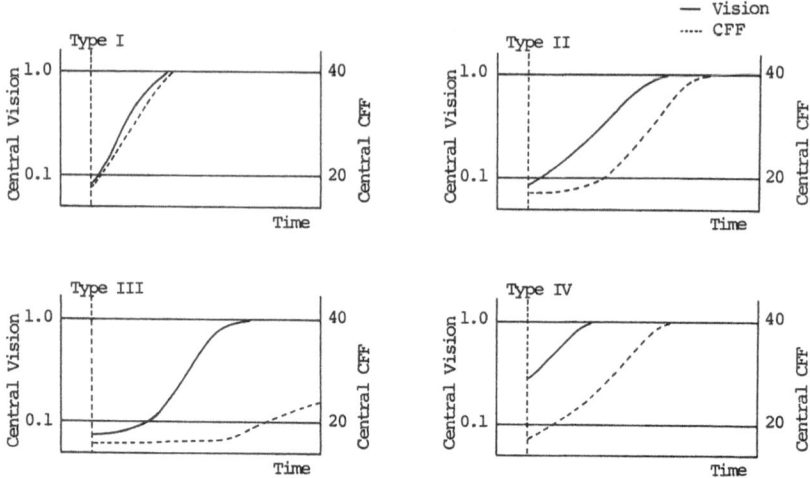

Fig. 4. Various types of course of recovery of vision and CFF in optic neuritis.

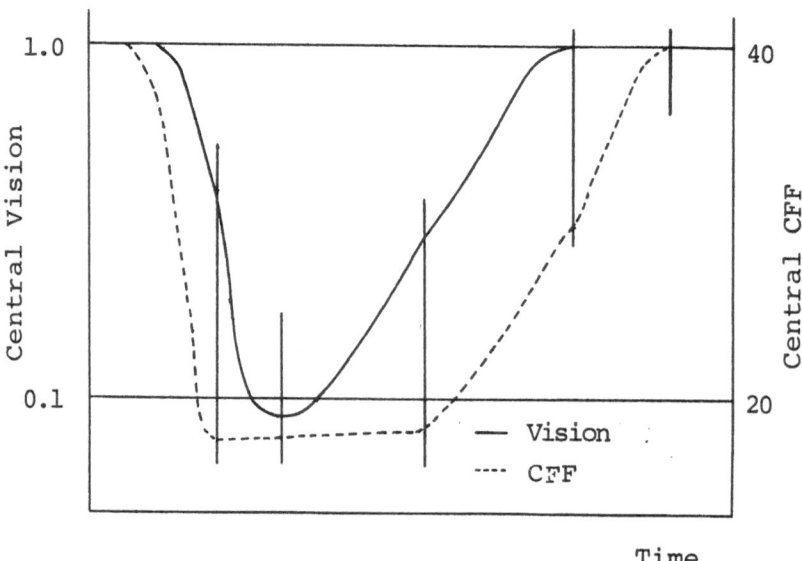

Fig. 5. A schematic drawing of course of vision CFF in optic neurits.

field. A flicker attachment, originally designed by Dr. Nakabayashi (1967) was inserted in the optical pathway of Autoplot Tangent Screen made by Bausch and Lomb.

Patients were chosen from those who visited the outpatient clinic and neuro-ophthalmology clinic of our institutions during the past 8 years.

RESULTS AND DISCUSSION

Figure 2 is a typical case of optic neuritis in which kinetic Goldmann perimetry failed to detect central scotoma. However, in central flicker field studies we detected central scotoma. The central vision was 0.3 and central CFF was 15 Hz. We could easily come to a diagnosis of optic neuritis. Figure 3 is a typical course of recovery of vision and CFF in optic neuritis. Following steroid therapy, vision was recovered first, followed by the recovery of CFF. After one month and a half, the patient complained of blurring of vision. Although there was very small reduction of visual acuity, CFF was reduced remarkably, indicating that there was recurrence of optic neuritis. As far as we rely on central vision and ordinary kinetic perimetry and campimetry, it is not easy to detect very early changes of optic nerve lesion or recurrence of optic neuritis.

Various types of recovery of central vision and central CFF are shown in figure 4. Figure 5 is a schematic drawing of the course of recovery of vision and central CFF in optic neuritis. Vertical lines indicates the time of observation. If we see a patient in a very early stage, we can detect dissociation of vision and CFF as shown in type IV. If we see a patient at the time of lowest vision and CFF, the course of recovery and CFF may vary from case to case. This observation of dissociation of vision and CFF is most important in the diagnosis of optic nerve diseases in their early stages.

Normal values ranges from 40 to 50 Hz and the lowest limit is 35 Hz. If central CFF is less than 25 Hz, we can definitely make a diagnosis of optic nerve disease even though vision is restored within a normal range. Therefore, the 'flicker test' is equally or even more important than the examination of pupillary reflex.

Based on our experience in the past 8 years, we can conclude that the 'flicker test' is useful in the diagnosis of optic neuritis and papillits, toxic amblyopia, optic nerve injury, compression of the optic nerve by the tumor. This test is also useful in the differential diagnosis of atrophic stage of papilledema, optic atrophy and disc pallor only, amblyopia, refractive anomaly, disturbance of accommodation, hysteria and simulation.

SUMMARY

We developed an apparatus for the measurement of central CFF and used this on over 10,000 cases during the last 8 years. It was confirmed that CFF is remarkably decreased in optic nerve or 3rd neuron diseases and this 'flicker test' is the most reliable test to be used in the diagnosis of optic nerve diseases in neuro-ophthalmological practice.

REFERENCES

Matsuda, H. & Nakabayashi, M. Studies on a newly devised flicker campimeter. *Clin. J. Ophthal.* 21: *673-677* (1967).

Mizukawa, T., Nakabayashi, M., Manabe, R., Otori, T. & Kosaki, H. Studies on flicker fusion fields by an iso-frequency method. *Med. J. Osaka Univ.* 11: *155-164* (1960).

Mizukawa, T., Nakabayashi, M., Manabe, R. & Otori, T. Clinical studies on the visual field. *Clin. J. Ophthal.* 22: *253-267* (1968)

Authors'. address:
380, Nishiyama, Sayama-cho,
Minami-Kawachigun, Osaka Prefecture
Japan 589

DISCUSSION OF THE SESSION ON
NEURO-OPHTHALMOLOGY

CHAIRMAN: H. BYNKE

Bynke: I suggest that we divide the discussion into three parts. *The first*: questions to Dr. Frisén about his introductory paper and the *second*: questions to Dr. Isayama about his paper. And in the *third* part, if we have time, some questions to subsequent speakers.

Hayreh: Dr. Frisén I am talking more about the text of the paper which came through rather than the speech which I was actually discussing with you yesterday.

In the opening sentence of your paper you said that lesions of anterior visual pathway may be associated with fundus abnormalities in several ways but most commonly through interference with axoplasmic flow transport mechanism and through descending degeneration of the axons.

From all the available evidence so far, we know that the conduction in the axon is along the membrane. The axoplasmic transport itself has very little to do with the conduction of the impulse. This has very important implications, for example: does obstruction of the axoplasmic flow transport interfere with the function?

The implication goes on to glaucoma and people feel that since raised intra-ocular pressure reduces the axoplasmic flow transport, the visual field defects in glaucoma can be explained on the basis. But all the available evidence from experimental studies and from clinical observations of patients with optic disc oedema due to raised intracranial pressure, lasting for months and months and even years, indicates that there is no detectable visual functional change with axoplasmic flow transport. I know Dr. Frisen said that perhaps our methods are not sensitive enough to test early functional defects but within the limitation and within the available technique so far we know that it does not interfere with the function.

And the following point I like to talk about is a paper where he showed some patients with Leber's optic atrophy with hyperemia of the nerve fibers. One sees that, but every patient with Leber does not have that. So that is not universily applicable to patients with Lebers optic atrophy.

Frisén: Well, I am not as much bothered about this disproportion as regards axonal constipation and visual testing as Dr. Hayreh is. However, it is disturbing that we cannot show functional correlates of disturbed axon flow.

Perhaps we can bring this up in a couple of years time and solve it then. Concerning the appearance of retinal nerve fiber layer hyperemia in Leber's optic neuropathy I cannot add very much from my own experience as I have not seen many cases but I would guess that the time factor is very important here. The disease of course has a quite protracted course and if you come into the clinical picture several weeks or perhaps a few months after the beginning of visual impairement I think it would be reasonable to expect that hyperemia is absent. I would think it would be characteristic of the acute phase.

Fankhauser: Dr. Frisén's paper was of particular importance for the kind of thinking I'm practising because it very strikingly shows that pre-information is crucial for the detection of scotomata, as most scotomata are extremely difficult to detect unless you have pre-knowledge and pre-information. This is very easily obtained by the method of Dr. Frisén and hence with this information of knowing where they may be, you can detect them with a much higher degree of probability just by increasing scandensity and alternating the measuring error across these areas where you have found them on the photographs.

Bynke: I have a question myself to Dr. Frisén but it is about the same thing that has been discussed already. I have often been confused by all these old patients who have a seemingly diffuse loss of nerve fibers, but we cannot find any field defects in them and I know that the opinion of Dr. Frisén is that our methods are not very sensitive. Are you sure that everything that looks like nerve fibers degeneration is that thing, it may be something else, possibly?

Frisén: I think that this is a point that is very well taken. Of course what appears to be retinal nerve fiber layer concerns not only the nerve fibers but there is a great abundance of small vessels in the same area and what we are witnessing in the fundus is not only loss of nerve fibers but also loss of supporting tissues, particularly small vessels. We have much to learn in this regard. It is also my impression that we loose nerve fibers as the years pass by and that it is much more difficult or much more seldom that you see a prominent nerve fiber layer in the aged. It is much easier to witness these things in the young people. I think this is a reflection of what is going on in the body of all of us, in all parts of the body, the continuing loss of neural structures and the reason for having difficulties in picking up this diffuse atrophy of the neural apparatus resides primarily in our poor definitions of what is normal. We don't know very well what characterizes a normal visual field; we have quite big tolerance limits and apparently accept pronounced deterioration of function without calling it decisively abnormal and this actually goes back to the fact that we don't really know what we measure in perimetry. We don't understand the anatomical basis of simple contrast sensitivity. If we used a measure that was sensitive to the density of working units we would be in a better position to reveal the diffuse loss of neural channels. I had the opportunity of speaking of this in Marseilles, namely peripheral visual acuity. Acuity is the only known visual function that has a well understood anatomical basis and a diffuse loss of channels must lead to a loss of acuity.

Greve: I presume that the nerve fiber bundle defects, the slits, are irreversible. It is well known that in the demyelinating disease, multiple sclerosis, in early stages specially, there is a great fluctuation of defects. These defects may be reversible to an enormous extent. Could I ask Dr. Frisén what he sees in these cases? There seems to be tendency in his paper that the present perimetric methods are not sensitive enough. What is the correlate of your funduscopy in these cases of early defects in multiple sclerosis both central and in the Bjerrum area?

Frisén: This is a very important question and brings up the difficulties in defining the various types of optic neuropathies as we may see in the demyelinating disease but in principal we have two major varieties! *First* the acute demyelinating optic neuropathy that we often discover in younger patients, that really I believe is primarily demyelinating in nature and where the visual deficit has to do with disturbed conduction in morphological intact neural channels and the restitution of function to normal levels is possible just because the anatomical groundwork is still there. The axons can go on working properly once the conduction deficit is normalised. This is not so with the *second* variety of demyelinating optic neuropathy, the one that we see in patients that have had demyelinating disease for several years or several decades, patients that have a chronic progressive optic neuropathy with progressive deterioration of function. These are the patients that loose nerve fibers. They show no reversibility in my experience.

Enoch: I was going to make certain comments in response to Dr. Otori's paper but I think that in this discussion as it evolves with Greve and Frisén, this may be the point to make the comment.

In the rather strange nature of division of responsibility of these meetings I will be giving a paper Tuesday on the Int. Ophthalmological Optics Conference. Normally I would personally object to comments such as I am making but I think it is quite pertinent to this discussion. Some years ago we described the so called fatigue or saturation like effect relating to repeated static perimetric tests and we have simply asked the question what happens in e.g. a person with demyelinating disease or possible demyelinating disease if you increase the level of intensity of the adaption or the test by an enormous amount, let us say a thousand times more than cupula of the perimeter. It turns out we had a resolution test that did this. We used a five degree target and could measure the resolution in time in an intense adapting field.

We had a patient who had just recovered from a first incident of probable multiple sclerosis. His visual acuity had returned to about 20/20. And now by using an intense background his visual resolution fell within a minute or two from 20/20 to 28/100 or even less.

It is fascinating that if you test the second eye of this individual, where there have been no visual symptoms at all, you see exactly the same thing only in a slightly less degree. We have seen this happen in quite a number of patients.

We also have cases I might add where there are no symptoms in either eye but probably multiple sclerosis showing comparable effects.

Frisén: Dr. Enoch, I think this nicely demonstrates the need for testing methods that put a greater stress on the visual system than does simple comparison sensitivity. Although it bothers me a bit to think about what people using dazzling tests would say about this kind of results, as the dazzling tests the recovery of vision following a bright adaptation of the macula-is usually considered a sign of macular disease.

Tagami: Regarding unilateral visual field defects in chiasmal lesions, you show in your paper diffuse atrophy of nerve fiber bundles in perimetrically normal eyes. But by using serious visual field examination, for example a Tübingen static central field, didn't you detect field defects corresponding to the nerve fiber bundle defects?

Frisén: No I did not. And I think this is once again due to the large tolerance we have with regards to normal limits.

Bynke: I think we have to conclude this subject. There is often a very good correspondence between the nerve fiber degeneration and the visual field defects. This is natural but it is also natural that this correspondance is not always there. It can be an early damage that has produced a visual field defect and not yet any defect of the nerve fiber bundles of course. I think that this subject is very important and that we all should look more after nerve fiber degeneration than we did before. My study of these things in Bill Hoyt's department has convinced me that we can train. I could not see much at first but after a few months of training it goes better.

So it is important also for making a prognosis. For example Dr. Frisén and Dr. Lundström have shown that nerve fiber degeneration is very valuable to make a prognosis in cases of supra-sellar tumors. With advanced nerve fiber degeneration and visual field defects the prognosis is not so good. If the nerve fibers are not injured but there are large visual field defects the prognosis may be much better. So this is an important matter in neuro-opthalmology and specially for the anterior visual pathway. Now we must end this part of the discussion now but hopefully we can come back.
can come back.

Our next subject is Dr. Isayama's paper.

Dannheim: I found it interesting that Dr. Isayama showed a few diagrams of the transcranial operation procedure. This might induce several side-effects specially for the prognosis of the recovery of visual damage and this was the reason we confined our material to the transnasal access only to be sure that there is not much of a side-effect due to displacing the chiasm while removing the tumor.

Isayama: I have much experience after the operation; for example, if during the fronto-temporal approach beneath the chiasm the vessels were damaged, serious damage of the visual field occured.

In some cases of for instance craniopharyngeoma tumor cells may involve the optic nerve and if they are removed a serious damage may occur. Transnasal approach is better for that point of view, I think.

Bynke: I can confirm that atypical defects are often found in pituitary adenomas and that the localising value may be very small in some cases.

We had a rare case of pituitary adenoma, a man of 63 years, and this is the only case I have seen with an inferior attitudinal hemianopia in both eyes. Inferior altitudinal hemianopia in one eye is not so rare, but the bilateral type is infrequent. The chromophobe adenoma had a very large supra-sellar portion.

In another case, a woman of 45 with Nelson's syndrome the adenoma was mainly intra- and infrasellar. There was no large suprasellar extension in this case and in spite of this the defects are the same. They are very similar in both cases. The mechanism behind the field defects could not be revealed at the operation in any of these cases, but it was supposed that the anterior cerebral artery had compressed the optic nerves on both sides. But we are not sure that this is true. Dr. Isayama had at least one case with an overlying anterior cerebral artery that had compressed one optic nerve.

I have seen such cases too, but many of them had a classical bitemporal hemianopia. So I am not sure that this is the cause of this type of defects but of course it may be. What is your opinion Dr. Isayama? Do you think that this fur you found in the optic nerve caused by the artery overlying the nerve is significant in this connection?

Isayama: You mean whether this type of altitudinal defects can be caused by optic nerve damage? I think the compression of optic nerve causes a central scotoma will appear. It is very difficult to explain such altitudinal ningeal vessels. These vessels enter the optic nerve perpendicularly. In the centre of the nerve the vessels are rather scarse and if compression occurs a central scotoma will appear. It is very difficult to explain such attitudinal change by direct chiasmal pressure. I think compression of the anterior cerebral artery will cause this damage.

Bynke: What I mean is that we often find compression by this arteriy and a fur in the nerve during operation, but that many of these patients have no altitudinal defects. They have bitemporal defects. So my question is about the significance of these findings.

Isayama: In my opinion the altitudinal defect caused by this arterial compression is irregular and not so completely altitudinal.

Bynke: Dr. Dannheim, we have discussed yesterday cases with blind eyes on one side and then you said you have seen cases that took two or three years before they developed temporal hemianopia in the contralateral field. These cases are very important. Dr. Isayama's cases were as far as I could understand supra-sellar meningiomas. This occurrence is typical of supra-sellar meningiomas. Is that your opinion too, Dr. Dannheim? Or have you seen such things in pituitary adenomas and cranipharyngeomas.?

Dannheim: The visual fields and computer-tomograms of 4 out of 20 patients, who's visual loss caused severe diagnostic problems, are presented:

1. 37 year old male, episode of failing vision in one eye previously, diagnosed as retrobulbar neuritis and 'successfully' treated with steroids. Admission because of recurrence with bilateral loss of vision. Visual fields revealed a severe bitemporal defect with crossing of the midline. Full recovery of visual acuity after drainage of a large cystic craniopharyngeoma, but still some relative bitemporal defects.

2. 22 year old male with sudden onset of marked visual loss in one eye diagnosed as optic neuritis. Repeated examination disclosed an upper temporal dense defect including the center in the affected eye and circumscript nerve-fibre defects in the 'good' eye. Partial recovery of the visual field, full recovery of vision after removal of a large prolactinoma.

3. 67 year old female, severe progressive loss of vision in one eye and slight relative defect in the temporal field of the other eye, especially present as a disturbance of sensation of supraliminal stimuli. Symptoms interpreted as ischemia of the chiasm, since skull x-rays, CT and angiography failed to show any compressing lesion. CT was repeated 2 weeks later, when the 'good' eye presented a sudden deterioration of the temporal visual field and visual acuity. The tiny tumor, which now was found, turned out to be a glioma of the chiasm. Slight recovery was noticed postoperatively.

4. 55 year old female, severe unilateral visual loss had been diagnosed as neuritis, since skull x-rays – twice performed – was inconspicuous of a tumor. 9 months later the field of the 'good' eye revealed minimal changes in isopters and disturbance of sensation in the temporal hemifield. CT proved a presellar meningeoma. After removal of the tumor this better eye recovered completely, the practically blind eye recovered partially with a temporal and inferior altitudinal hemianopia.

1. Monocular or binocular loss of vision without ophthalmoscopically visible explanation must be suspected as an intracranial tumor, as long as it can not be excluded by thorough x-ray studies including CT.

2. Juvenile age may favour the diagnosis of optic neuritis, but pituitary adenomas or craniopharyngeomas are also frequent in this age group.

3. Recovery of vision with or without steroids may favour the diagnosis 'neuritis', but it is also observed with different tumors.

4. Arguments against neuritis are more or less simultaneous affection of both eyes and absence of spontaneous recovery.

5. Monocular visual loss requires an accurate evaluation and follow up of the good eye's visual field even after years.

6. Plain skull x-ray findings may be minimal or absent even with dramatic loss of vision in meningeomas and gliomas of the optic nerve and chiasm.

7. The vertical borderline of disturbance is the prominent feature of the visual field with intracranial lesions. In discrete lesions it may be present only as a change in sensation without alteration of isopters. In advanced cases or in a far anterior localisation the vertical borderline may be obscured or replaced by central scotomata or nerve defects, which might be misinterpreted as optic neuritis.

8. Additional, independently present feature like refractional changes of isopters, amblyopia or a history with an injury just prior to the onset of symptoms may cause immense diagnostic difficulties.

References:

Dannheim, F. Visual fields before and after transnasal removal of a pituitary tumor. Correlation of topographical features with sensorial disturbance for liminal and supraliminal stimuli. 3rd Internat. Visual Field Symposium, Tokyo 1978 (same volume).

Frisén, L., Sjoestrand, J., Norrsell, K. & Lindgren, S. Cyclic compression of the intracranial optic nerve: Patterns of visual failure and recovery. *J. Neurol., Neurosurg. Psychiat.* 39: *1109-1113* (1976).

Greve, E.L. & Raakman, M.A.C. On atypical chiasmal visual field defects. *Docum. Ophthal. Proc. Series* 14: *315-325* (1977).

Knight, C.L., Hoyt, W.F. & Wilson, C.B. Syndrome of incipient prechiasmal optic nerve compression. Progress toward early diagnosis and surgical management. *Arch. Ophthal.* 87: *1-11* (1972).

Greve: The paper of Dr. Isayama and the comment of Dr. Dannheim confirm the study that we have presented on our last symposium in Tübingen. In our series of 37 patients with chromophobe adenoma, 10 presented with atypical defects, of which 3 had unilateral central defects and 2 were unilateraly blind. Even more important was that the average time between the first visual complaint and the diagnosis was on an average 13 months in the atypical VF cases with extremes of many years. Neuritis was the most frequent first (and wrong) diagnosis made. These findings stress the necessity of careful VFE not only of the affected eye but of the other eye and a careful follow-up at regular intervals of patients with retrobulbar neuritis e causa ignota.

Friedmann: Would the speakers who have dealt with the removal of the compressive lesions indicate how long after the removal they continue to do visual fields and on whom should this responsability devolve. We found that by following up patients for years after removal we have detected 4 or 5 recurrences and the problem is who goes on doing these visual fields: the neuro-surgeon, the neurologist or the ophthalmologists? My question is: how long do you go on and who should take this responsability?

Frisén: 1) forever. 2) ophthalmologist.

Verriest: In my experience too the ophthalmologist must do it because the neurologist will not do it.

Bynke: I have seen recurrences of pituitary adenoma after very long time; the longest case had a recurrence after 25 years. We examine the visual fields in patients operated for pituitary adenoma at least once a year for the rest of their lives.

I think it is now time to make a summary of this topic. It is very difficult to do that because this topic is very large. My conclusion is that the field defects found in pituitary adenoma and in cranio-pharyngioma are often very similar. We cannot as ophthalmologists make a differential diagnosis of these two tumor types. But on the other hand the supra-sellar meningioma often gives very asymmetric field defects. They are much more asymmetric in many cases than they are in pituitary adenomas and cranio-pharyngeomas. This may help us to say what type of tumor we have but the ultimate diagnosis of the tumor type must be made by the X-ray specialists and also at the operation. In many cases the diagnosis is not clear until we have opened the skull and seen what it is.

That was a very short conclusion of this matter and now I will ask you if you have any questions to the subsequent lecturers.

Drance: I like to ask the neuro-ophthalmologists a question with regards to these ischemic neuropathy papers which were very beautiful and I find it agrees so closely with what we find. However there is in the definition of ischemic optic neuropathy as Dr. Aulhorn mentioned and as the neuro-ophthalmologists and neurologists usually practise a built-in difficulty and that is that the patient has to present with symptoms and therefore we are only looking at severe extensive ischemic optic neuropathies. In the glaucoma patients we follow every 3 to 6 months routinely we therefore see much smaller changes which were not present in Dr. Aulhorn's material. I suspect very strongly that the little hemorrhages that have now been seen by so many people at the optic nerve head in the presence or absence of elevated intra-ocular pressure are probably the minor forms of ischemic optic neuropathy which Dr. Aulhorn stated she did not have in her material. The question therefore is: there is something wrong with the definition of ischemic optic neuropathy as it is currently held by ophthalmologists, neuro-ophthalmologists and neurologists.

Hayreh: Yes, this is the problem because neuro-ophthalmologists believe in the massive swollen disk and the whole lot of it. They are not interested in the small things. A very small lesion like the type Drance has described, they don't see very often because the patients really don't have the symptoms and that is why they are not accustomed to see any of the more early type like persons who are interested in glaucoma or in the optic nerve. I don't know whether the definition of ischemic optic neuropathy is wrong.

The question is what you want to see and what type of patients are seen. I have seen many patients with a full blown ischemic neuropathy. I saw a lady two months ago. Seven years ago she developed an ischemic optic neuropathy in one eye. She was seen first by the neurologist and by the time she was seen the disc became atrophic and they started working neurosurgically and ultimately they did craniotomy on that lady. And they found something around the chiasmal region which they diagnosed as chiasmal arachnoiditis and then about three months ago she developed it in the second eye. And when I saw her, she had a classical ischemic optic neuropathy and she underwent unnecessary craniotomy and the whole lot. So this was a lady who had a frank anterior ischemic optic neuropathy and I think it is the diagnostic ability of people that maters.

108

SUMMARY OF SESSION I: NEURO-OPHTHALMOLOGY

CHAIRMAN: H. BYNKE

We are now going to finish the neuro-ophthalmological session. Let me first express our gratitude to prof. Matsuo and his team. Their generosity and hard organizing work have made this symposium possible. Be sure, prof. Matsuo, that we enjoy very much to stay as your guests here in Tokyo.

I have chosen to divide the main topic, that is visual field defects in lesions of the infrageniculate pathway, into two subtopics. The first about retinal nerve fibre degeneration is modern and must always be considered in this connection. The second about tumours of the sellar region is old but nevertheless so important that it cannot be excluded when we discuss the infrageniculate pathway. Excellent surveys of these subtopics have been given by our introducers prof. Frisen and prof. Isayama.

Our knowledge about lesions of the infrageniculate pathway and their clinical correlates has been deepened by the valuable contributions of Tagami, Hayreh, Frisén, Vestergren-Brenner, Dannheim, Aulhorn and Otori. But of course many problems remain unsolved. For example, why may the visual field be normal or almost so with a fundus picture that cannot be separated from a moderate, diffuse loss of the nerve fibre layer? Is this explained by inadequate perimetric methods, as has been suggested by Frisén, or possibly by a false interpretation of the fundus picture? Another problem is the incomplete correspondence between the appearance of the field defects and the exact location of the suprasellar tumour, as has been demonstrated by Isayama. Is this due to impairment of an individually variable vascular supply of the chiasma?

The unsolved problems will stimulate us to proceed with our research. There is no doubt that we will understand these and other things better in the future. We are very grateful to the introducers, to the subsequent lecturers and to everybody who has participated in the discussions. Thank you!

Docum. Ophthal. Proc. Series, Vol. 19

EARLY GLAUCOMATOUS VISUAL FIELD DEFECTS AND THEIR SIGNIFICANCE TO CLINICAL OPHTHALMOLOGY

PAUL R. LICHTER & CAROL L. STANDARDI

(Michigan, U.S.A.)

ABSTRACT

A consecutive series of primary open angle glaucoma patients was evaluated to determine the earliest glaucomatous visual field defect. One hundred twelve fields were considered worthwhile for detailed analysis. The fields were performed on a Goldmann perimeter utilizing static-kinetic techniques.

Although paracentral defects and isolated nasal steps were found to occur early in the pattern of glaucomatous field loss, the very earliest defect may be a difference between the two eyes on field comparison. Where glaucomatous damage is suspected, but where the individual visual fields are normal, a comparison of the fields between the two eyes should be made to detect differences such as in blind spot size or isopter extent particularly where identical threshold targets were used. The nucleus of a defect occurring within nasal steps also occur early as do other specific defects such as dense paracentral nuclei within relative arcuate defects. These early defects should be detectable in clinical practice where careful perimetric techniques are utilized. It is, however, important that methodology be emphasized in reports of field findings.

INTRODUCTION

Visual field defects are the *sine qua non* of glaucoma by the most stringent definitions. Thus, the earlier a defect in the visual field is detected, the earlier one can be certain that a given patient's optic nerve is susceptible to damage from a specific pressure. However, detection of early glaucomatous visual field defects is dependent on appropriate examination techniques and knowledge of the kinds of defects to expect. Defects found using sophisticated equipment and time-consuming examinations might not be found using more conventional techniques. Thus, when describing early field defects, one must keep in mind the methods used to detect them. The present study has evaluated early glaucomatous visual field defects in a clinical setting.

MATERIALS AND METHODS

A consecutive series of 148 patients with primary open angle glaucoma was evaluated. Each patient underwent a thorough ophthalmologic evaluation with particular attention paid to optic discs and visual fields. Visual field

* This study was supported by the University of Michigan, Glaucoma Research and Development Fund.

111

testing was performed on the Goldmann perimeter utilizing a modification of screening methods described by Armaly (1969) and by Rock et al. (1971.

Each patient had a visual field defect considered to be glaucomatous in origin. Visual field defects of an extensive nature were then excluded leaving only defects considered to be of value in determining the earliest glaucomatous visual field changes. A total of 112 fields met these criteria and were analyzed further.

Determination of the status of the visual field was made by subjective parameters. Comparison was made between the visual field findings and optic disc evaluation. Where the optic discs were symmetrical and appeared definitely physiologic, visual fields with defects were looked upon with suspicion. However, such defects were not automatically considered spurious. If a definite field defect existed, it was counted as such despite the appearance of the optic disc.

The visual fields were sorted into categories. Where the visual field was found complicated due to disease unrelated to glaucoma, the field was excluded from the study.

RESULTS

Nineteen patients (38 eyes) had abnormal optic discs with visual fields which appeared normal when evaluating each separately. However, we de-

(a)

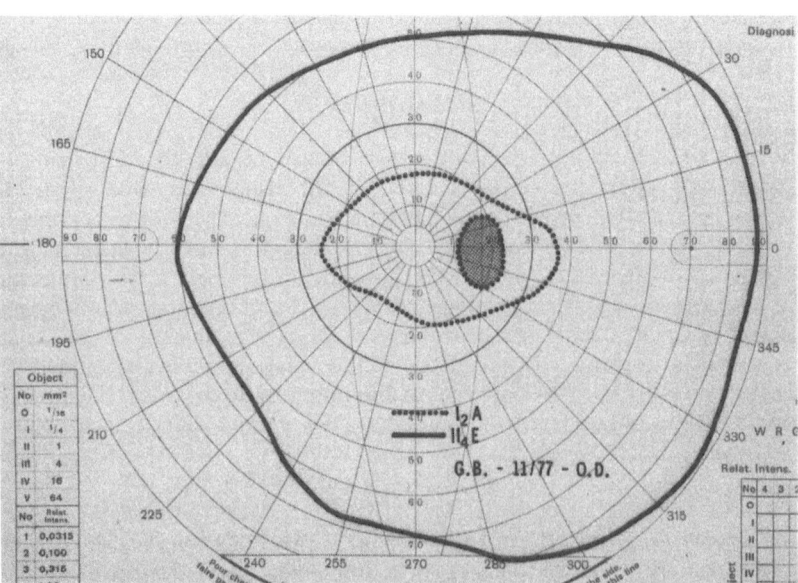

Fig. 1. (lichter). Right (a) and left (b) visual fields from same patient recorded at same visit. This patient had a disparity in optic disc appearance with the more damaged optic disc on the same side as the larger blind spot.

112

cided to compare the two eyes to see if differences could be detected which might suggest a very early field defect.

Eight of these 19 patients showed no difference in the fields of the two eyes. Eleven of the patients had a difference in the fields. The more abnormal field corresponded to the more abnormal optic disc on nine of these patients, but on the remaining two, did not correspond. Of this latter group of 11 patients, ten showed a difference in the size of the blind spot between the two eyes (Fig. 1). One had definite constriction of the nasal field.

The remaining 74 visual fields demonstrated defects which contributed further to a determination of the earliest types of defects. These were separated into groups as follows:

Group 1 (8 eyes 10.8%) — isolated paracentral defect; one eye had two defects making a total of nine defects. (Fig. 2).

Group 2 (14 eyes 18.9%) — nasal step; four eyes had an advanced nasal step with an associated relative arcuate defect. Ten eyes had an isolated nasal step (Fig. 3).

Group 3 (8 eyes 10.8%) — the nucleus of a nasal scotoma adjacent to the horizontal meridian lying between 10 and 20 degrees from fixation within a nasal step (Fig. 4).

Group 4 (16 eyes 21.6%) — the nucleus of a defect occurring within 5 degrees of fixation plus baring of the blind spot and/or an arcuate defect (Fig. 5).

(b)

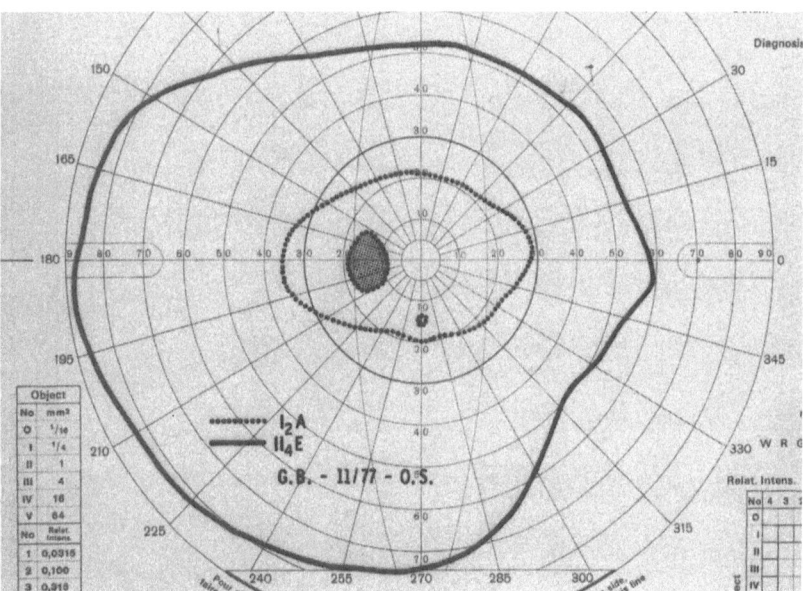

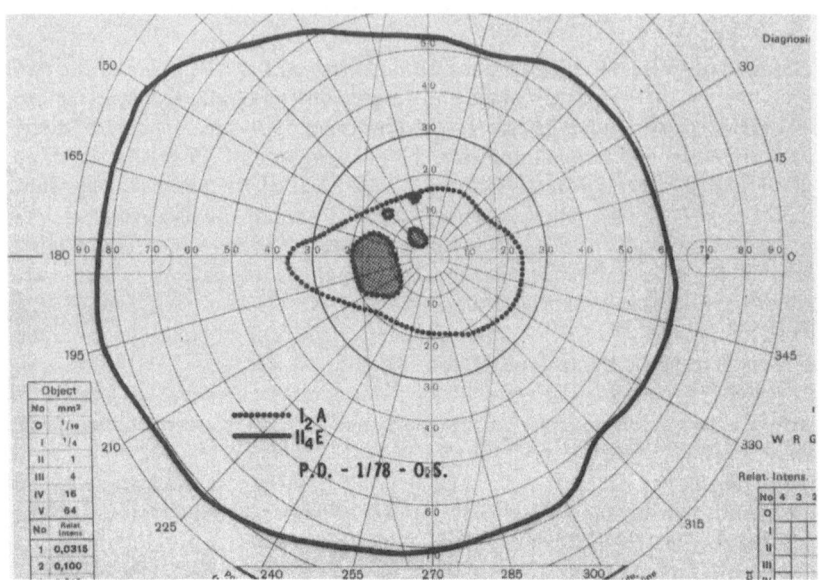

Fig. 2. (Lichter). Example of paracentral defect.

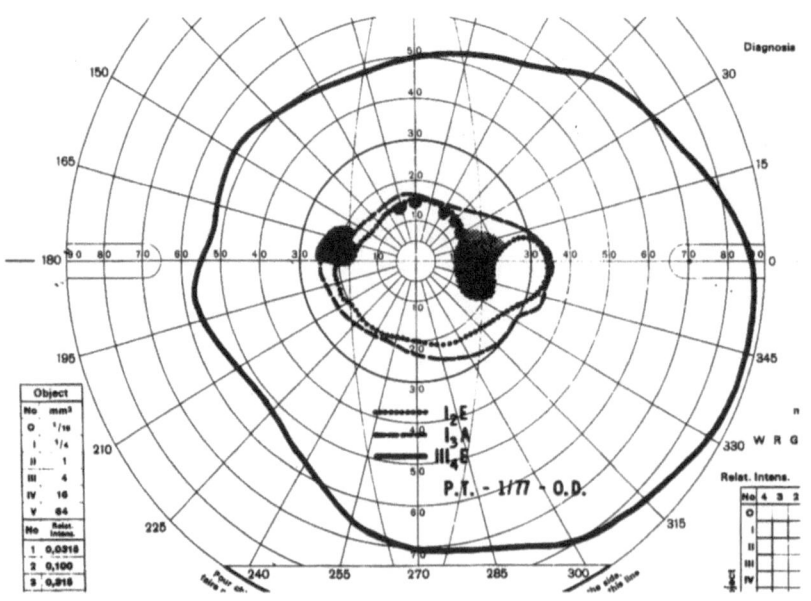

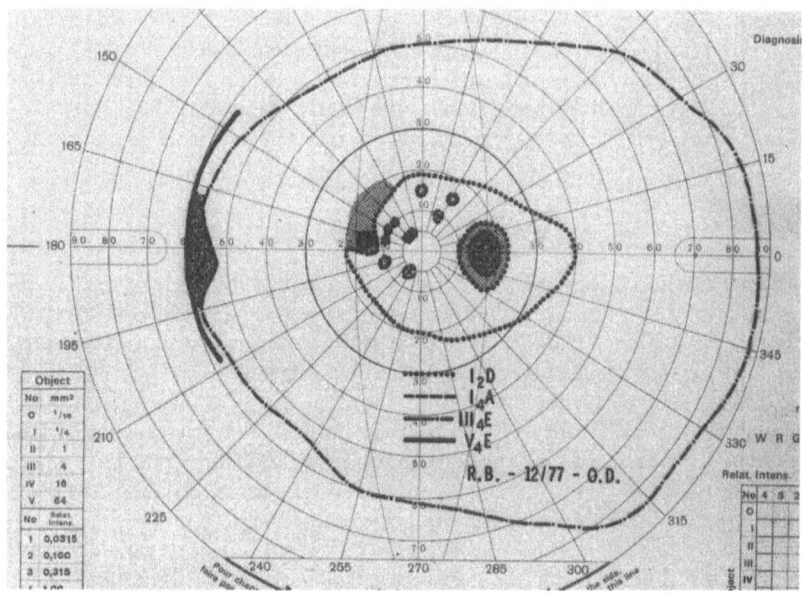

Fig. 4. (Lichter). Nucleus of a defect within a nasal step.

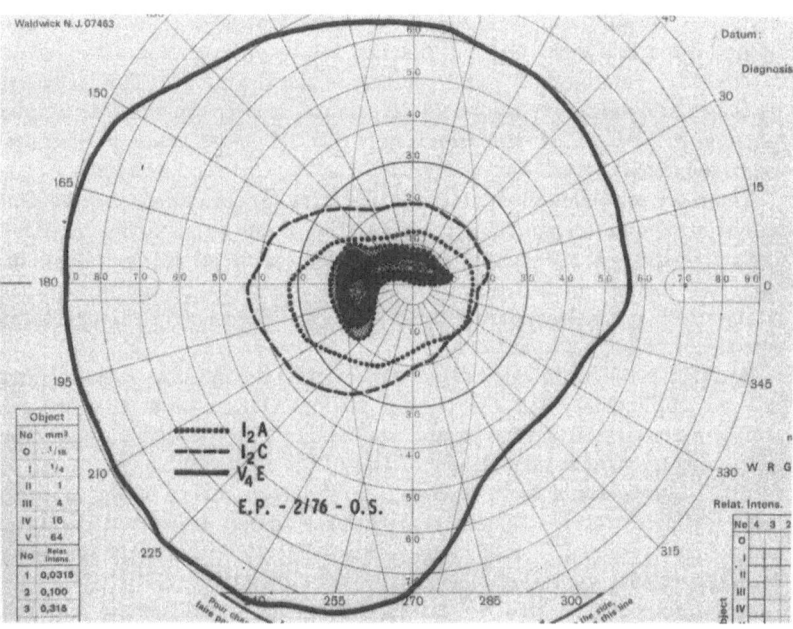

Fig. 5. (Lichter). Large nucleus of a defect a large portion of which is within 5 degrees of fixation associated with a relative arcuate defect.

115

Group 5 (21 eyes 35.5%) − the nucleus of a defect outside of 5 degrees of fixation plus baring of the blind spot and/or an arcuate defect (Fig. 6).

Group 6 (7 eyes 9.5%) − unusual defects; two eyes had a temporal step; one eye had a superior depression similar to a vertical step (Fig. 7).

Three eyes had an elongated blind spot; one eye had a large inferonasal depression.

DISCUSSION

Much attention has been paid to determining the beginning defect in the evolution of glaucomatous visual field loss. Aside from research interests, knowledge of what to look for can assist the clinician in discovering glaucomatous damage at its earliest stage. Aulhorn & Harms (1967) have reviewed the history of early defects in their thorough study of the subject. They concluded as did Drance (1969) that the earliest glaucomatous visual field defects were isolated 'spot-like' scotomas in the Bjerrum area. They stated that an enlarged blind spot and a constricted field are rarely the first defects to appear. A nasal step almost never occurred by itself.

It is important to note, however, that Aulhorn & Harms were careful to point out that methodologic differences in performing the field test can account for variations in findings. They preferred profile perimetry over isopter perimetry.

Determining the earliest visual field defects in glaucoma can be done in several ways. First, all patients with ocular hypertension (i.e. no field defects) can be followed carefully for development of a field defect. This method has a low yield. Second, one can follow patients with field defects in only one eye looking for early defects in the second eye. Third, one can dissect existing glaucomatous field defects to discover the most dense portions of the defect on the assumption that the most dense portion was where the defect began. This assumption may be incorrect, however.

There are problems encountered in searching for the earliest defects. One cannot always be certain that an early defect is due to glaucoma. Artifacts and other diseases can account for such defects. It is helpful to evaluate the optic disc in all cases. Where a field defect appears in the presence of symmetrical, normal appearing optic discs, the field defect should be suspect as not belonging to glaucoma.

Another problem in early defect detection is the method of testing used and the applicability for the clinical setting. Our method, although not profile perimetry, is a very careful static-kinetic test which is more time consuming than fields taken in the offices of the average clinician.

Still another problem in detecting early defects relates to the fact that many patients who get glaucomatous damage already have visual field loss when first examined. Therefore, it is impossible to determine if their field defect represents the earliest changes.

Our results suggest that the earliest glaucomatous field defect may be a subtle difference in the visual field between the two eyes where either field by itself may be interpreted as normal. This difference may include a larger

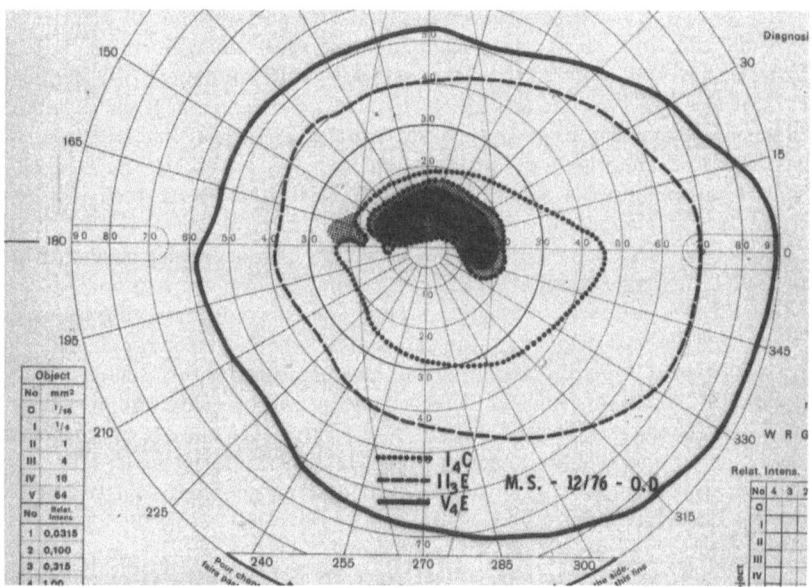

Fig. 6. (Lichter). Nucleus of a defect beyond 5 degrees of fixation associated with a relative arcuate defect.

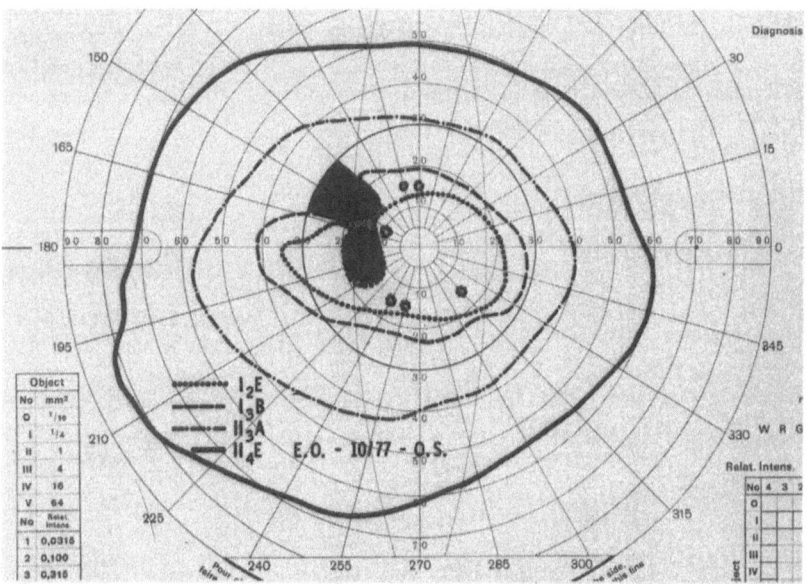

Fig. 7. (Lichter). Unusual wedge-type defect above the blind spot and not connected to it.

117

blind spot or a more constricted field on one side with use of identically selected and utilized targets. Although blind spot 'enlargement' and field 'contraction' can occur in normal eyes, one would not expect two identical eyes of the same patient to show differences in this regard. It seems logical that since comparison of optic discs can be so helpful in distinguishing normal from abnormal, so too can field comparison be equally valuable. This is particularly the case where the individual optic disc or the individual visual field may appear normal.

Other defects occur with varying frequency. An isolated paracentral defect or an isolated nasal step is quite common. Also seen frequently are paracentral nuclei within relative arcuate defects with or without nasal steps. This perhaps emphasizes the paracentral origin of arcuate defects.

A particular type of defect seems to be a nasal step with a nucleus defect within the step. This nucleus defect is just above or below the horizontal meridian. The search for the nucleus of a field defect may be important in that it may imply where the defect began. If this is true, particular attention should be paid to the region of the horizontal meridian between 10 and 20 degrees from fixation.

Of interest is a recent report by Werner & Drance (1977) where 22 field loss eyes were studied retrospectively for early field defects. Thirteen of the 22 eyes showed subtle nonspecific localized scatter or depressions in the field prior to developing a definite defect. In 12 of the 22 eyes, a nasal step was the first definitive field defect while in 10 eyes, paracentral scotomas appeared first. These findings are quite consistent with our results. It suggests that subtle, nonspecific field changes should not be dismissed as spurious. We would only emphasize the need to compare fields of the two eyes.

With a careful examination, using standard equipment and techniques, early glaucomatous field defects can be discovered in the everyday practice of ophthalmology. Knowing where to pay particular attention in the examination and interpretation should prove helpful.

REFERENCES

Armaly, M.F. Ocular pressure and visual fields. *Arch. Ophthalmol.* 81: *25-40* (1969).
Aulhorn, E. & Harms, H. Early visual field defects in glaucoma. Glaucoma Symposium. Tutzing Castle S. Karger Basal/New York 1967, P. 151-186.
Drance, S. The early field defects in glaucoma. *Invest. Ophthalmol.* 8: *84-91* (1969).
Rock, W.J., Drance, S.M. & Morgan, R.W. A modification of the Armaly visual field screening technique for glaucoma. *Canad. J. Ophthalmol.* 6: *283-292* (1971).
Werner, E.B. & Drance, S.M. Early visual field disturbances in glaucoma. *Arch. Ophthalmol.* 95: *1173-75* (1977).

Authors' address:
University of Michigan
Department of Ophthalmology
Room C6058, University Hospital
Ann Arbor, Michigan-48109
U.S.A.

THE EARLY VISUAL FIELD DEFECT IN GLAUCOMA AND THE SIGNIFICANCE OF NASAL STEPS

STEPHEN M. DRANCE, MEG FAIRCLOUGH,
BEVERLEY THOMAS, GORDON R. DOUGLAS,
REMO SUSANNA

(Vancouver, Canada)

ABSTRACT

The earliest field defects in chronic simple glaucoma are important in order to understand the pathogenesis of the disease and develop screening methods for early detection of damage. The nasal step has not been studied and defined in non-glaucomatous people. Patients who had no field defect and then developed one were studied to ascertain the earliest field defects. Normal eyes had the nasal periphery and mid-periphery studied by kinetic and static perimetry. The results show that paracentral scotomata, nasal steps in periphery and centre can be the first signs of damage either alone or in combination. Temporal sector defects occasionally also occur initially. More than one nerve fibre bundle can be affected from the outset. Nasal steps greater than 4° occur very rarely in normals, particularly if all points are tested more than once.

INTRODUCTION

The realization that intraocular pressure, though obviously important in the production of glaucomatous damage, is not an efficient predictor of subsequent visual field defects, has resulted in screening of the visual field and meticulous examination of the optic nerve in all patients at risk. Examination by means of static perimetry of large populations with elevated intraocular pressure has led Aulhorn to conclude that paracentral scotomata constitute 70% of early field defects and that in 29% peripheral nasal field defects accompany these paracentral scotomata, but in only 0.7% of patients was the peripheral nasal field defect found to be the only visual field defect. Armaly examined the fields of patients with elevated pressures and 87% were discovered to have paracentral scotomata while 1.9% had peripheral nasal field defects as their only sign of field damage. LeBlanc & Becker have more recently reported that peripheral nasal field defects were more common and occurred as the only manifestation in 11% of fields. An understanding of the earliest disturbances in the visual field is important not only for an understanding of the pathogenesis of glaucomatous defects but also for the development of screening procedures which have to be designed not to miss field defects which indicate glaucomatous damage. In a previous

* This work was supported in part by the Medical Research Council of Canada Grant MT 1578, and in part by the E.A. Baker Foundation for Prevention of Blindness, Canadian National Institute for the Blind.

119

study we (Werner, Drance & Schulzer (1977) have shown that nearly half of definitive nerve fibre bundle defects in chronic open angle glaucoma are preceded by localized areas of increased scatter of responses in the area which subsequently develops the defects. Such areas of scatter also occurred in some patients who did not develop visual field defects. These disturbances are therefore only warnings of subsequent damage and must lead to meticulous and repeated plotting of the visual field particularly in the areas concerned. There is very little in the literature on the occurrence of nasal steps in normal people who undergo screening perimetry.

The present study examines the sites of early, definitive visual field disturbances in patients who were at risk but had normal visual fields and then developed definitive, reproducible nerve fibre bundle disturbances. A careful evaluation of the extent of nasal steps in people with normal fields was also carried out.

PROCEDURE

Early Field Defects

Thirty-five eyes of 30 patients were studied. All developed a definitive, reproducible nerve fibre bundle defect (reproducible nasal steps either greater than 5° or more than .5 log unit in depth, paracentral scotomata deeper than .5 log unit, and sector-shaped scotomata in other parts of the field). All patients had at least 2 visual fields without central and peripheral field defects and developed scotomata during the course of observation which could be reproduced on at least 2 successive occasions. The scotomata were classified into relative and absolute paracentral scotomata, central or peripheral nasal steps, sector defects, and various combinations of these.

Nasal steps

Fifty-one eyes of 51 people with normal ocular examination including a normal optic nerve head and no obvious local pathology were studied. One eye of each person to be studied was randomly chosen. If the person had not had a previous visual field plotted, 2 visual field examinations were carried out, one as an educational one, and only the results from the second were included in the study. In each patient the smallest stimulus which plotted the absolute nasal periphery was found. With this stimulus 10 kinetic thresholds 5° above and 5° below the horizontal meridian were plotted. Ten static differential thresholds were measured 5° above and ten 5° below the horizontal meridian 5° within the most peripheral nasal isopter. The stimulus which would delineate the isopter closest to 20° nasal from fixation was found and used to plot 10 kinetic readings 5° above and ten 5° below the horizontal. Ten static differential thresholds were then measured on the nasal side 5° above and 5° below the horizontal 15° from fixation. In each person the oblique meridian on the nasal side was chosen and 10 static differential thresholds were measured along it 10° from fixation. All central tests were done with the best correction with the appropriate addition for the distance of the Goldmann perimeter. Peripheral points were tested without correction.

For each of the 51 eyes the kinetic differences were ascertained by calculating the mean of the 10 responses above and the mean of the 10 responses below the horizontal and subtracting the value obtained below from that obtained above. The means of 51 patients above and below the horizontal were checked for statistical significance using a paired t test and the variance of the individual differences was calculated and the standard deviation computed. The absolute differences were in fact the 'nasal steps'. The same statistical technique was used for the log 10 of the static differential thresholds and their differences above and below the horizontal. The means of the log 10 of the differential thresholds for each of the 51 was obtained above and below the horizontal and the differences between those 2 values calculated. The means of the thresholds above and below the horizontal meridian were compared using the paired t test and the variance and standard deviation of the individual differences was calculated.

The range of the 10 kinetic readings above and the 10 kinetic readings below the horizontal was used so as to get the extremes of the maximum possible nasal steps. The chance of such a maximal nasal step occurring in a single pair of measurements would be only 2:100 providing all the readings were different but increases with repetition of observations.

RESULTS

Early Field Defects

Twenty-seven (77%) of the 35 eyes developed a paracentral scotomata when the field was first discovered to have a defect (Fig. 1). In 9 (26%) the paracentral scotoma was the only initial field defect; 8 of these paracentral defects were relative and 1 was absolute. Twenty-six (75%) of the 35 patients showed a nasal step when the field was initially discovered defective. In 7 (20%) of them the nasal step was the only initial defect and in 2 (6%) the nasal step could only be found in the peripheral field.

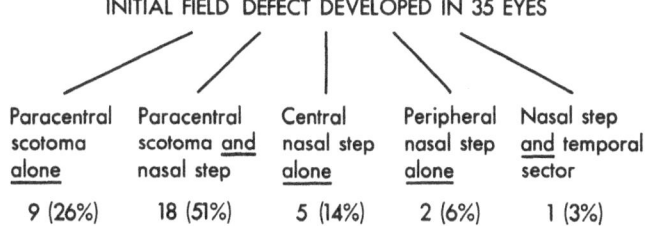

INITIAL FIELD DEFECT DEVELOPED IN 35 EYES

Paracentral scotoma alone	Paracentral scotoma and nasal step	Central nasal step alone	Peripheral nasal step alone	Nasal step and temporal sector
9 (26%)	18 (51%)	5 (14%)	2 (6%)	1 (3%)

Fig. 1. Distribution of the initial field defects in 35 glaucomatous eyes.

Of the 35 eyes there were thus 9 (26%) manifesting only paracentral defects when first discovered and 7 (20%) who developed nasal steps central or peripheral as the only initial defect. The remaining 19 (54%) eyes had a combination of a paracentral defect with a nasal step or sector defect when the visual field defect first developed. In 13 (Fig. 2) the nasal step and the paracentral scotoma were manifestations of a disturbance of the same nerve fibre bundle (Fig. 3) but in 5 a paracentral scotoma was in the opposite half of the field (Fig. 4) to the nasal step so that more than one nerve fibre bundle was involved even at the onset and in 1 the nasal step was accompanied by an unrelated temporal sector defect. Of these 5, 2 showed a temporal field defect in addition to the paracentral scotoma and/or corresponding nasal step and 1 showed an inferior paracentral scotoma with a superior nasal step.

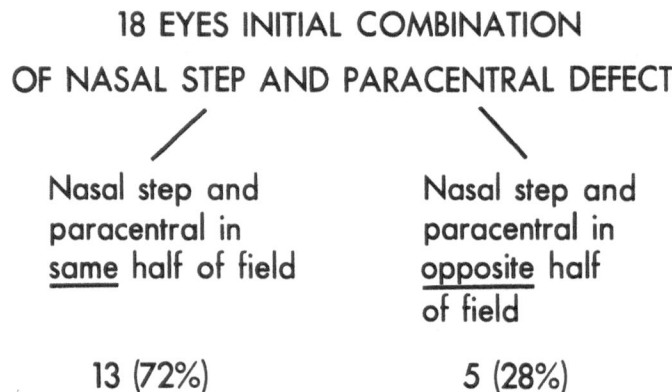

Fig. 2. Distribution in upper or lower field of multiple initial field defects.

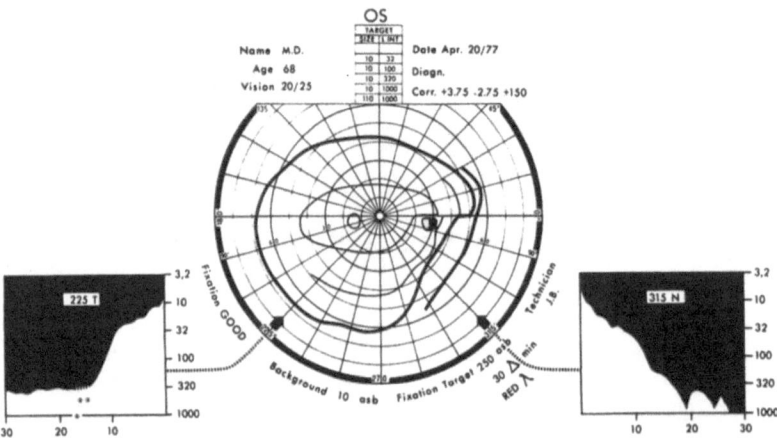

Fig. 3. Early visual field defect showing that the entire nerve fibre bundle can be affected from the outset of a defect.

122

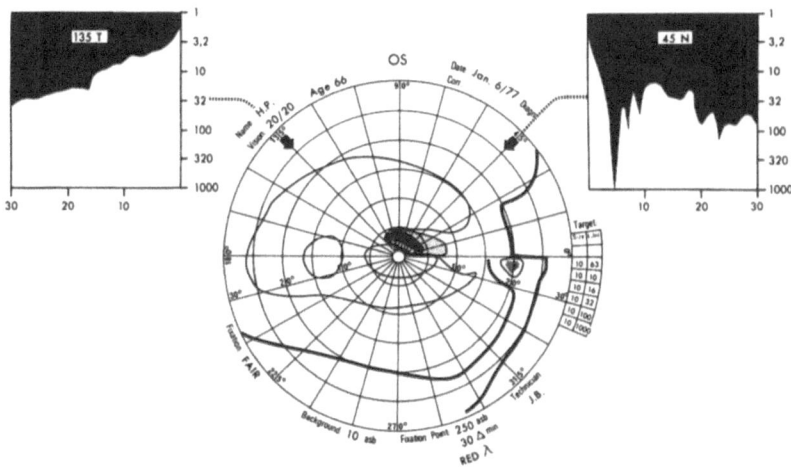

Fig. 4. Earliest field defect showing that more than one bundle can be affected from the outset of the field abnormality.

Peripheral kinetic nasal step

The mean nasal boundary 5° above the horizontal of the 51 eyes was 55.87° (SD 3.57°), whereas the mean boundary 5° below was 55.47° (3.99°). The paired t test shows these differences not to be statistically significant even at the 10% level of confidence (Table 1). The variance of the individual differences was 4.20 and the standard deviation was 2.05°. Thus the individual differences were normally distributed with a mean of 0° and a standard deviation of 2.05° (Table 2). One would therefore predict and expect that measuring the nasal steps, ie., the absolute value of the individual difference, of fresh individuals from the population at large would result in an average nasal step of 1.64° and only 5% of people from that population would show a nasal step larger than 4.1°. The actually observed mean 'nasal step' of the 51 eyes, which we examined, was 1.34° (Fig. 1).

Table 1. Means of 10 Thresholds 5° Above and Below Nasal Horizontal Meridian.

	Peripheral Kinetic	Central Kinetic	Peripheral $\log_{10}$ Diff. Threshold	Central $\log_{10}$ Diff. Threshold
Above Horizontal Mean	55.87° SD 3.57	20.08° SD 1.65	3.43 SD 0.32	1.76 SD 0.19
Below Horizontal Mean	55.47° 3.98	19.829° 1.73	3.44 0.36	1.77 0.22
Paired Test	1.41	2.17	0.243	0.37
	N.S. at 1%	N.S. at 1%	N.S. at 1%	N.S. at 1%

123

Central nasal steps

The mean nasal boundary of the central isopter 5° above the horizontal in the 51 eyes was 20.08° (SD 1.65°) whereas 5° below it was 19.83° (SD 1.73°). These differences were not significant at the 1% level of confidence (Table 1). The variance of the individual differences was .69 and the standard deviation .83°. The central differences would therefore be normally distributed round a mean of .25° with a standard deviation of .83° (Table 2). The calculated predicted absolute nasal step of fresh patients from a population at large would be on the average .52° and only 5% of that population would have a nasal step greater than 1.62°. The actually observed mean nasal 'step' was .66°.

Peripheral Static Differential Thresholds

The mean $\log_{10}$ differential threshold 5° above the horizontal was 3.43 (SD .32) whereas below it was 3.44 (SD .36). These differences of the means were not statistically significant (Table 1). The variance of the individual differences above and below the horizontal was .13 and the standard deviation .36. These differences were normally distributed round a mean of 0 with a standard deviation of .13 (Table 2). The calculated predicted difference in the $\log_{10}$ of the peripheral differential thresholds above and below the horizontal would be on the average of .29 and only 5% of the population would be expected to have a difference in the $\log_{10}$ of the differential threshold above and below the horizontal greater than .26. The observed mean $\log_{10}$ differential threshold of the 51 eyes was .22.

Central Differential Thresholds

The mean $\log_{10}$ differential threshold 5° above the horizontal was 1.76 (SD .19) and below 1.77 (SD .22). These differences were not statistically significant (Table 1). The variance of the individual differences above and below the horizontal was .01 and the standard deviation .11. The individual differ-

Table 2. Results of Individual Differences Between Thresholds 5° Above and Below Horizontal Meridian.

	Peripheral Kinetic	Central Kinetic	Peripheral $\log_{10}$ Diff. Threshold	Central $\log_{10}$ Diff. Threshold
Variance of Individual Differences Above-Below	4.2	0.69	0.13	0.01
S.D.	2.05°	0.83°	0.36	0.11
Expected Above-Below Difference	1.64°	0.52°	0.29	0.09
Observed Difference	1.34°	0.66°	0.22	0.08

124

ences were normally distributed around a mean of 0 with a standard deviation of .01 (Table 2). The calculated predicted difference of the $\log_{10}$ of the central differential threshold above and below the horizontal for fresh people being tested would be .09 and only 5% of the population would have a difference in the $\log_{10}$ of the differential threshold above and below the horizontal of greater than .22. The observed mean difference of the $\log_{10}$ differential threshold of the 51 eyes was .08.

DISCUSSION

The present study confirms that the earliest visual field defects in chronic open angle glaucoma can be either paracentral scotomata or nasal steps in the central isopters or the peripheral isopters or both. The present study also suggests that when a visual field defect is first discovered, in a field which was previously quite normal, the damage may be extensive enough from the beginning to involve an entire nerve fibre bundle as evidenced by the association of a paracentral scotoma with a nasal step in the first field showing abnormality and that in 3 to 6 months in a previously normal field, more than one nerve fibre bundle may be involved. Whether such nerve fibre bundles are affected simultaneously, or very shortly one after the other in separate episodes occurring within the time interval between 2 successive fields, i.e. 3 to 6 months, is not clear, as one would have to do perimetry almost weekly to ascertain this point. It is significant that in 2 patients there was a characteristic nasal step and/or paracentral scotoma associated with a temporal visual field defect at the time of the first field disturbance. This indicates that temporal field defects can occur early in the disturbed field in association with other field defects. These findings substantiate the need for the modifications which we (Rock, Drance & Morgan 1973) (Brais, Drance 1972) made to Armaly's selective central screening. With the original method one would miss a group of patients whose field disturbances would not be picked up by screening only the classical central and nasal peripheral part of the visual field. In people with no ocular disease, very small nasal steps can be plotted but in 95% of normals such steps are smaller than 5° when the nasal isopter is plotted by more than a single estimation above and below the horizontal meridian. The chances of getting a lerger nasal step, when none is present, on a single pair of measurements do exist but are less than 2: 100. A nasal step should be checked by numerous and repeated plots of the affected area.

REFERENCES

Armaly, M.F. Selective perimetry for glaucomatous defects in ocular hypertension. *Arch. Ophthalmol.* 87: *518-524* (1977).
Aulhorn, E. & Harms, H. Early field defects in glaucoma. Glaucoma Symposium, Tutzing Castle, Ed. Leydhecker, Karger, Basel (1966) p. 151.
Brais, P. & Drance, S.M. The temporal field in glaucoma. *Arch. Ophthalmol.* 88: *518-522* (1972).

LeBlanc, R.P. & Becker, B. Peripheral nasal field defects. *Am. J. Ophthalmol.* 72: *415-419* (1971).

Werner, E.B., Drance, S.M. & Schulzer, M. Early visual field defects in glaucoma. *Arch. Ophthalmol.* 95: *1173-1175* (1977).

Authors' address:
Department of Ophthalmology
University of British Colombia
2550 Willow Street
Vancouver - 8 B.C.
Canada

126

Docum. Ophthal. Proc. Series, Vol. 19

A CRITICAL PHASE IN THE DEVELOPMENT OF GLAUCOMATOUS VISUAL FIELD DEFECTS

E.L. GREVE, F. FURUNO & W.M. VERDUIN

(Amsterdam, The Netherlands)

ABSTRACT

The results of a retrospective and prospective investigation on the development of glaucomatous visual field defects (GVFD) are reported. A series of patients that had documented normal fields developed GVFD. A significant number of patients go through the stage of fluctuating wedge-shaped (w.s.d.) before the stage of a fully developed GVFD. The fluctuating w.s.d. and its theoretical and practical significance is described. The authors feel that a fluctuating w.s.d. may indicate that the optic nerve fibers are in a critical stage of functioning.

There is an increasing interest for the detection of the earliest manifestations of glaucomatous damage. An important reason for this is that the existence of glaucomatous damage is a factor that may influence the start of medical therapy. Also the presence of glaucomatous damage influences the amount of reduction of intraocular pressure (IOP) that one wishes to achieve. The difference between glaucoma suspects (ocular hypertensives) and patients with established glaucoma depends on the presence of glaucomatous damage. In the last years we have come to realize that one cannot base therapeutical decisions on IOP alone. There are too many factors (riscfactors) that also play a part in the process that leads to glaucomatous damage.

The detection of early glaucomatous damage is highly dependent on visual field examination because the only other possibility, evaluation of the excavation, presents serious intra- and interobserver difficulties (Greve & Verduin 1977). Of course the findings of a suspect excavation should lead to a visual field examination.

Other methods that examine visual function, e.g. colour vision, gratings, critical flicker fusion frequency, Westheimer functions etc. have been claimed to provide earlier indications of glaucomatous deterioration of visual function. Some of them will be discussed during this symposium. However promising, they have not (yet) been evaluated sufficiently to be used in practice. At present we have to rely on the manifestations of nerve fiber bundle defects (NFBD).

The early defects that are described here are a product of static perimetry. The normal variation of threshold measurements in static perimetry is 0.3 log. units (Greve 1973). In this case a sensitivity reduction of 0.5 log. units is pathological unless it is caused by an angioscotoma. Based on these considerations we have defined an early defect as a defect having a minimum intensity of 0.5 log. units and a minimal width of $3°$ in the upper part (Greve 1973; Greve & Verduin 1977). We have called this a wedge-shaped defect (w.s.d.).

Glaucomatous defects are nerve fibre bundle defects (N.F.B.D.) and we prefer to demonstrate the presence of w.s.d. as a sort of fan in the course of the nerve fibre (see fig. 6). Early defects in the $30°$ radius visual field have also been described as isolated paracentral scotoma for maximum luminance (Aulhorn & Harms 1966) and in the form of increased variation of measurements in static perimetry (Rønne 1909).

Isolated peripheral (outside $30°$) nasal steps have been found with different frequency depending on the authors and the method of examination they used (Armaly 1972; Drance 1969; LeBlanc & Becker 1971; LeBlanc 1977; Rønne 1909; Werner & Drance 1977). Enlargement of the blind spot and baring of the blind spot without further static perimetric confirmation are no longer acceptable as early glaucomatous defects.

METHODS

Since 1969 our clinic uses the following examination procedure: In the detection phase multiple stimulus static perimetry in the $25°$-radius visual field with a maximum of 150 stimuli is used and the periphery is investigated by means of kinetic perimetry; in the assessment phase meriodional single stimulus static perimetry is used with steps of 1 degree in a defect-area. This procedure of examination is time consuming. The method can only be carried out with the help of excellent technical ophthalmic assistants. In this way the early defects described in this article can be found and followed.

PATIENTS

For this study three groups of patients were selected from our glaucoma patients documentation system. One of the conditions for selection was that adequate visual field examination had been carried out.

Group 1. In this group of 40 eyes of 33 patients there were 19 patients (23 eyes) that developed a visual field defect after a previously documented normal visual field (group 1a). There were 7 patients (9 eyes) that developed only a w.s.d. after previously documented normal visual field (group 1b). There were also 7 patients (8 eyes) that developed a defect for maximal luminance after a stage of a w.s.d. (group 1c).

Group 2. This group consisted of 40 eyes of 28 patients that already had NFBD in the visual field. In another previously normal area of the visual field, a new early visual field defect was discovered as an extention of the already existing NFBD.

The first two groups were evaluated retrospectively.

Group 3. In this group were 20 eyes of 16 patients wherein only a w.s.d.

was found. The first patients of this group have been followed prospectively since 1975.

In our total collection of thousands of glaucoma patients we could find only 3 visual fields with isolated peripheral nasal steps.

DESCRIPTION OF THE GROUPS

In group 1a the development of visual field defects after a normal visual field took place in 11 of the 19 patients via an intermediate stage of w.s.d. In 8 of the 11 patients it could be demonstrated that, after a previously normal visual field, a w.s.d. developed which subsequently disappeared and was reproduced again in a later examination (fig. 1 and 2). Only after this stage of a fluctuating w.s.d. (fig. 3) did a visual field defect of greater intensity develop. In the other 8 patients a visual field defect of greater intensity developed without the intermediate stage of a w.s.d. The stage of a w.s.d., however, can be missed by our detection procedures and also in the period between two successive examinations. The average time between the

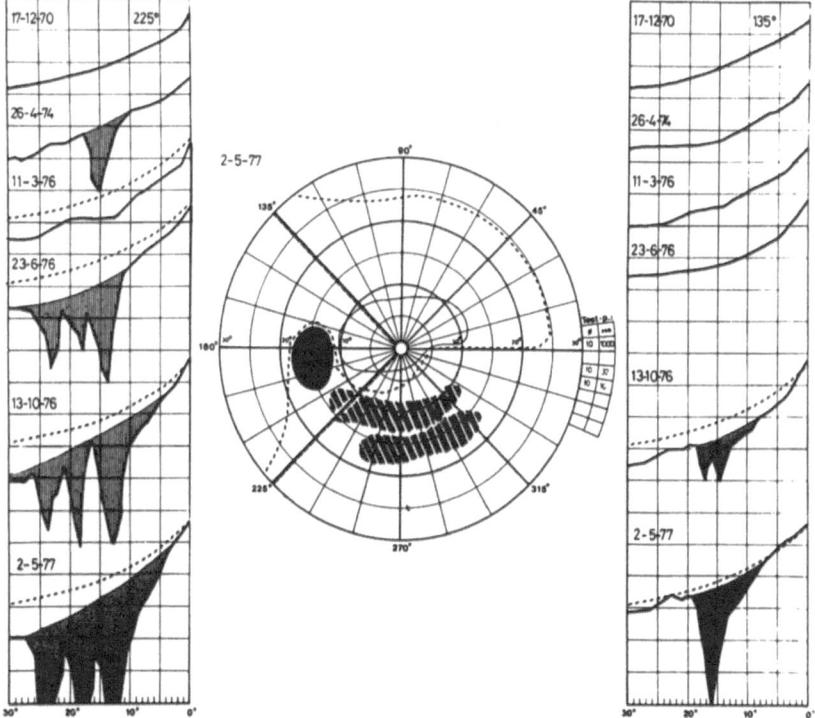

Fig. 1. , VF of the left eye of a glaucoma-patient that had no VFD in 1970. He developed a w.s.d. in 1976 (225° meridian) which disappeared on a subsequent examination, but reappeared again later, to develop in a VFD for max. L.

129

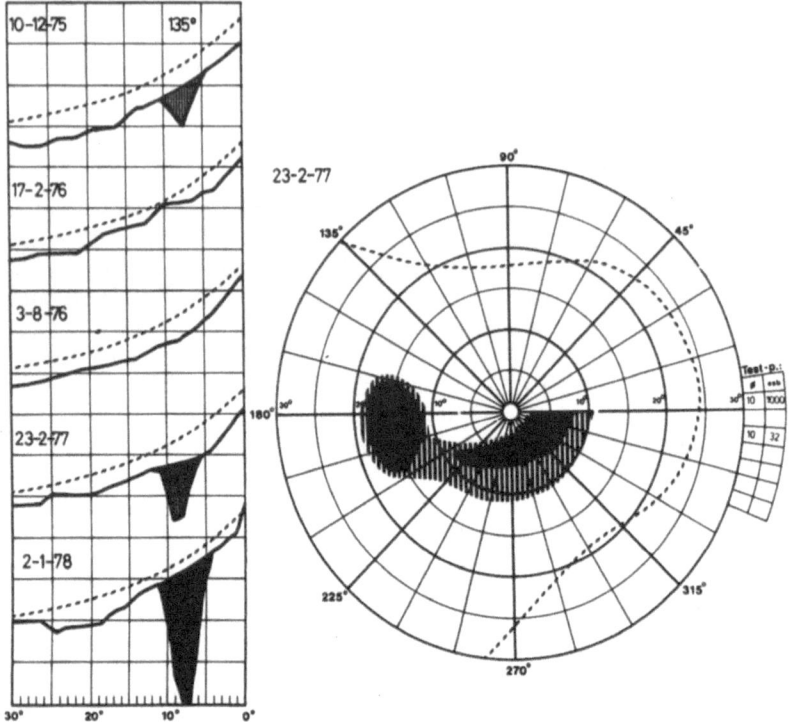

Fig. 2. VF of the left eye of a glaucoma-patient that had an arcuate defect in the lower half of the visual field. He developed a w.s.d. in 1975, which disappeared (135° meridian). In 1977 it reappeared and developed into a VFD for max. L.

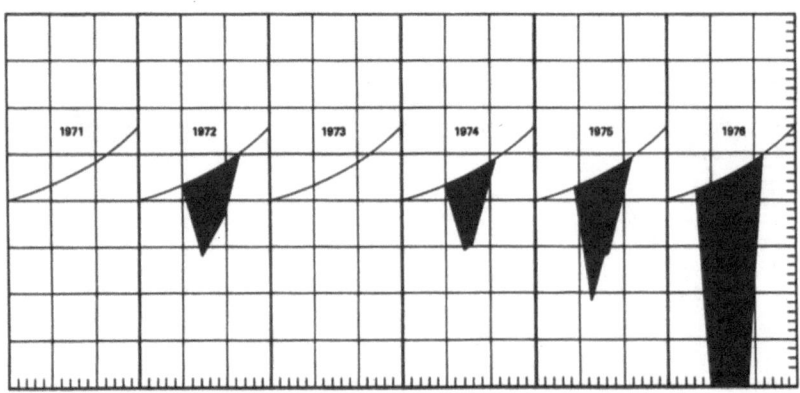

Fig. 3. Schematic drawing of a fluctuating wedge shaped defect (w.s.d.). In 1972 the w.s.d. appeared, but disappeared again in 1973. The defect for maximum luminance in 1976 developed after reappearance of the w.s.d.

130

detection of w.s.d. and the development of a defect of greater intensity was $2\frac{1}{2}$ years. This period of time is no more than a rough estimate because not all patients in this retrospective investigation were examined with the same intervals. In group 1b a w.s.d. developed after a documented normal visual field. In these 7 patients the w.s.d. was examined in several meridians in the course of the same nerve fibre bundle (fig. 4).

In group 1c the w.s.d. had already been found in the first examination. In the follow-up period a defect of greater intensity developed from the w.s.d. In one of the patients the w.s.d. disappeared first before a defect of greater intensity developed. This is the stage of a fluctuating w.s.d. as mentioned in group 1a.

Group 2. This group consisted of the well-known and accepted NFBD. This group has been taken up in the study to demonstrate that in the course of existing partial NFBD a w.s.d. can develop in an area that was previously normal. In this case the w.s.d. clearly is part of the NFBD (fig. 5).

Group 3. This group consisted of 16 patients whereby during the first examination only a w.s.d. had been found. In the majority of these patients a w.s.d. could be demonstrated in succesive meridians in the course of the

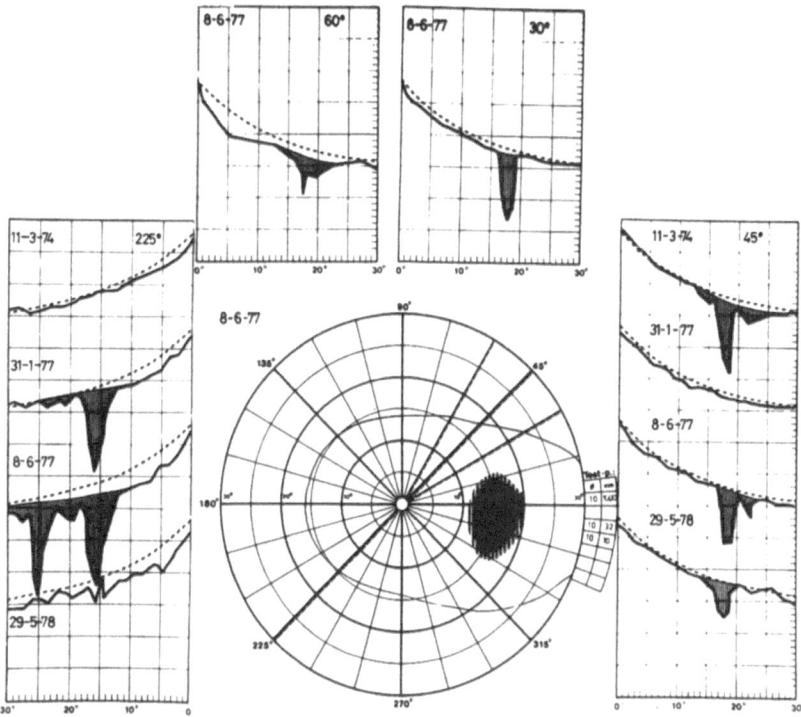

Fig. 4. VF of the right eye of a glaucoma-patient showing a fluctuating w.s.d. in the 45° meridian which can be followed in the course of the N.F.B. in the 30° and 60° meridian. Note also the w.s.d. in the 225° meridian that disappeared in 1978.

fibre bundle. This group has been followed prospectively in order to study the time period of the development of glaucomatous defects. In the follow-up period 3 patients have already developed defects of greater intensity out of a w.s.d.

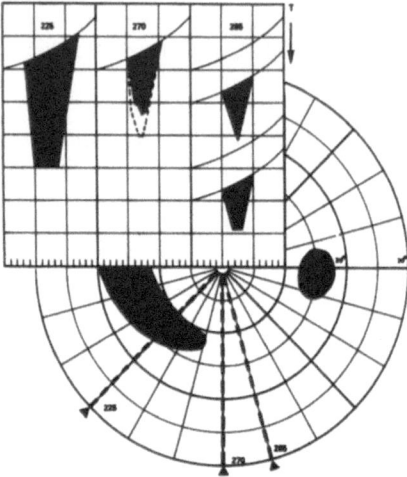

Fig. 5. Schematic drawing of a partial nasal nerve fiber bundle defect. It has a maximum intensity in the 225° meridian. It is relative in the 270° meridian. The 285° meridian shows a fluctuating w.s.d. as a relative cecopetal extension of the same NFBD. On succesive examinations the w.s.d. appears, disappears and reappears.

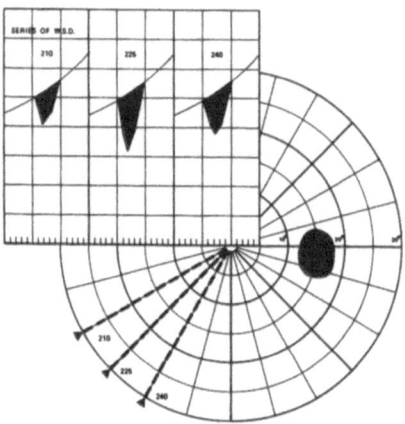

Fig. 6. Schematic demonstration of a series of w.s.d. in adjacent meridians, following the course of a retinal nerve fiber bundle.

132

DISCUSSION

Visual field defects in glaucoma are probably caused by lesions of nerve fibre bundles at the optic disc. NFBD are, as it is well known, not typical for glaucoma but may occur in other non-glaucomatous diseases, specially in the ischemic optic neuropathies.

This investigation reports on a group of patients that developed a glaucomatous VFD after a documented normal visual field. The group was examined at regular intervals with sophisticated techniques. It was established that a w.s.d. can be a phase in the development of G.V.F.D. It is now clear that a stage of relative defects may precede the development of defects for maximum luminance (wrongly called absolute defects).

A w.s.d. is a significant reduction of sensitivity that can be found by means of static perimetry and that can be well defined. W.s.d. may occur as: 1. an isolated defect; 2. a series of defects in the course of the nerve fibre bundles; and 3. as part of an already existing partial NFBD.

In the case of an isolated defect it is not sure that we are really dealing with an NFBD. If sucessive meridians on each side of the first meridian are examined it can be demonstrated whether the isolated w.s.d. is part of a NFBD or not (fig. 6).

Of the patients that we studied, group 1 demonstrates that a w.s d. can be a stage in the development from a normal visual field to a visual field defect of greater intensity. Moreover, this group and group 2 demonstrates that in the intermediate stage there may be intermittent presence of the w.s.d. We have called this a fluctuating w.s.d. The finding of a w.s.d. may indicate that this eye is still in a reversible stage of glaucomatous damage.

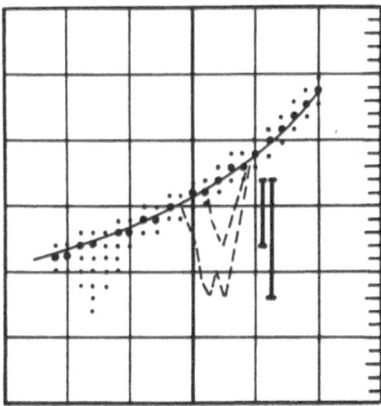

Fig. 7. Schematic representation of the relation between a w.s.d. and increased variation. On the right hand side two w.s.d. are demonstrated (broken lines) with intensities of 0.5 and 0.9 log. units. At the left hand side increased variation is indicated by an increased number of small dots. A line drawn through the lowest dots will form a w.s.d.

On the one hand the w.s.d. may be reversible and on the other hand it is clear that from a w.s.d. defects of greater intensity can develop. Group 2 shows that a w.s.d. can develop in a course of well-known and accepted NFBD. This is another reason to accept a w.s.d. as one of the earliest manifestations of glaucomatous damage. In group 3 the w.s.d. was the only visual field defect. This group will be followed in a prospective investigation which will provide quantitative knowledge about the number of defects that develop from w.s.d. and about the time period between the existence of a w.s.d. and the development of a defect of greater intensity. It is interesting that 3 patients of this group have already developed a defect of greater intensity from their w.s.d.

A series of w.s.d. is the earliest NFBD that can be demonstrated with our techniques. The isolated paracentral defects for maximal luminance are a later stage that the w.s.d. The increased variation of measurements in static perimetry that we, like Werner and Drance, regularly find is also an early sign of glaucomatous damage. Increased variation however is a criterium that is more difficult to handle. Increased variation may be the same as a w.s.d. as shown in fig. 7. If one draws a line through the lower extremes of the variation one gets a w.s.d.

Our concept of the first three phases in the development of a glaucomatous NFBD is as follows (fig. 8):

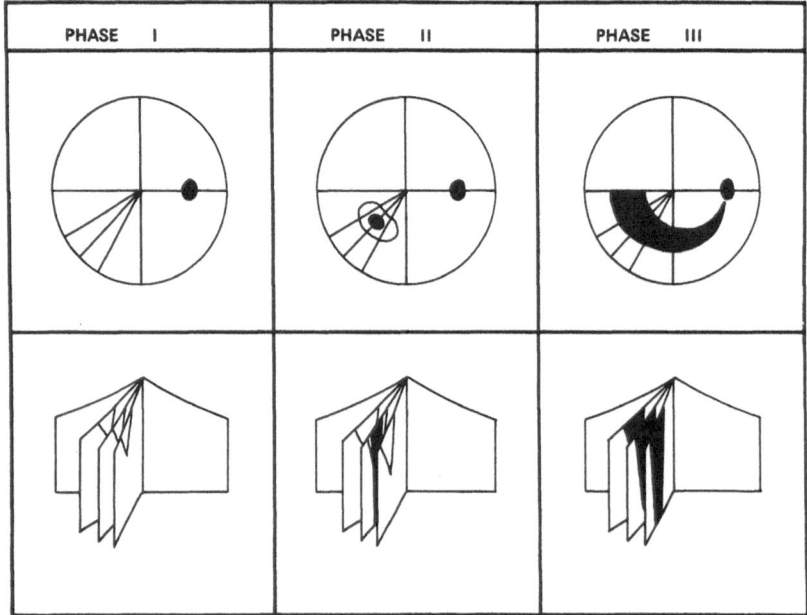

Fig. 8. Schematic representation of the development of a paracentral nerve fiber bundle defect (NFBD). Phase I shows a series of w.s.d., in phase II the intensity of the defects increases and in phase III a full arcuate NFBD has developed.

134

Stage 0. No defects.
Stage I. Series of fluctuating w s.d.
Stage II. Development from w s.d. to a defect for maximum luminance.
Stage III. Fully developed arcuate NFBD.

Stage I. means probably that the area where the fluctuating w.s.d. has been found will develop a defect of greater intensity in the foreseable future. It seems likely that a w.s.d. indicates that the critical IOP of this eye has been exceeded. The fact that the w.s.d. can be reversible makes this first phase a very interesting phase for therapeutical decisions. The findings of a series of fluctuating w.s.d. means that the glaucomatous eye is in a critical phase of unstable functional equilibrium. This could be in many cases an excellent moment to start medical therapy. A carefull follow-up of the series of w.s.d. will tell us whether the new level with medical therapy of IOP is over or under the critical IOP.

One of the problems of the treatment of glaucoma without visual field defects is that the time between the increase of the IOP and the development of visual field defect is unknown. If we could show that a certain period of time exists between the development of a w.s.d. and the subsequent development of a defect of greater intensity, then the phase of fluctuating w.s.d. is highly interesting for the treatment of glaucoma suspects. Considering this it is interesting that in the group of patients that developed a defect of greater intensity from a documented normal visual field through the phase of a fluctuating defect, the average time between the stage of a w.s.d. and the defect of greater intensity was $2\frac{1}{2}$ years. If this observation is confirmed by a prospective investigation, the stage of a fluctuating w.s.d. is indeed a critical phase in the development of glaucomatous defects.

CRITICAL CONSIDERATIONS

This investigation does not present data on frequency of occurence of w.s.d. in normal subjects. In our experience one rarely finds a w.s.d. in normal subjects, however, we have no data available of a large study of normal subjects.

It is important to know how often a defect of greater intensity develops from the w.s.d. in untreated glaucoma patients. Moreover, it is important to know what the length of time is between the development of w.s.d. and a defect of greater intensity. It is expected that these questions can be answered in the near future.

There is the question whether the finding of a w.s.d. is dependent on the procedure of examination. Short-term reproducibility of a w.s.d. has received our attention. The pathogenesis of the development of a w.s.d. is unknown.

REFERENCES

Armaly, M.F. Selective perimetry for glaucomatous defects in ocular hypertension. *Arch. Ophthal.* 87: *518* (1972).

Aulhorn, E. & Harms, H. Early visual field defects in glaucoma. In: Glaucoma Symposium, Tutzing Castle, Ed. Leydhecker, Karger, Basel. p. *151* (1966).

Drance, S.M. The early field defects in glaucoma. *Invest. Ophthal.* 8: *84* (1969).

Greve, E.L. Perimetry in Glaucoma: with special reference to some early glaucomatous defects. Irish Faculty of Ophthalmology-Yearbook 1973: *pg. 12 + 13*.

Greve, E.L. Single and Multiple Stimulus Static Perimetry in Glaucoma, the two phases of visual field examination. *Docum. Ophthal.* 36: *1-355* (1973).

Greve, E.L. & Verduin, W.M. Detection of early glaucomatous defects: I. Visual field investigation. *Docum. Ophthal. Proc. Series* 14: *103-114* (1977).

Greve, E.L. & Verduin, W.M. Detection of Early Glaucomatous Defects: II. Cupping and Visual field. *Docum. Ophthal. Proc. Series* 14: *115-120* (1977).

LeBlanc, R.P. & Becker, B. Peripheral nasal field defects. *Amer. J. Ophthal.* 72: *415* (1971).

LeBlanc, R.P. Peripheral nasal defects. *Docum. Ophthal. Proc. Series* 14: *131* (1977).

Rønne, H. Ueber das Gesichtsfeld beim Glaukom. *Klin. Mbl. Augenheilk.* 47: *12* (1909).

Werner, E.B. & Drance, S.M. Early visual field disturbances in glaucoma. *Arch. Ophthal.* 95: *1173* (1977).

Authors' address:
Eye Clinic of the University of Amsterdam
Wilhelmina Gasthuis
1e Helmersstraat 104
1054 EG Amsterdam
The Netherlands

Docum. Ophthal. Proc. Series, Vol. 19

ANALYSIS OF PATIENTS WITH OPEN-ANGLE GLAUCOMA USING PERIMETRIC TECHNIQUES REFLECTING RECEPTIVE FIELD-LIKE PROPERTIES

JAY M. ENOCH & EMILIO C. CAMPOS

(Gainesville, Florida U.S.A.)

ABSTRACT

Several lines of research have been drawn together in this brief paper. Perimetric tests of receptive field-like functions localized in the inner retina are unequivocally altered in open angle glaucoma. In 49 out of 49 cases changes in the sustained-like function were shown to occur. These changes in measured function may or may not parallel alterations in the visual field. The visual field tends to vary substantially in time in the population sampled. The disease process may be amenable to treatment, if evidence for remissions in functional properties remains.

INTRODUCTION

The receptive field is defined as the area of the retina from which measured discharges or potentials of a neuron may be influenced. In this laboratory sustained-like and transient-like psychophysical functions believed to reflect receptive field-like properties have been employed for several years for testing clinical populations (Enoch 1978, Enoch, Berger & Birns 1970, Enoch & Johnson 1976, Enoch & Lawrence 1975, Enoch, Lazarus & Johnson 1976, Enoch & Sunga 1969, Enoch, Sunga & Bachmann 1970, Frankhauser & Enoch 1962, Johnson & Enoch 1976, Sunga & Enoch 1970). Both can be tested perimetrically. There is evidence that the sustained-like function is already organized at the outer plexiform layer, whereas the transient-like function is apparently first organized in the inner plexiform layer (Enoch 1978). On the basis of an extensive series of studies the sustained-like function is altered by pathology of the inner *and* outer plexiform layers while the transient-like function apparently is only affected by inner plexiform layer anomalies (Enoch 1978).

In this paper we will discuss data obtained from patients with open angle glaucoma, including a group of 49 patients where the sustained-like function and kinetic perimetry (and many other tests) were tested monthly and

* This research has been supported in part by a National eye Institute Research Grant No. EY-01418 (to JME), NIH, Bethesda, Maryland, in part by a Fellowship supported by Fight-for-Sight, Inc., to ECC), New York City, in tribute to the memory of Hermann Burian, M.D., and in part by National Eye Institute Contract No. NIH 71-2514 to Bernard Becker, M.D., Washington University, St. Louis, Missouri.
** Dr. Campos is on leave of absence from the University of Modena.

followed over a one-year period. Some sample cases will be considered. Examples of patients where both the sustained- and transient-like functions were tested will be described.

METHOD

The procedure is in essence the one described by Enoch (1978). It is noteworthy that all tests are performed on modified commercially available perimetric devices. We used a Goldmann perimeter manufactured by Haag-Streit (Bern).

The *sustained-like function* is obtained by varying the size and luminance of a continuously visible background field upon which is displayed a small, fixed luminance, slowly flashing stimulus.

Field I: A small, regularly flashing test field (140 msec/per second) is centered on the point in the visual field to be tested. The (static) threshold of Field I against the standard general surround field (the cupola) is determined and then set at a fixed 'criterion' luminance above this threshold (usually 0.8 log units). Field I is provided by the standard pantograph arm on the Goldmann perimeter. The available model has a flicker attachment which served as chopper.

Field II This is the background field, continuously presented and centered about Field I, with its area being altered step-wise over a large range down do that of Field I. To bring Field I to threshold the luminance of Field II is varied with a neutral density filter wedge by either the subject or examiner. A modified Haag-Streit fixation projector has been employed to form Field II.

Field III: The cupola of the Goldmann perimeter forms the surround field which is held at the standard luminance value (31.5 apostilbs = 10.02 cd/m^2) throughout testing. This field minimizes artifactual responses and controls light adaptation. The stimulus array was located at 5° on the 0° half meridian on the Goldmann perimeter and an auxiliary fixation projector was used. When studying lesions causing relative field loss or field loss without sharp boundaries, test loci were selected in or near areas of relative scotoma. Control data were obtained from uninvolved points in the same eye at the same distance from the fovea.

A typical sustained-like function (Fig. 1) is V- or U-shaped, with a center-like and a surround-like component. The magnitude of the effect increases with eccentricity from fixation. *Only* the surround-like component is affected in pathology.

The *transient-like function* measures the difference in luminance between a stationary and a rotating windmill necessary to bring flashing Field I to threshold. The same criterion level is used. Fields I and III are the same as used for sampling the sustained-like function. Four vaned windmills of convenient sizes for each retinal location are substituted for the round discs in the projector of Field II. Field II rotation is obtained by means of a Dove prism (8 ON and OFF transitions/second are used). The magnitude of the transient-like effect increases with eccentricity (Fig. 1). In the presence of pathology the difference in luminance for the stationary and moving wind-mill (Field II) necessary to bring Field I to threshold approaches zero.

To obtain reliable results it is essential to correct blur. This is achieved by using classical stigmatoscopy methods (the lens power producing the minimum increment threshold for Field I on Field III. (Ames & Glidden 1928, Frankhauser & Enoch 1962). Each value is the average of ascending and descending judgments. This method provides a check on the reliability of the test and the criterion of judgment of the patient.

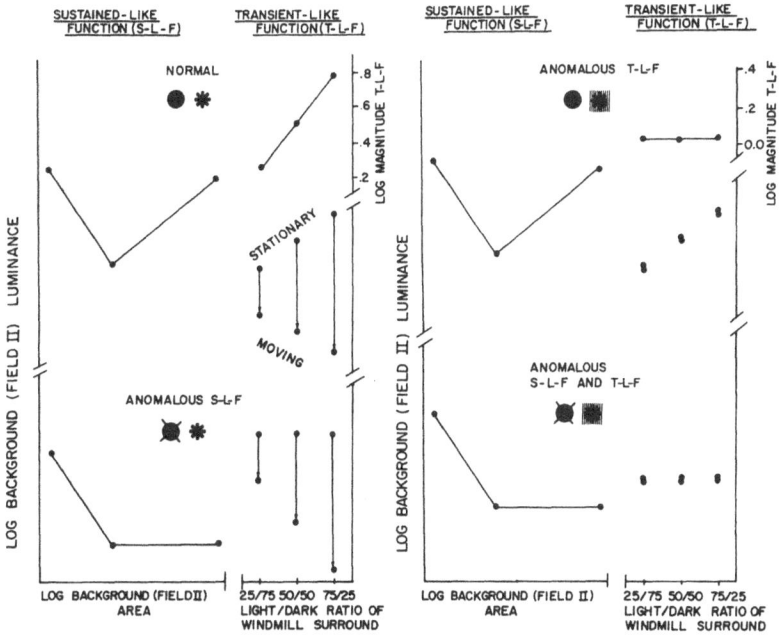

Fig. 1. The log of the luminance of Field II (ordinate) is plotted against the log of its area (abscissa) for the sustained-like function. Ordinates are the same for the transient-like function. The abscissa in this case indicates light/dark ratio (duty cycle) of wind-mill surround zone. A normal sustained-like function has a V or U shape. In pathology the surround-like or inhibition-like component is flattened. The transient-like function is represented by the vertical arrow which connects the measured values of luminance for the stationary and moving windmill, needed to bring Field I to threshold. In pathology the difference of the measured values tends to go to zero. The line which connects the values of the luminances for the stationary windmills with 25/75, 50/50 and 75/25 light/dark zones provides a control for the sustained-like function (for details see Enoch 1978). A filled circle indicates a normal sustained-like function; a crossed circle represents an abnormal sustained-like function; a circle crossed only by one stripe represents a reduced sustained-like function. A normal transient-like function is indicated by an asterisk, whereas an asterisk hidden by a graticle or grating pattern shows an abnormal transient-like function.

139

Forty-nine out of 49 open angle glaucomatous patients (100%) with visual field loss tested each month for one year showed changes in the sustained-like function when tested in or near areas of relative visual field loss (Enoch 1978). In some instances, the sustained-like function was at first normal, then became abnormal, and then returned to normal. In other cases, it remained abnormal during the entire test period. Moreover, fluctuations of various types were observed both in the visual field and the sustained-like function. The right eye findings of patient JR are presented in Fig. 2-1. The sustained-like function tested at 15° eccentricity on the 240° half-meridian was abnormal for the year tested. The visual field, however, showed interesting changes over the same period. At first, the field was almost normal, with a relative scotoma in the infranasal quadrant, in which the sustained-like function was tested (Fig. 2-1). Note, in Fig. 2 the second number represents the month in the year sequence. Three months later the field deteriorated (Fig. 2-4) with a slight improvement the sixth month (Fig. 2-6). This was followed by deterioration (Fig. 2-7), improvement in (Fig. 2-8) and a final deterioration which remained stable for the rest of the year (Fig. 2-10).

In the case of patient AB, the data in the left eye are considered. The sustained-like function was tested at 15° eccentricity on the 285° half meredian. At first the 1/3e and 1/2e isopters were considerably restricted (Fig. 3-1). The point where the sustained-like function was tested and found to be abnormal lay just on the border of the 1/3e isopter. The next month a noticeable improvement took place so that the test point was on the border of the I/2e isopter, but was still abnormal (Fig. 3-2). A further improvement of the field was accompanied by a normalization of the sustained-like function (Fig. 3-4). The fifth month the field deteriorated again but the sustained-like function remained normal (Fig. 3-5) until the seventh and eighth month when a slight improvement in field was recorded (Fig. 4-7). Then there was deterioration of the field (Fig. 4-8). The field improved again but the sustained-like function now was abnormal (Fig. 4-11) and reduced (Fig. 4-12).

In patient MA two test points in the right eye were followed: 15° eccentricity on the 45° half meridian (Point 1) was tested for the entire year, and 12° eccentricity on the 44° half meridian was added during the last nine months (Point 2). Initially, Point 1 was normal and the visual field did not show significant changes (Fig. 5-1). During the fifth month a relative scotoma appeared in the supero-nasal quadrant. Point 1 was normal, but when the patient was tested at Point 2 the sustained-like function was abnormal (Fig. 5-5). In the sixth month Points 1 and 2 were outside the 1/2e isopter but the findings were the same (Fig. 5-6). The field remained quite stable until the ninth month. At that time both test points exhibited an abnormal sustained-like function (Fig. 5-9). This condition persisted relative to the sustained-like function for the remainder of the test period while the field improved slightly (Fig. 5-10 and 5-12).

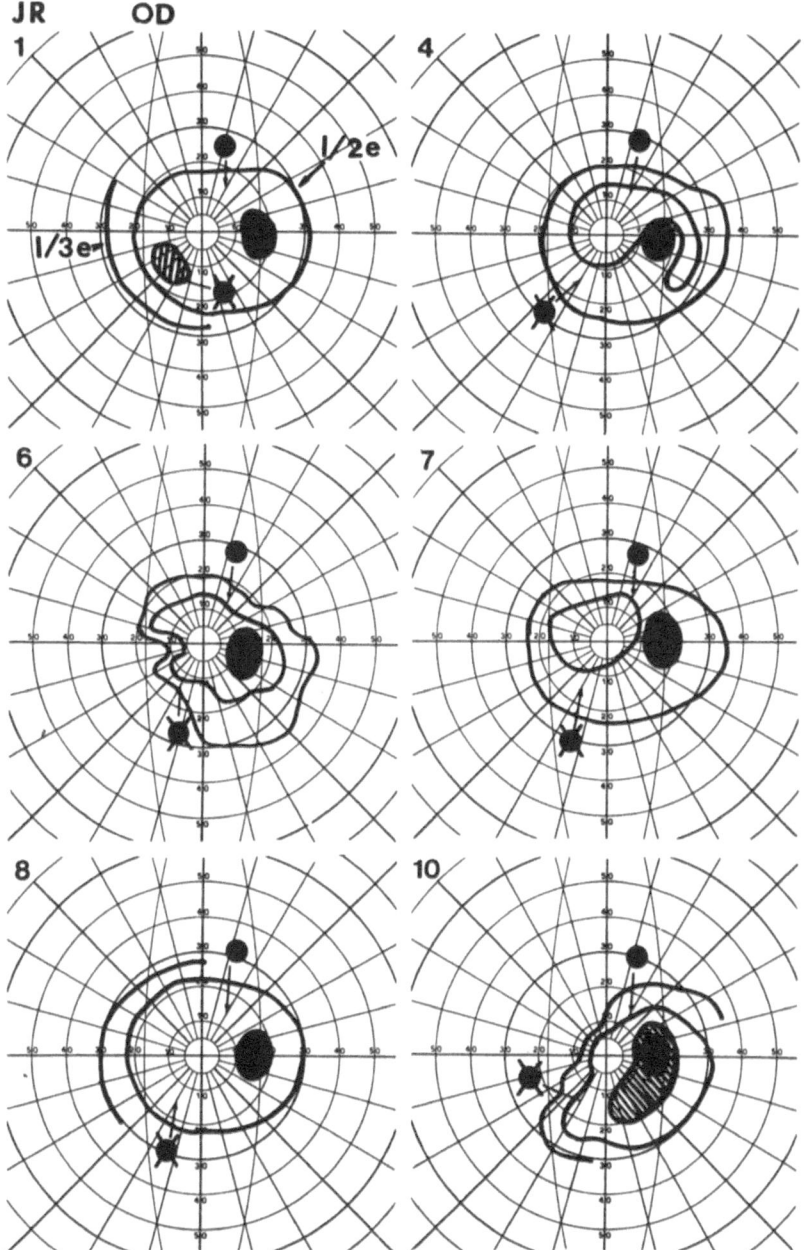

Fig. 2. Visual fields and sustained-like function measurements in patient JR. The second number represents the month in the year test sequence. The symbols for the sustained-like function are the same as in Figure 1.

Finally, two cases are reported where the sustained- and transient-like functions were tested in individuals with open angle glaucomatous visual field losses. Both the sustained- and transient-like functions were abnormal at 6° eccentricity on the 45° half meridian of the right eye of patient YB. The control point (6° eccentricity on the 225° half meridian) was normal (Fig. 6). Note, the point at 6° eccentricity on the 45° half-meridian lay outside of a nerve fiber bundle defect. The patient had been remiss in taking her medications and at the time of testing IOP was greater than 40mmHg.

Patient VC's data from the right eye are particularly interesting (Fig. 7). The sustained- and transient-like functions were abnormal at 3° eccentricity on the 45°, 0° and 225° half meridians. The two functions were normal at a control point chosen at 3° eccentricity on the 135° half meridian. Note, where the points on the 225° and 0° half meridians fall in areas of nerve fiber bundle defects the test point on the 45° half meridian is located in an apparently normal zone.

AB 1   OS

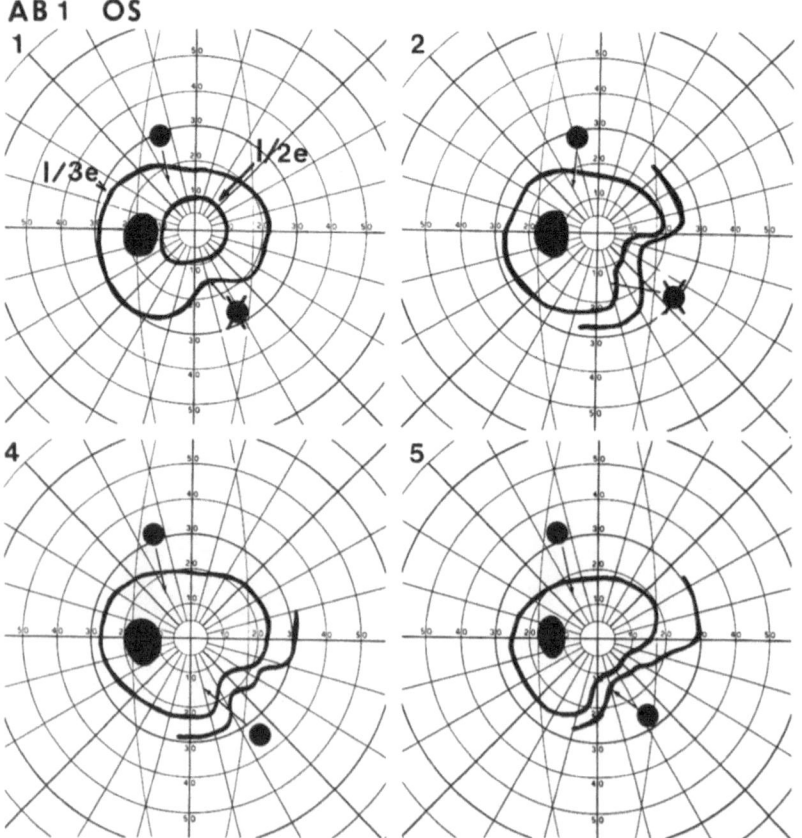

Fig. 3. Visual fields and sustained-like function findings of the first five months of the year test sequence in patient AB. Symbols are the same as in the previous figures.

142

DISCUSSION AND CONCLUSIONS

1. 1. All glaucomatous patients with visual field losses followed over a one-year period had changes in the sustained-like function. The later fluctuated showing remissions and exacerbations. In some cases sustained-like functions lagged field changes, in others they appeared first.

2. The visual field, as tested with kinetic perimetry, also changed in time. These data are of clinical interest. They suggest that once the stage of the disease is able to provoke visual field losses, the latter are presumably not the expression of a localized lesion, but a substantial portion of the nerve fiber layer can participate in the process. Furthermore, it seems that these fluctuations need not be directly related to introcular pressure variations (see Table I, II, III).

3. In patients where the transient-like function was tested, the latter

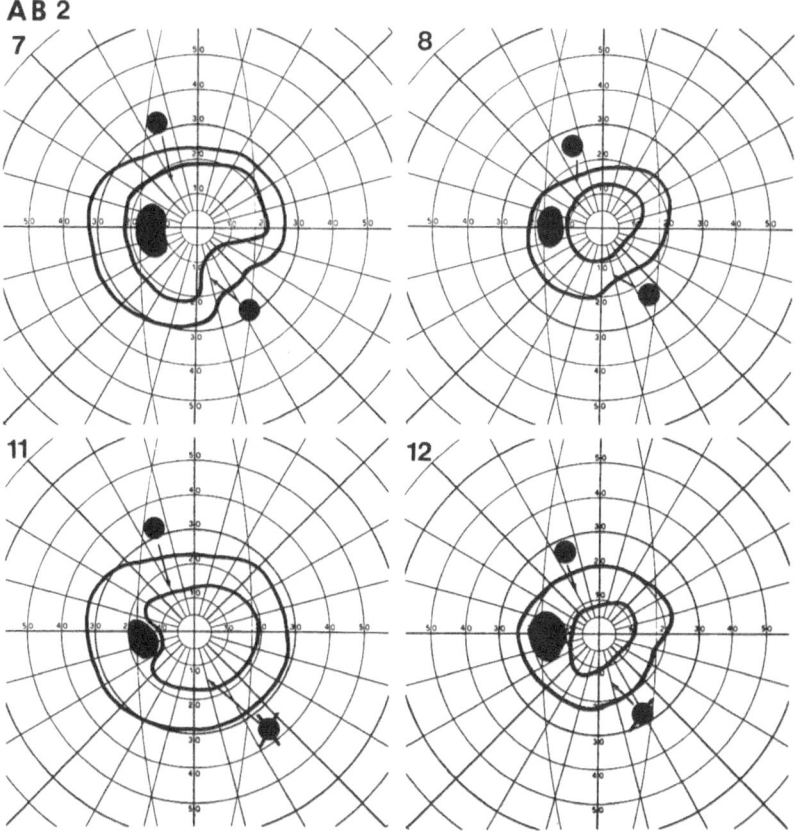

Fig. 4. Visual fields and sustained-like function findings during the second half of the year test sequence in patient AB. Symbols are the same as in the previous figures.

143

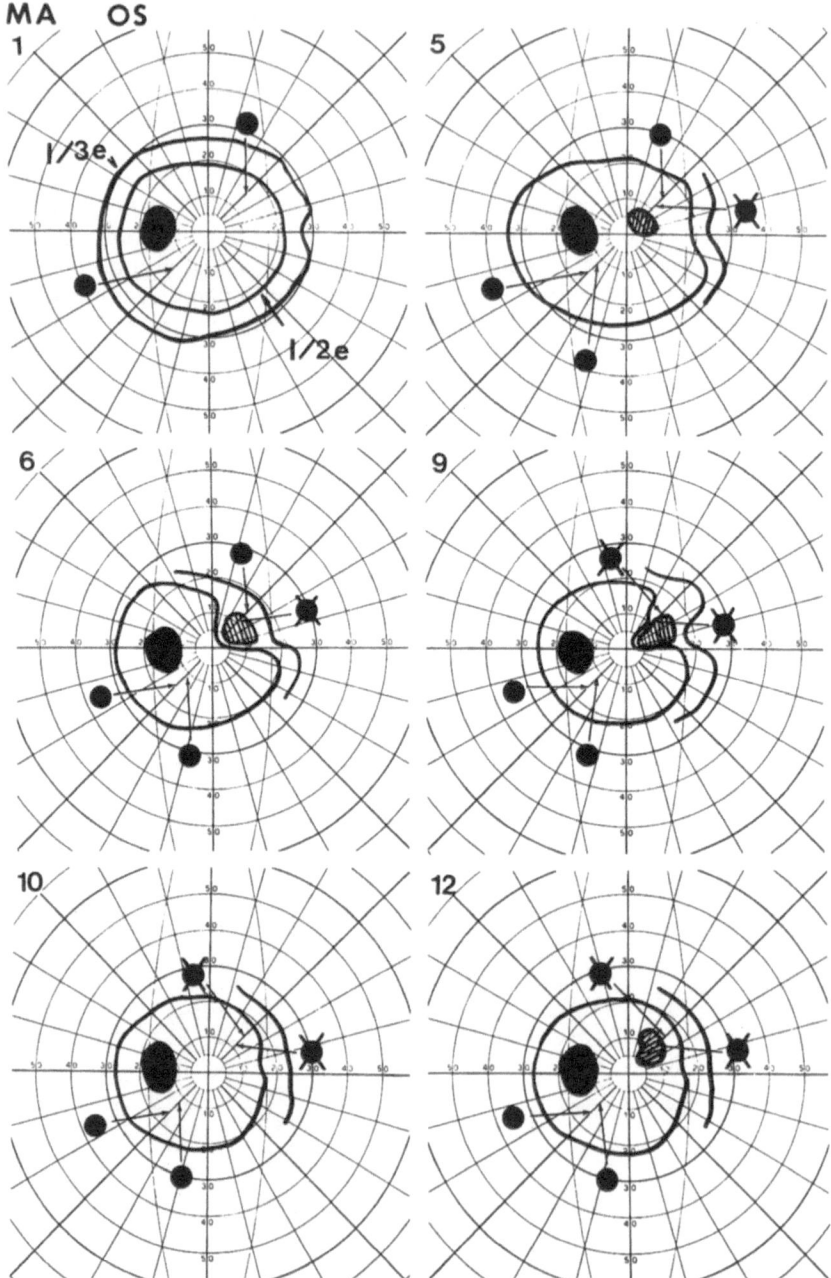

Fig. 5. Visual fields and sustained-like function findings in patient MA. Symbols are the same as in the previous figures.

Table 1. JR OD

Month	I.O.P. mm HG	Visual Field	Sustained-like Function
1	34	Small Changes	Abnormal
2	28	Stable	Abnormal
3	–		
4	30	Deteriorated	Abnormal
5	31	Stable	Abnormal
6	26	Improved	Abnormal
7	32	Deteriorated	Abnormal
8	35	Improved	Abnormal
9	30	Stable	Abnormal
10	29	Deteriorated	Abnormal
11	32	Stable	Abnormal
12	32	Stable	Abnormal

Table 2. AB OS

Month	I.O.P. mm HG	Visual Field	Sustained-like Function
1	22	Isopters Restricted	Abnormal
2	25	Improved	Abnormal
3	25	Stable	Stable
4	19	Improved	Normal
5	22	Deteriorated	Normal
6	22	Stable	Normal
7	20	Improved	Normal
8	18	Deteriorated	Normal
9	21	Stable	Normal
10	20	Stable	Normal
11	23	Improved	Abnormal
12	20	Deteriorated	Reduced

Table 3. MA OD

Month	I.O.P. mm HG	Visual Field	Sustained-like Function Point 1	Point 2
1	16	Almost Normal	Normal	
2	18	Stable	Normal	
3	20	Stable	Normal	
4	18	Stable	Normal	
5	10	Deteriorated	Normal	Abnormal
6	18	Deteriorated	Normal	Abnormal
7	14	Stable	Normal	Abnormal
8	20	Stable	Normal	Abnormal
9	20	Stable	Abnormal	Abnormal
10	16	Improved	Abnormal	Abnormal
11	17	Stable	Abnormal	Abnormal
12	17	Stable	Abnormal	Abnormal

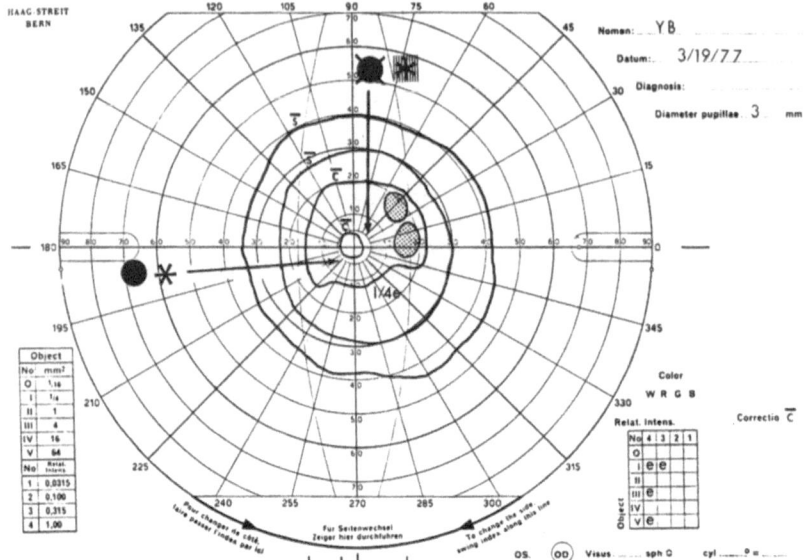

Fig. 6. Visual field and data obtained from tests of the sustained-like and transient-like functions in patient YB. Symbols are the same as in the previous figures.

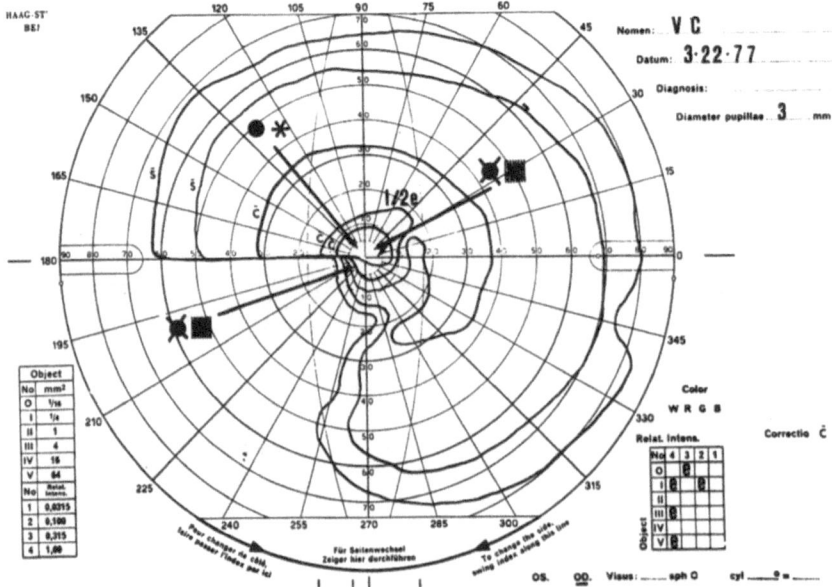

Fig. 7. Visual field and data obtained from tests of the sustained-like and transient-like functions in patient VC. Symbols are the same as in the previous figures.

146

was almost always abnormal if the sustained-like function was abnormal. At this time it is not clear if one or the other function is affected first. We believe we are sampling both functions at the inner plexiform layer. There is separate evidence (Enoch 1978) indicating that the alterations in these two response functions have origin prior to the myelinated portion of the optic nerve and that the functional changes measured are synaptic in origin.

4. Since both the sustained- and transient-like functions have been found to be abnormal in areas outside fiber bundle defects in open angle glaucoma, it becomes important to consider whether these parameters can be used as indicators of eventual visual field losses.

5. The sustained- and transient-like functions have been shown to be two independent functions, i.e., they may separately change in the sense of deterioration and/or improvement. If the aforementioned functions stay abnormal for a prolonged period of time, the prognosis seems to be less favorable (e.g., see Fig. 2). However, when fluctuations are shown, i.e., improvements and deteriorations, the likelihood of a successful treatment would seem to remain.

6. Whether or not functions reflecting retinal receptive field-like properties prove to be directly predictive of probable visual field loss, they provide us with added and somewhat independent useful information on the severity of this disease. Their being affected in 100% of a sample of 49 cases of open angle glaucoma must be regarded as highly significant.

7. The behavior of the visual field in time deserves further comment. A diagnosis of visual field loss is often made and accordingly a therapy prescribed on the basis of a single analysis. This kind of approach warrants review, particularly on the basis of our findings. Careful tests were always performed by the same well-trained technician. The variations are therefore considered to be significant. Their meaning has still to be clarified and many factors may be involved. Furthermore, it may be argued that the fluctuations of the visual field may be used also as a diagnostic tool. Indeed, once the pathology is already far advanced, only progressive deterioration in the field will be observed. The presence of fluctuations, i.e., regressions and exacerbations, may be a sign that the system still has a reasonable recovery potential. Apart from these considerations, the practical consequence which can be drawn from our findings is that an evaluation of a visual field in a glaucomatous patient is possible only after having examined a number of independently determined sequential records.

Obviously, added cases have to be tested and followed in time with both functions. The selection of the test points needs to be improved. Clearly, it is difficult to assess the status of the visual field on the basis of a small sample of test points. A test strategy based on the frequency of involvement of different areas of the visual field in glaucoma is advisable, e.g., making use of the distribution of areas of glaucomatous involvement described by Aulhorn & Karmeyer, 1977.

ACKNOWLEDGEMENTS

The authors wish to express their appreciation to Mrs. Beverly Lawrence of the Department of Ophthalmology, Washington University School of Medicine, St. Louis, who offered technical assistance on this program and who carefully collected and collated much of the data presented here.

The authors also extend their thanks to Bernard Becker, M.D., for permission to use new data collected under a NEI contract to the Washington University Glaucoma Center, St. Louis, Mo.

REFERENCES

Ames A. & Glidden G. Ocular measurement. *Trans. Section Ophthal. p. 102* (1928).

Aulhorn E. & Karmeyer H. Frequency distribution in early glaucomatous visual field defects. 2nd Int. Visual Field Symposium. Tübingen (West Germany), September, 1976. *Doc. Ophthalmol.* Proc. Ser. 14: *75-83* (1977).

Enoch J.M. Quantitative layer-by-layer perimetry. The Francis I. Proctor Medal Lecture of the Association for Research in Vision and Ophthalmology, 1977. *Invest. Ophthalmol.* 17: *199-251* (1978).

Enoch J.M., Berger R. & Birns R. A static perimetric technique believed to test receptive field properties: Extension and verification of the analysis. *Doc. Ophthalmol.* 29: *127* (1970).

Enoch J.M., Berger R. & Birns R. A static perimetric technique believed to test receptive field properties: Responses near visual field lesions with sharp borders. *Doc. Ophthalmol.* 29: *154* (1970).

Enoch J.M. & Johnson C.A. Additivity of effects within sectors of the sensitization zone of the Westheimer function. *Am. J. Optom. & Physiol. Optics* 50: *350* (1976).

Enoch J.M. & Johnson C.A., Fitzgerald C.R. Human psychophysical analysis of receptive field-like properties: V. Adaptation of stationary and moving windmill target characteristics to clinical populations. *Doc. Ophthalmol.* 41: *347* (1976).

Enoch J.M. & Lawrence B. A perimetric technique believed to test receptive field properties: Sequential evaluation in glaucoma and other conditions. First Int. Visual Field Symposium, Marseille (France), May 1974. In 'L'annee Therapeutique et Clinique en Ophthalmologie'. Tome XXV. Fuery Laney, Marseille, 1974, pag. 215. Published also in *Am. J. Ophthalmol.* 80: *734* (1975).

Enoch J.M., Lazarus J. & Johnson C.A. Human psychophysical analysis of receptive field-like properties. I. A new transient-like visual response using a moving windmill (Werblin-type) target. Sensory Processes. 1: *14* (1976).

Enoch J.M. & Sunga R.N. Development of quantitative perimetric tests. *Doc. Ophthalmol.* 26: *215* (1969).

Enoch J.M., Sunga R.N. & Bachman E. Static perimetric technique believed to test receptive field properties. I. Extension of Westheimer's Experiments on spatial interaction. *Am. J. Ophthalmol.* 70: *113* (1970).

Enoch J.M., Sunga R.N. & Bachman E. Static perimetric technique believed to test receptive field properties. II. Adaptation of the method to the quantitative perimeter. *Am. J. Ophthalmol.* 70: *126* (1970).

Frankhauser F. & Enoch J.M. The effects of blur upon perimetric thresholds. A method for determining a quantitative estimate of retinal contour. *Arch. Ophthalmol.* 86: *240* (1962).

Johnson C.A. & Enoch J.M. Human psychophysical analysis of receptive field-like properties. II. Dichoptic properties of the Westheimer function. *Vis. Research* 16: *1455* (1976).

Johnson C.A. & Enoch J.M. Human psychophysical analysis of receptive field-like properties. III. Dichoptic properties of a new transient-like psychophysical function. *Vis. Research* 16: *1463* (1976).

Johnson C.A. & Enoch J.M. Human psychophysical analysis of receptive field-like properties. IV. Further examination and specification of the psychophysical transient-like function. *Doc. Ophthalmol.* 41: *329* (1976).

Sunga R.N. & Enoch J.M. A static perimetric technique believed to test receptive field properties. III. Clinical trials. *Am. J. Ophthalmol.* 70: *244* (1970).

Authors' adress:
Department of Ophthalmology
and Center for Sensory Studies
University of Florida
Box J-284, JHMHC
Gainesville, Florida 32610
U.S.A.

149

LIMINAL AND SUPRALIMINAL STIMULI
IN THE PERIMETRY OF CHRONIC
SIMPLE GLAUCOMA

F. DANNHEIM

(Hamburg, GFR)

ABSTRACT

Supraliminal, evenly moving targets appear as altered in areas of absolute or relative glaucomatous visual field defects. Discrete changes of sensation of supraliminal stimuli may be found even in patients with practically normal fields according to conventional static and kinetic perimetry. Those minimal glaucomatous perimetric alterations are often located in the nasal field adjacent to the horizontal meridian. Since they may pass over to definite scotomata they are indicative of an earlier stage of glaucomatous functional damage.

INTRODUCTION

In the past 2 years we have been applying not only static and kinetic perimetry in patients with chronic simple glaucoma, but also supraliminal moving targets. The second method proved valuable especially in cases with discrete sensoric alterations (Dannheim 1977, 1978). The aim of this report is to give some details of the procedure and it's results.

METHOD

Peripheral and central kinetic visual fields were tested using a TÜBINGER and a modified RODENSTOCK perimeter with 3.2 cd/m^2 background luminance. It was attempted to present the kinetic targets from different directions in random order (Heijl & Krakau 1977). The isopters had been carefully traced near the nasal horizontal meridian not to miss even a tiny nasal step.

In many instances static perimetry was now applied in doubtful areas of the visual field either meridionally in the BJERRUM-area or circularly in the search of discrete nasal steps.

For an evaluation of sensation a target of 10' was chosen about 0.3 to 0.6 log. units above threshold. This target was manually moved centripetally along the vertical and the 2 oblique meridians with a constant speed of 2° to 4° per second. Following this a circular course was used nasally between 10° and 30°, temporally at 30°. Such an evaluation of sensation required about 3 to 5 minutes per eye.

A good cooperation was as essential as a precise instruction of the patient that the whole perimetric procedure is being turned upside down: If he until now had to watch for the appearance of a target he was now supposed to report on a lack in the subjective appearance of the steadily moving target – a short flicker only, a loss in brightness or a change in the sharpness of contour. The effect of desaturation of colored stimuli was not used routinely. The subjective disappearance of the target in the blind spot was an indicator for the reliability of responses. A moving visible target is of course a temptation to be followed instead of the fixation spot (Heijl & Krakau 1977). But most patients were able to fulfill this requirement after a short time of training. Since it is difficult to keep such a steady fixation for a longer time a close observation of the eye being tested was necessary as well as a pause every now and then. In cases with changes of sensation the test was repeated in this area of the field and in adjacent areas for evaluation of the exent and topographic arrangement of the sensoric alteration.

RESULTS

2 out of 38 patients with circumscript field defects due to chronic simple glaucoma have been selected to illustrate that a test with supraliminal targets may reveal even earlier or more discrete sensoric alterations than conventional static and kinetic perimetry.

I.N., record No. 61458, 43 year old lady, chronic glaucoma known since 6 years. OD with marked loss of rim tissue.

Kinetic perimetry of the right eye (Fig. 1, left) shows no obvious alteration, whereas static perimetry of the upper half is a little suspect, in the lower half of the field normal. Changes of sensation are definitely present above fixation (given as hatched), below fixation only very faintly in a region, where the crossing target showed a short flicker only. Half a year later (Fig. 1, center) definite alterations were present in static perimetry, both above and below fixation, a relative scotoma had developed in kinetic perimetry on meridian 90°. The area of disturbance in sensation has enlarged especially below fixation. 2 weeks later (Fig. 1, right) the intraocular pressure was 10 mm Hg lower. The changes for supraliminal stimuli are about the same. Static and kinetic perimetry reveals a slightly lower over all sensitivity, whereas the defective areas have improved a little – if at all.

I.R., record No. 82973, 51 year old lady, chronic glaucoma known since 7 years. Optic disc in both eyes with definite loss of rim tissue.

The peripheral fields (Fig. 2) show a symmetrically arranged discrete nasal step in the mid periphery. Zones of disturbance of sensation are present binasally and bitemporally (hatched). The central field of the right eye (Fig. 3) has been presented earlier (Dannheim 1977, 1978). The nasal step is visible in the isopters between about 15 and 30°. Circular static perimetry was located 15° paracentral as to hit an area just at the border between disturbed and normal function. It revealed for white and colored stimuli no substantial alterations, except for a minimal increase in variation of single responses in some instances only. Sensation of supraliminal stimuli – however – was definitely disturbed in a sector reaching as far centrally as 10°. This effect is marked in the static plot as hatched.

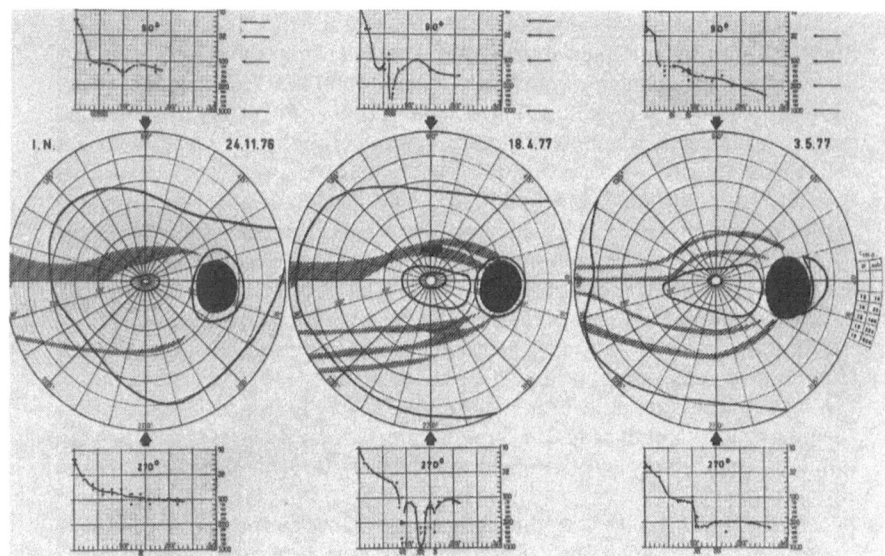

Fig. 1. Glaucomatous visual field with disturbance of sensation progressing to relative defects. Description in the text.

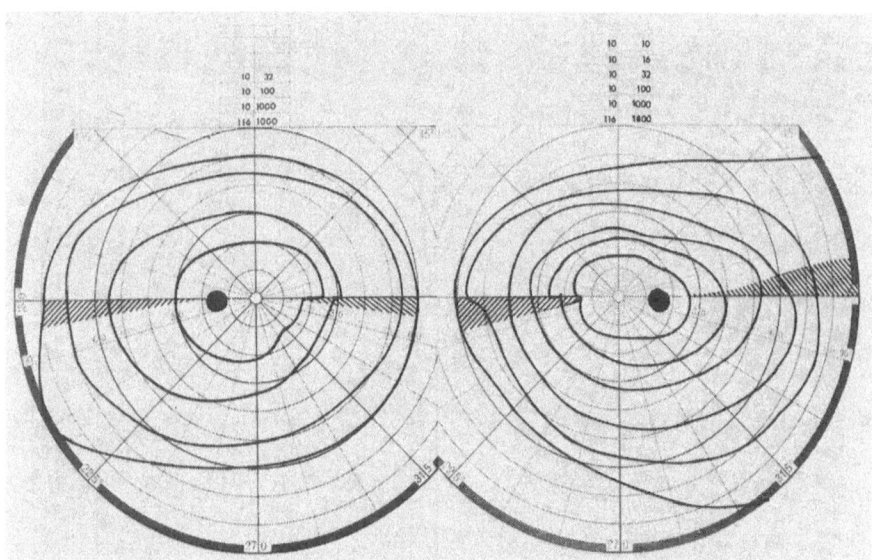

Fig. 2. Peripheral visual fields of chronic glaucoma: Bilateral discrete nasal step combined with symmetrical zones of changes of sensation nasally and temporally.

In the following time pressure control of this right eye was not satisfying. 3 months later the findings were constant. 11 and 21 months later, however, the nasal step was more marked as before, reaching now from about 10 to 45° paracentral (Fig. 4). The isopters of the temporal field do show some impression now. Circular static perimetry 15° nasally has a definite depression at the location where formerly only the supraliminal stimuli had indicated some pathology. The tongue-shaped area with disturbed sensation has moved right into the center. Circular static perimetry 5° paracentrally is normal even in locations where the supraliminal stimulus appears as altered subjectively. Circular static perimetry 30° temporal, however, shows both changes for liminal and supraliminal targets.

The right eye of this lady, where the intraocular pressure was controlled after surgery, had discrete nasal steps to start with (Fig. 1) as in the fellow eye. In the last 2 tests 2 years later (Fig. 5) this field was normal according to static and kinetic perimetry. Supraliminal stimuli, however, reveal a very similar pattern as in the other eye indicative of the same disease – just less advanced.

34 of our 38 patients with circumscript glaucomatous alterations had changes of sensation in the nasal field near the horizontal meridian in at least one eye. 2/3 of these cases had nasal steps in the corresponding field (Fig. 2, 3, 4), whereas in the others the visual field seemed normal according to threshold perimetry (Fig. 5). Circumscript alterations in the nasal field were in more than half of these 34 cases the dominating or the only glauco-

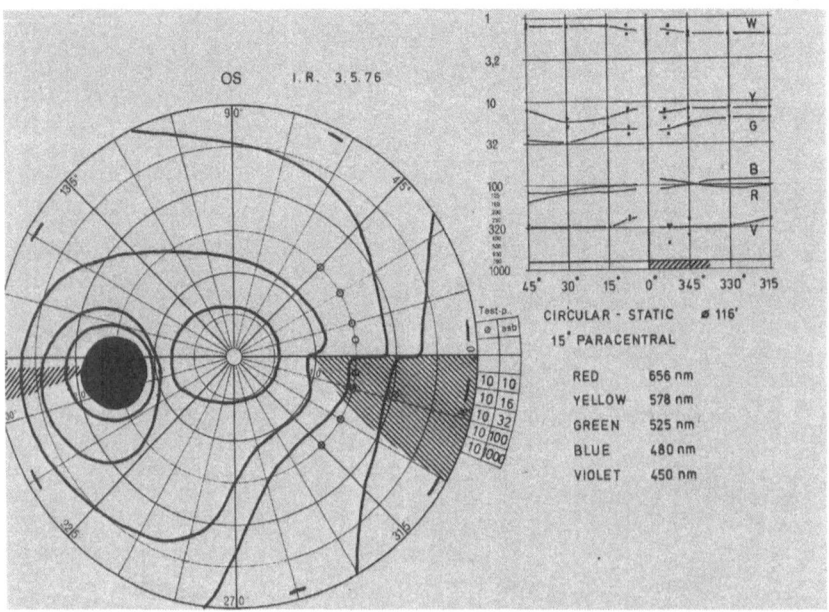

Fig. 3. Central static and kinetic field of the left eye from fig. 2. Description in the text.

154

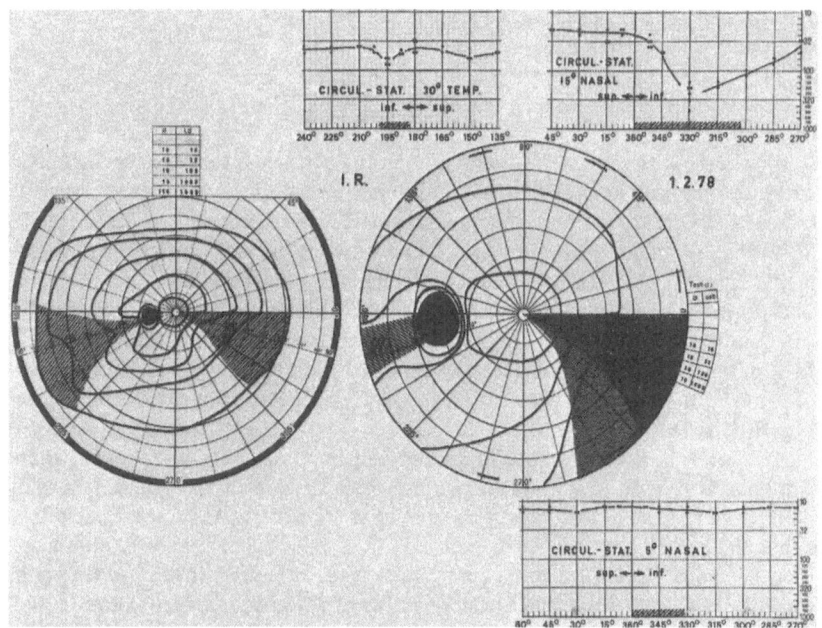

Fig. 4. Peripheral and central static and kinetic field from fig. 3 with progression of changes of sensation into relative defects.

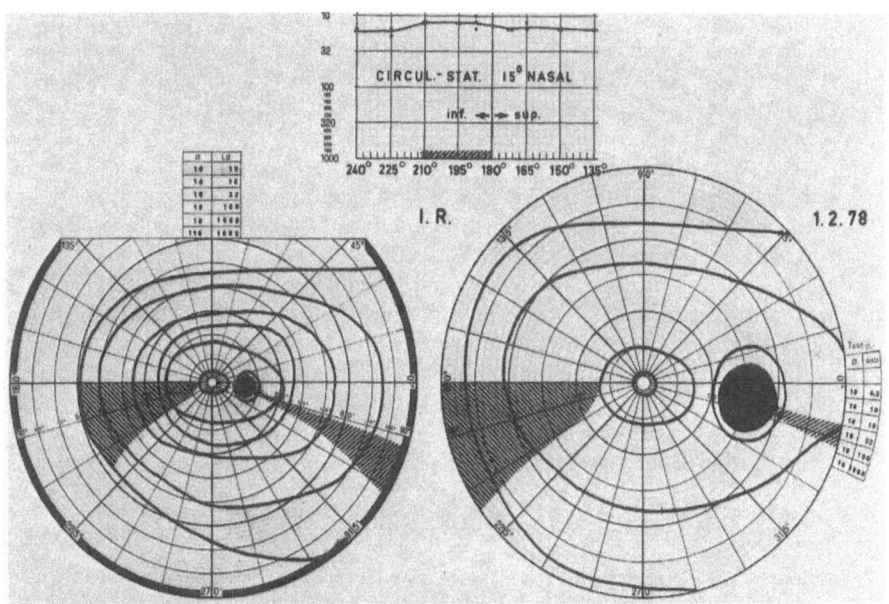

Fig. 5. Peripheral and central static and kinetic field of the right eye from fig. 2 with regression of the nasal step, but persistent disturbance of sensation.

155

matous perimetric changes (Aulhorn & Karmeyer 1977, Leblanc 1977, Dannheim 1977, 1978).

DISCUSSION

If a patient with chronic simple glaucoma turns out to have visual fields without changes in static and kinetic perimetry but with alterations of sensation as presented here the question arises whether or not this alteration is due to glaucomatous damage. The following might support this statement: Typical changes of sensation were never present in a group of about 200 normals, and only observed in patients with damage of the optic nerve. In some patients the fellow eye had well established glaucomatous defects. In 2 patients a progression from a change of sensation only to a change also of threshold perimetry was observed, and in 2 patients a regression in the opposite direction could be traced.

But why is the threshold of perception in some cases unchanged when the sensation of supraliminal stimuli indicates already discrete glaucomatous damage? First of all one must consider, that static and kinetic perimetry is a subjective, relatively unprecise method. It may well be, that very fine bundles of nerve fibres, already being damaged, do not show up even with repeated static testing, since the stimulus always hits adjacent, unaffected areas of the field. A tiny supraliminal moving target, however, will stimulate all retinal locations consecutively along a certain trail. Even a scotoma as narrow as a larger retinal vessel may be picked up in patients with good responses. Changes of sensation, however, must not necessarily precede the changes of threshold perimetry over long periods of time: 2 of our patients which developed defects in a formerly unaffected field within the last 2 years showed both changes of threshold perception and sensation of supraliminal targets at the same time, as fields where taken at about 6 months intervals.

The second explanation for the discrepancy between sensation and perception is more speculative: In sensation of supraliminal moving white – or even colored – stimuli higher sensoric functions are involved as compared to perception of threshold stimuli. Those more complex abilities might be affected selectively. These questions must be worked up in further studies as well as the question of regression of visual field damage, which may be observed in some cases of chronic glaucoma.

ACKNOWLEDGEMENT

I am greatly indebted to Prof. Drance for critical comments.

REFERENCES

Aulhorn, E. & Karmeyer, H. Frequency distribution in early glaucomatous visual field defects. *Docum. Ophthal. Proc. Series* 14: *75-83* (1977).
Dannheim, F. In: *Docum. Ophthal. Proc. Series* 14: *160-161* (1977).

Dannheim, F. Zur Perimetrie beim Glaukom. Schwellennahe und überschwellige Reize. *Klin. Mbl. Augenheilk.* 1978 173: *232-237* (1978).

Heijl, A. & Krakau, C.E.T. A note on fixation during perimetry. *Acta Ophthal.* (Kbh) 55: *854-861* (1977).

Leblanc, R.P. Peripheral nasal field defects. *Docu. Ophthal. Proc. Series* 14: *131-133 (1977).*

Author's address:
Universitäts-Augenklinik
Martinistr. 52
2000 Hamburg 20
GFR

Docum. Ophthal. Proc. Series, Vol. 19

ACQUIRED DYSCHROMATOPSIAS
THE EARLIEST FUNCTIONAL LOSSES IN GLAUCOMA

R. LAKOWSKI & S.M. DRANCE

ABSTRACT

Large losses in colour vision equivalent to the acquired dyschromatopsias seen so frequently in glaucoma patients with extensive field losses should be seriously considered as indicating a risk of open angle glaucoma when found in ocular hypertensive patients.

Patients with normal fields, but increased intraocular pressures (ocular hypertensives), both not receiving and receiving topical medication (OHnT, OHT) were compared with glaucoma patients at three levels of field damage (CS1, CS2, CS3) on a battery of colour vision tests. These tests include the Farnsworth-Munsell 100-Hue test and the Pickford-Nicolson anomaloscope. All clinical vision results are compared to equivalent age controls. Results on the 100-Hue test show a difference between the controls and the OHnT, with a dramatic increase in score (worsening discrimination) in the OHT group. The CS1, CS2, and CS3 groups show a progression in score along with severity of field damage. A comparison with the 95th percentile for the control group shows 19% of OHnt and 50% of OHT scores beyond this limit, and a progression in the CS groups to 74% of CS3 beyond the 95th percentile for normals.

P-N anomaloscope results include matching ranges on each of three equations, expressed in just noticeable differences. Losses amounting to tritan and tetartan defects are found in OHT and all CS groups, with scores significantly higher than normal in all groups.

INTRODUCTION

It is a main thesis of this paper that large losses in colour vision equivalent to the acquired dyschromatopsias seen so frequently in glaucoma patients with extensive field loss should be seriously considered as indicating an increased risk of developing open angle glaucoma when found in ocular hypertensive patients. Thus, colour vision results should be included when considering susceptibility to field damage resulting from intraocular pressure.

In our original data (Lakowski et al, 1972) on a limited number of ocular hypertensive eyes (with normal visual fields), it was shown that their performance on colour vision tests was significantly poorer than that of equivalent controls. Thus, although acuity tests showed only a marginal variability, colour vision tests indicated large variations in performances from near 'perfect' to anomalous, dichromatic, or almost achromatic. It was then suggested that such extreme losses could be used to predict subsequent glaucomatous field defects.

We now present more extensive colour vision data from about 250 ocular hypertensive eyes and from about 200 glaucomatous patients analysed according to the extent of visual field loss. In addition we have studied a small group of ocular hypertensive patients who developed the earliest signs of field losses within five years of testing.

It is hoped that this extensive data can be accepted as evidence that extreme colour vision losses (equivalent to tritanopia) are indicative of damage and that they can also be looked upon as most probably predicting subsequent field losses in open angle glaucoma.

METHOD

Description of the clinical population

The patients selected for this study had to satisfy certain ocular criteria which included good acuity (20/30 or better), normal maculae, no retinal detachments or lens opacities, no pseudo-exfoliation or drusen of the disc. All glaucoma subjects and one group of ocular hypertensive subjects were on miotics.

Ocular hypertensives (OH) are classified as patients with open angles, normal acuity, normal discs, and full visual fields (as indicated from kinetic perimetry tested with the Goldmann perimeter) who have had repeated intraocular pressures above 21 mm Hg. We divided the OH into 2 groups: (a) ocular hypertensives not on topical medication, that is OHnT, and (b) ocular hypertensives on therapy, denoted here by OHT. It is assumed, for the sake of this subdivision, that those on therapy have had higher pressures.

Three stages of chronic simple glaucoma are distinguished: (i) CS1 patients with early field losses, peripheral nasal step, central nasal step, or both central and peripheral step; (ii) CS2, patients with arcuate field losses (with and without nasal step); (iii) CS3, patients with extensive field loss, or central temporal islands including altitudinal losses. No patients with con-

Table 1. Statistical summary of the five groups of glaucomatous eyes.

Stages of Glaucoma	Number of Eyes	AGE Mean	Mean Acuity Decimal
OHnT	145	59.5	0.91
OHT	103	62.8	0.85
CS1 (mild)	63	59.3	0.86
CS2 (medium)	66	64.4	0.74
CS 3 (severe)	65	63.7	0.71

* This work was supported by MRC grant No. 4342.

genital or closed angle glaucoma or with low tension glaucoma have been included.

Six variables were collected and analysed for each of the five groups of glaucomatous eyes; size of subsample, age, acuity, 1OP at time of colour vision testing and maximum recorded IOP, pupil diameter at test, and macular sensitivity (see Table 1).

Mean IOP at the time of testing varied only from 19.5 to 22.7 over the five groups, and maximum IOP varied from 26.0 to 30.7. Pupil diameter in OHnT was 4.3 mm, and in the other groups 2.5 mm. Macular sensitivity ranged from 3.1 asb in OHnT to 8.6 asb in CS3.

Testing procedure

Routine clinical examination included perimetric fields (kinetic and static by means of Tübingen and Goldmann perimeters), and intraocular pressure was obtained by Goldmann aplanation tonometer. An extensive battery of colour vision tests included tests of colour confusion, colour discrimination and metamerism. However, only results from the Farnsworth-Munsell *100-Hue test*. Table 2 indicates mean values plus variance for six groups, anomaloscope) will be presented as those tests distinguish clearly between various stages of glaucoma and are thus diagnostically useful.

RESULTS

For the sake of brevity only the results from the 100-Hue test will be discussed in detail, and the only P-N anomaloscope data used will involve examining the discrimination data derived from analysis of matching ranges. *100-Hue test.* Table II indicates mean values plus variance for six groups, the five glaucomatous sub-groups and the age control group. There is a difference in error score between the age control group and OHnT and a dramatic increase in error scores between the OHnT and OHT group, and a gradual increase in error score with increasing severity of field loss is also seen. Despite the large variance for the glaucomatous sub-populations, most of the differences between the means for the 100-Hue test are significant at $p < .01$ or $p < .05$ levels. Only the difference on the 100-Hue between the OHT and CS2 is not significant (NS). The variance in 100-Hue scores between Normal controls and OHnT and OHT groups is shown in figure 1.

Table 2. Means for 100-Hue scores.

| | | Stages of Glaucoma | | | | |
	Age Controls	OHnT	OHT	CS1	CS2	CS3
Mean	88	119	182	145	215	265
S.D.	35	77	106	96	129	150

Note the difference at the low score and between the conditions, and especially note the percentage of OHnT and OHT patients with scores over 150, that is, beyond the 95th percentile for an equivalent age normal population. There should be only 5% beyond this criterion level, but in OHnT there are 19%, and in OHT there are 50%.

A similar progression in 100-Hue scores occurs in the three CS groups, with most low scores occurring in the CS1 group. The percentage of scores beyond the 95th percentile for normals increases with severity of the field condition, CS1 has 34%, CS2 has 54%, and CS3 has 74% beyond this level.

P-N Anomaloscope

Results are quoted in discrimination units, the so-called 'just noticeable difference' units (j.n.d.), and are given as median values of matching ranges for the various sub-groups. Figure 2 shows that the red-green discrimination has the smallest significant changes when compared with age control population. The major losses for the glaucomatous population are in the yellow-blue and green-blue equations with the green-blue indicating tritan defects and the yellow-blue indicating tetartan defects. OHnT once again have distinctly higher scores than the normal population. The differences calculated from the *means* are statistically significant at $p < .01$ for both the red-green, yellow-blue, and green-blue equations. Of course the miotic effect exaggerates losses, and we can see an appreciable increase in the median values for OHT with losses of up to 40 and 50 j.n.d.s. for the green-blue and yellow-blue equations respectively. Finally, the CS3 median score is equivalent to a total lack of discrimination (the highest possible j.n.d. score) in the two

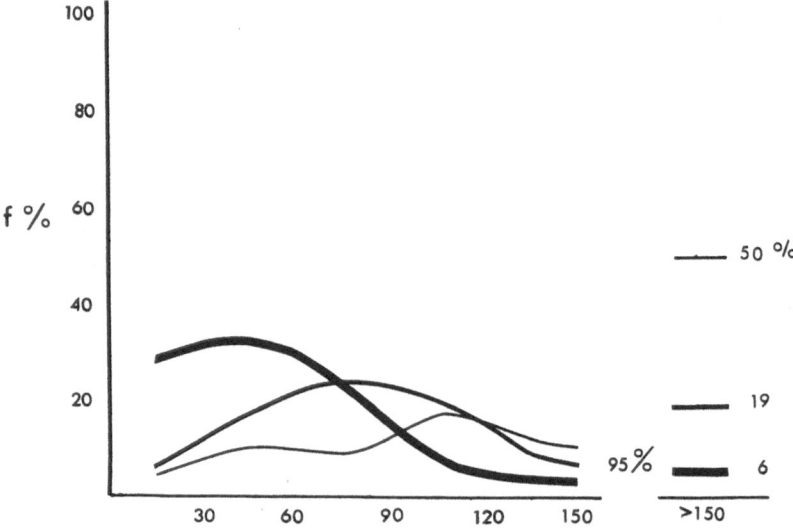

Fig. 1. Frequency distribution of 100-Hue scores for normal and ocular hypertensive patients.

162

MEDIANS

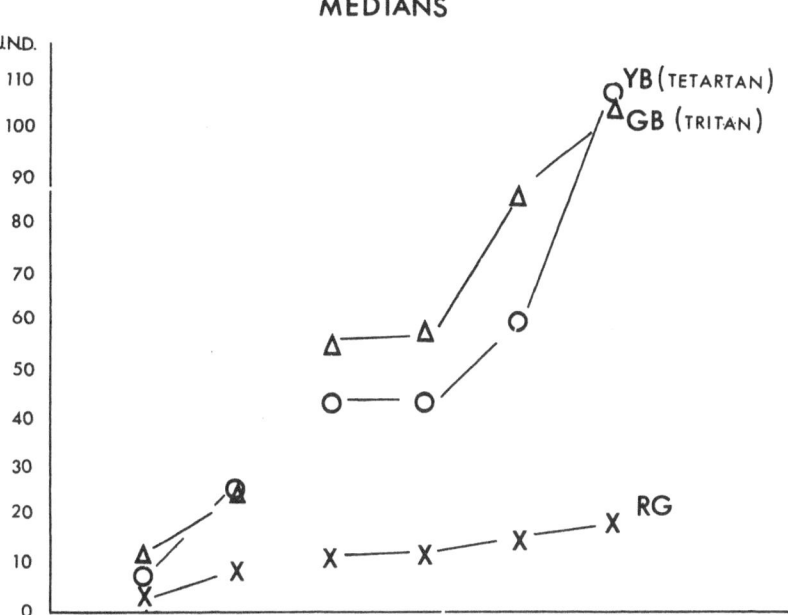

Fig. 2. Median for matching range in j.n.d. units for P-N anomaloscope.

equations. Such lack of discrimination if found in a congenital colour defective would amount to tritanopia at the dichromatic stage. Again, the differences between means in all equations between the age control population and the OHnT are significantly different at $p < .01$ level.

DISCUSSION

Data presented here show that the two most sensitive colour vision tests (100-Hue and P-N anomaloscope) reflect a deterioration of colour function with the increase in glaucomatous field. They also clearly show that OHnT patients with pupil diameters equivalent to the age control population are still significantly different at $p < .01$ in all colour modalities, and that they have significantly higher incidence of eyes with extreme colour losses than are found among the normal population, especially in the green-blue equation (the so-called tritan defects). Although the colour vision data comes from a study of discrimination at the foveal area, it corresponds to the extent of field loss which occurs extra foveally, and in spite of selection of good central visual acuities.

The colour vision data appears to provide additional information about the glaucoma patients. This is illustrated by the fact that extreme colour vision defects normally found in severe glaucomas (CS3) occur in about 20% of ocular hypertensives who have no field defects at all.

Can such information be of predictive value to the clinician? To assess this, we present preliminary data from an independent inquiry that is in progress at this time into the characteristics (in terms of colour visions tests) of subjects whose visual fields have deteriorated.

Transition from ocular hypertension to chronic open angle glaucoma. It is now almost five years since all our ocular hypertensive were colour tested and we are now attempting to see how many have developed glaucoma during that time. So far we have collected nine patients (9 eyes) in whom such a change has been recorded. Table 3 gives some indication of the colour vision performances of these patients in 1972 and how they compared with the whole group of OHT to which they then belonged. Their colour functions are also compared with those of the most extreme glaucoma group (CS3s). The variables compared include age, six colour parameters, etc. The first column indicates the means for these variables for the OHT group, the second column quotes means for the nine patients who were tested in 1972 and who subsequently changed from OHT category to CS1, and finally the last column shows the means of the CS3 group. It can be seen that those who developed glaucoma are older than those who showed no deterioration but no other parameters are different. If we now look at the colour vision variables we see that for the Ishihara and Dvorine PIC plates there is no significant difference between the means of the OHT group (as a whole) and those who developed glaucoma. It should be noted, however, that in the 100-Hue error scores and the P-N anomaloscope data there are significant differences in the value of the means at $p < .01$ for the 100-Hue means and at $p < .01$ and .05 for the yellow-blue and green-blue anomaloscope equations. It is also interesting to compare the means of

Table 3. Transition from OHT to CS1. 9 patients within 5 years of colour vision testing.

VARIABLES	OHT			OHT → CS1	CS3
AGE	63			73	63
IOP (at test)	21			24	23
IOP (maximal)	28			28	31
ACUITY	.83			.91	.71
MAC. SENS.	4.2			3.4	8.6
ISHIHARA	2	t sig.		2	9
DVORINE	3			4	9
100-Hue	182	← .05 →		256	265
P-N Anom.					
RG	20	← NS →		34	32
YB	54	← .01 →		90	83
GB	61	← .05 →		90	80

those who developed glaucoma with those of the advanced CS3 group, and here we see that they are almost identical.

Although these results should be treated with caution until more data is accumulated, yet the nine patients who developed glaucoma within five years testing, initially had extreme colour vision losses well above the means for the OHT group to which they belonged.

REFERENCE

Lakowski, R., Bryett, J. & Drance, S.M. A study of color vision in ocular hypertensives. *Canad. J. Ophthal.* 7: *86* (1972).

Authors' address:
Visual Laboratory
Department of Psychology
The University of British Columbia
2075 Wesbrook Place
Vancouver, B.C.
V6T 1W5
Canada

Docum. Ophthal. Proc. Series, Vol. 19

THE RELATION BETWEEN DEPRESSION IN THE BJERRUM AREA AND NASAL STEP IN EARLY GLAUCOMA (DBA & NS)

NARIYOSHI ENDO

(Tokyo, Japan)

ABSTRACT

In 1976 at Tübingen, we introduced a new front plate for detecting glaucoma through the analysis of central visual field (VF) in glaucoma with Friedmann VF Analyser (FVFA). On that occasion we tried to examine the relation between peripheral VF defects including nasal steps (NS), in early glaucoma.

First, we analysed 219 eyes (out of 765 glaucomatous VF) up to the stage of break through, already tested with the Goldmann perimeter (GP).

Then we found that 25% either had only a nasal step (NS) and/or an uncertain relation between depression in the Bjerrum area and NS.

Next, in order to make this clear, the following methods have been tested: 1) kinetic perimetry using GP (with Armaly & Drance's technique), 2) partial profile perimetry: nasal circularly at 40 degrees and along 2 meridians (15 degrees above and below the horizontal) using Tübinger perimetry and 3) testing by FVFA, including our new front plate.

From the results of 191 eyes, we will report the theme in detail, especially regarding early glaucomatous VF of 25 eyes.

INTRODUCTION

We reported on the visual field (VF) in glaucoma for the first time in 1966. Since then, we have empirically considered depression in the Bjerrum area (DBA) as the early VF changes in glaucoma (Matsuo & Endo, 1969; Matsuo et al., 1975; Shinzato, Suzuki & Furuno, 1976). From the viewpoint of emphasizing the central VF, we analysed the frequency of the VF changes in glaucoma by Goldmann perimeter (GP) and Friedmann Field Analyser (FVFA). We have constructed a new front plate, for the FVFA.

At the symposium in Tübingen, 2 years ago, it was discussed whether the early VF changes in glaucoma would be DBA or the nasal step (NS). This investigation attempts to study the relation between DBA and NS.

A. Results of a retrospective investigation using the Goldmann perimeter

Prior to starting the work, we reviewed the VF changes in glaucoma examined in 765 eyes since 1967 by GP. We defined the early changes as those that did not yet show a break-through. The relation between the central and peripheral fields was analysed in 219 eyes, as seen in Table 1.

DBA only was found in 85 eyes (39%) and this was the most frequent; a combination of DBA and NS was found in 78 eyes (36%); only NS was found in 19 eyes (9%), and the relation was unclear in 37 eyes (16%).

Table 1. Analysis of VF changes in early glaucoma.

A.	Depression of Bjerrum's Area	85 eyes	39%
B.	Rönne's Nasal step	19	9
C.	A? + B	14	6
D.	A + B?	23	10
E.	A + B	78	36
	Total	219	100

B. Results of a retrospective study including the new front plate

Since June 1977, the patients who first came to our clinic for examination for glaucoma, were examined according to the following testing methods:
1. Armaly & Drance's technique on GP.
2. Static perimetry with Tübinger perimeter (TP) particularly for detecting NS.
a. Circular static perimetry along the 40° parallel, between the upper and lower 45° oblique meridians at every 5°.
b. Meridional static perimetry 15° above and below the horizontal nasal meridian at every 5° from the center to the periphery. The background luminance used here was mesopic (0.032 asb).
3. Examination with the FVFA.
4. Quantitative perimetry with our new front plate: the background luminance used here was mesopic (0.032 asb).
5. The optic disk was photographed in mydriasis.

191 eyes of 96 patients were examined. Among them, 104 eyes had no VF changes. Among the rest of 87 eyes having some VF changes, 35 eyes had not been examined so sufficiently as described above; of the other 32 eyes, 7 eyes that already had a break-through were excluded; the 25 remaining eyes were used for this study.

In 13 cases, VF changes were detected by all the methods described above. The remaining 12 eyes were found to be in a prestadium, when defining the prestadium as the VF changes that were detected by only 2 or 3 methods. Details of the 25 eyes are given in Table 2 and 3.

Table 2. 9 patients, 12 eyes in prestadium of glaucoma.

	Methods				VF changes				Disc
	nP	F	T	G	dBa	NS	up	low	
1 − l	−	−	−	−	−	−	−	−	±
2 − l	±	−	−	−	±	−	±	−	±
3 − l	±	−	−	−	±	−	±	−	±
4 − R	±	−	−	−	±	−	±	−	±
3 − r	±	−	−	−	±	−	±	−	±
5 − R	±	−	−	−	±	−	±	−	±
6 − l	±	±	−	−	+	−	+	+	±
7 − r	±	−	±	−	+	±	+	−	±
8 − L	+	+	−	−	+	−	+	+	±
9 − r	±	−	+	−	+	+	+	−	±
9 − l	+	−	+	−	+	+	+	−	±
1 − r	±	±	+	+	+	+	+	−	+

Table 3. 7 patients, 13 eyes in early glaucoma.

	Methods				VF changes				Disc
	nP	F	T	G	dBa	NS	up	low	
10 − l	+	+	+	+	+	+	+	−	+
10 − r	+	+	+	+	+	+	+	−	+
11 − r	+	+	+	+	+	+	+	−	+
12 − L	+	+	+	+	+	+	+	−	+
6 − r	+	+	+	+	+	+	+	−	+
2 − r	+	+	+	+	+	+	+	−	+
13 − r	+	+	+	+	+	+	+	−	+
14 − R	+	+	+	+	+	+	+	−	+
13 − l	+	+	+	+	+	+	+	−	+
7 − l	+	+	+	+	+	+	−	+	+
11 − l	+	+	+	+	+	+	−	+	+
15 − L	+	+	+	+	+	+	+	+	+
16 − L	+	+	+	+	+	+	+	+	+

169

CASE REPORTS

Case 1.: a 52-year-old female. The visual acuity was 0.8. (1.0) on the right eye and 0.8 (1.0) on the left with light myopic astigmatism. The intra-ocular pressure (IOP) was 16 mmHg on the right and 20 mmHg on the left, and C value was 0.14 mm^3/min/mmHg on the right and 0.27 on the left. She was diagnosed as open angle glaucoma. The VF showed in the upper half of the left eye a slight depression as shown in Fig. 1.

Case 2.: a 30-year-old female. Visual acuity was 0.03 (1.0) on the right and 0.04 (1.0) on the left with myopic astigmatism. IOP was 22 on the right and 24 on the left. C value was 0.21 on the right and 0.14 on the left. She was diagnosed as open angle glaucoma. In the VF a NS was detected in both eyes as seen in Fig. 2.

ANALYSIS

The relation between DBA and NS will be discussed by the following two analysing methods:

I. The quantitative relations of the sensitivity in each quadrant were investigated on these eyes, as shown in Fig. 3 and 4. The result of a left eye were converted to that of a right one; each stimulus point of the 4 quadrants: nasal superior (NS), temporal superior (TS), nasal inferior (NI) and temporal inferior (TI) was plotted on the abscissa and the sensitivity at each point was plotted on the ordinate. Thus, the results were represented quantitatively. The result with FVFA in case 1 (Fig. 3) did not show any remarkable changes in both eyes, but with the new frontplate (NFP) showed relative depressions mainly on the left eye.

FVFA of case 2 (Fig. 4) shows depressions in the nasal superior part (NS) on the left eye and slight depressions in each quadrant on the right eye. Particularly, the nasal depression was large with the new frontplate. According to the analysis of these 25 eyes, the ND value at the depressive points with the new frontplate in prestadium was 1.2 at the lowest and the depression was 0.6 at the deepest. The value with FVFA was 1.4 at the lowest and the depression was 0.4 at the deepest. In an early stage, that is, in cases having clear NS, deep DBA already occurs. The value with NFP was 0.8 at the highest and the depression was 1.3 at the shallowest. The value with FVFA was 1.0 at the highest and the depression was 0.8 at the shallowest.

These relations helps to serve screening: that is, when FVFA is set at 1.2 and nP at 1.0 to measure, the presence or absence of NS can be revealed.

170

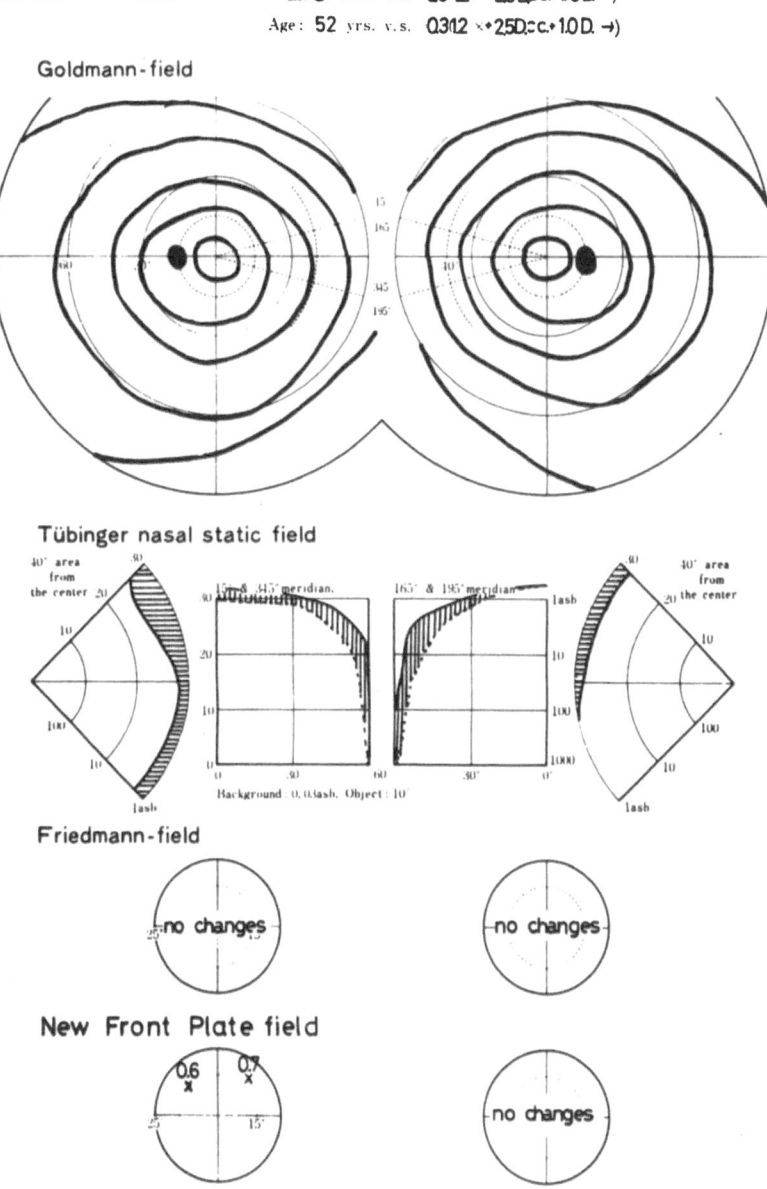

Case No. 9   Name: M. S.   □, ● 33cm v.d. 0.3(1.2 ×+2.5D ⊃c.+1.0D →)
Age: 52 yrs. v.s. 0.3(1.2 ×+2.5D ⊃c.+1.0D →)

Goldmann-field

Tübinger nasal static field

Friedmann-field

New Front Plate field

Fig. 1.   Visual field of case 1. See text.

Case No. 10 Name: F. K. □. ● 33cm v.d. −0.2(1.0 ×−3.0 D.)
                              Age: 30 yrs. v.s. −0.2(1.0 ×− 2.5 D.) ·

Goldmann-field

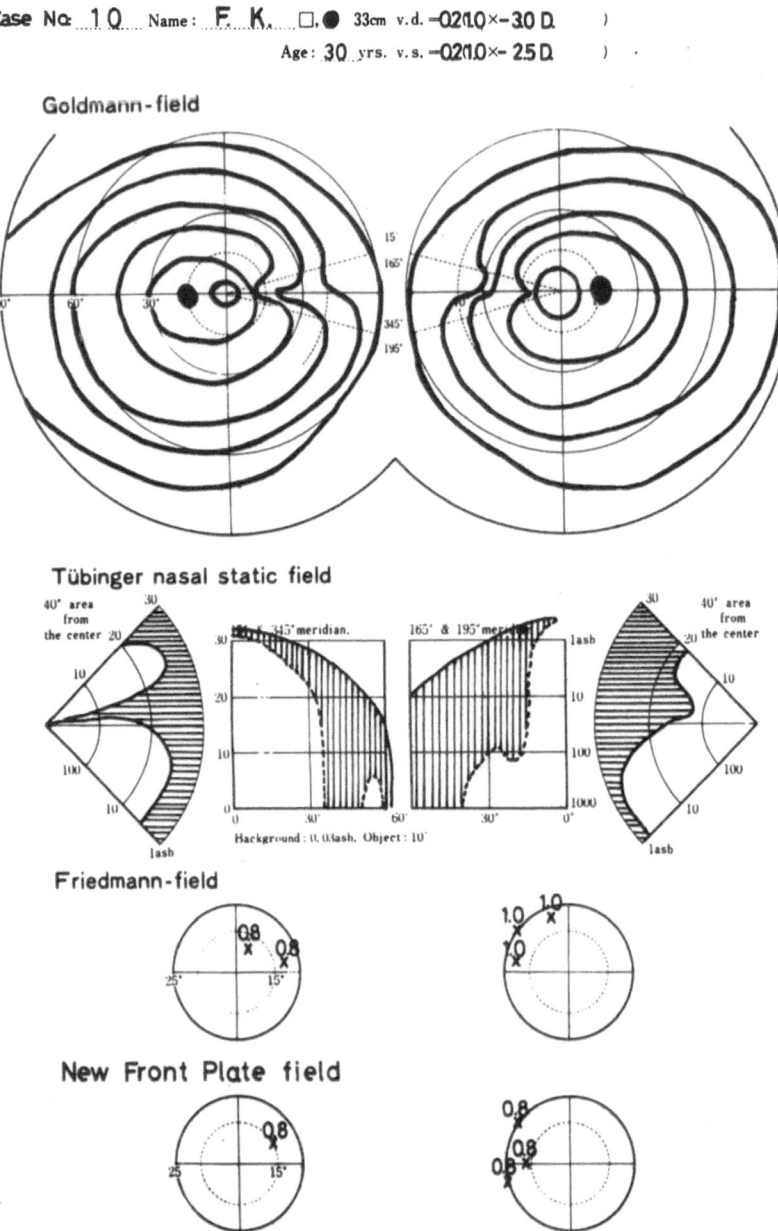

Tübinger nasal static field

Friedmann-field

New Front Plate field

Fig. 2. Visual field of case 2. See text.

172

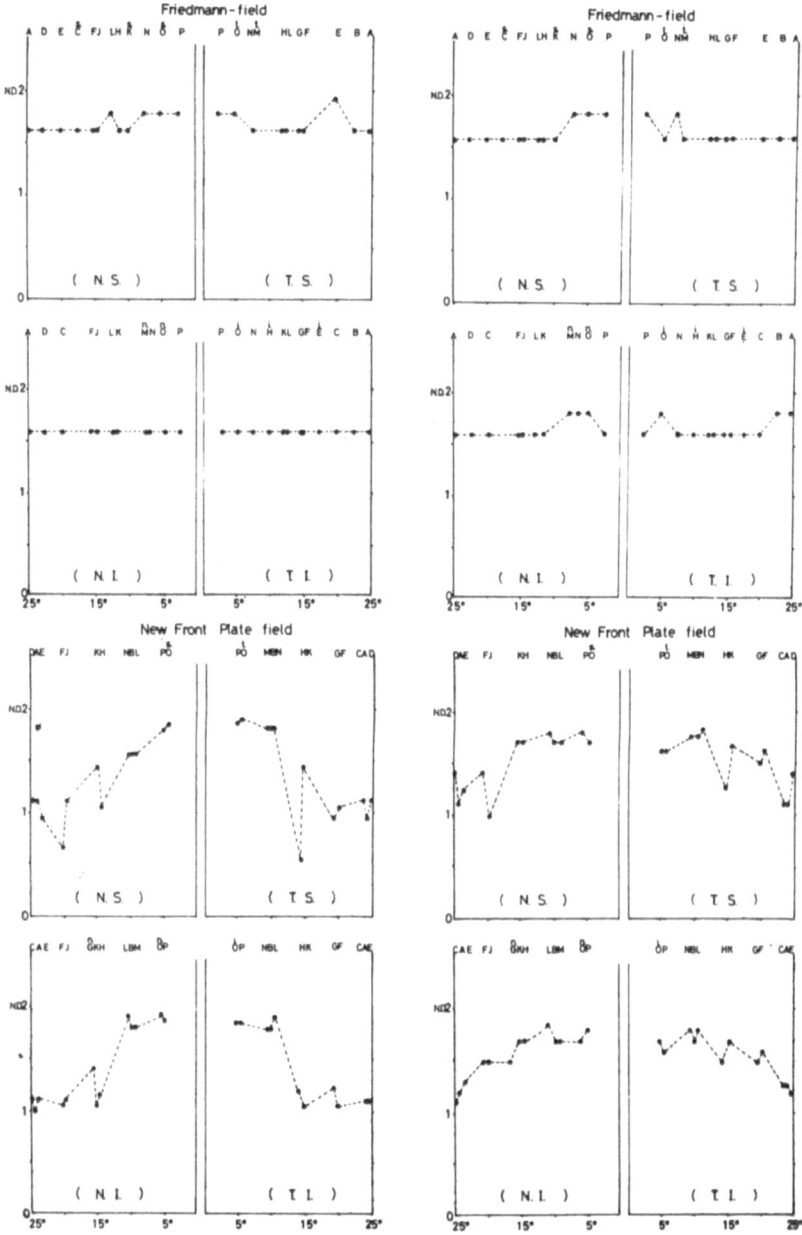

Fig. 3. Analysis of the results with FVFA and nP in case I.

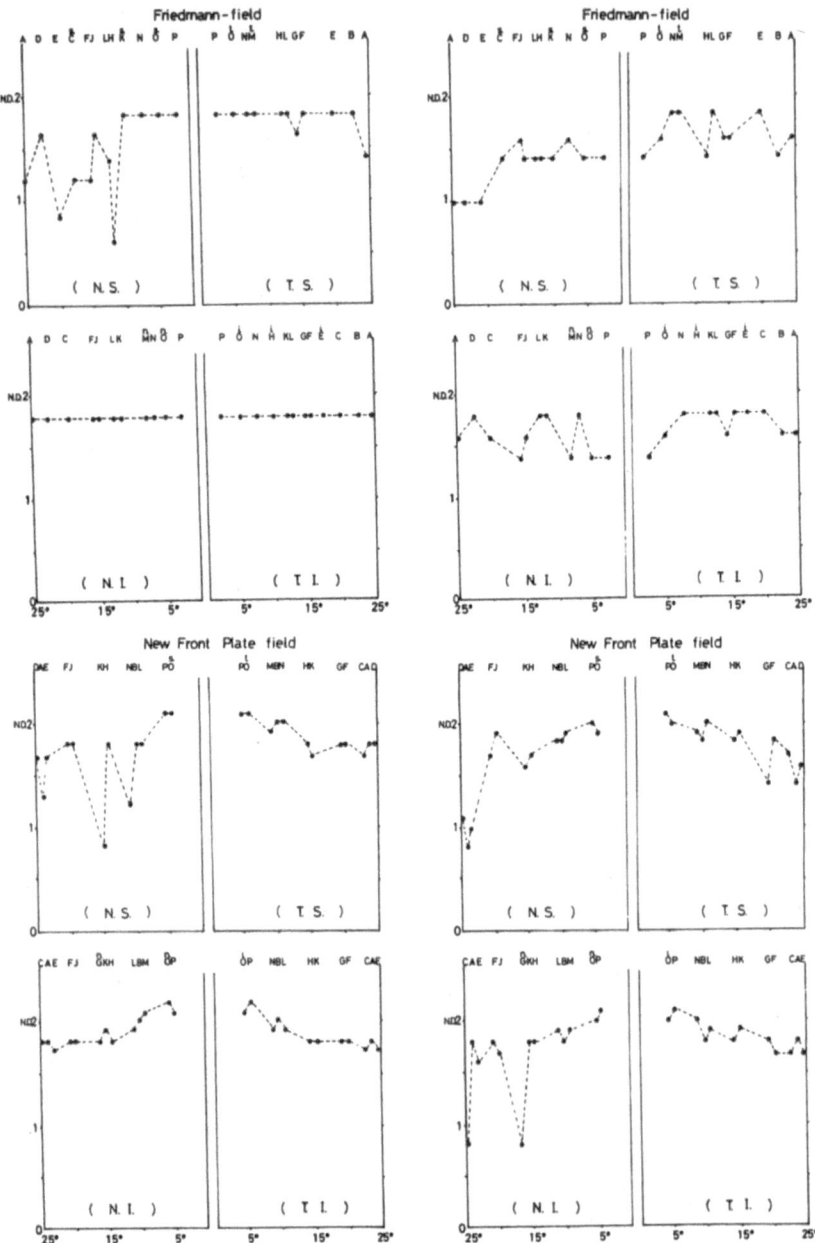

Fig. 4. Analysis of the results with FVFA and nP in case II.

II. The visual fields were divided into the upper and lower half fields and after being represented by the relation between DBA and peripheral nasal defect (PND), the depression was analysed. According to the results obtained, the quantitative relation of DBA depending on the presence or absence of PND is as follows:

1. with NFP, if the stimulus points of depressions of deeper than 0.5 log units are 14, PND exists; with FVFA, the number of it is 6.

2. with NFP, if the total of the depressions of deeper than 0.5 log units is 11, PND is present; with FVFA, the number of it is 4.

3. with NFP, if the total of depressions is 14, PND exists; with FVFA, the number of it is 13.

These figures will serve as a pilot for evaluating the results of quantitative perimetry.

DISCUSSION

There are many reports on early VF changes in glaucoma. Aulhorn and Armaly (1971) reported that PD exists most of the time with CD, although PD may be the only defect in less than 5%. But Becker (1971) and Leblanc (1976) stated the importance of PND and warned if too much weight is put upon CD, the early glaucoma might be missed, because 1/3 of it is only with PD. Drance (1969, Werner & Drance 1977) emphasized that the localized scatter or small depression are important in early changes. In our experiments we found similar results.

CONCLUSION

DBA without NS is quantitatively slight and has indistinct relation with NS. In other words, when having deep DBA, NS exists. And if the depressions of deeper than 0.5 log units can be seen within 15 degrees, PND exists.

ACKNOWLEDGEMENT

We wish to thank Prof. Matsuo, our director, for his kind and helpful instructions. Assistance of DRS. Tomtonaga (TP), Shinzato (nP), Suzuki (disc-photo), Matsudaira (GP), Furuno & Ogawa (analysis), Hara & Miss Harasawa (FVFA) are also appreciated.

In addition, we gratefully acknowledge the bounty from our alumni association and English instructions of Mrs. Kadomae, since 1st IPS in 1974.

REFERENCES

Armaly, M.F. Visual field defects in early open angle glaucoma. *Tr. Am. Ophth. Soc.*, 69: *147-162* (1971).

Becker, B. Peripheral nasal field defects. *Am. J. Ophth.* 72: *415-419* (1971).

Drance, S.M. The early field defects in glaucoma. *Invest. Ophth.* 8: *84-91* (1969).

Furuse, M. Clinical studies on the photometric harmony in the visual field. Report II: glaucoma. *Acta Soc. Ophthalm. Jap.* 70: *20-29* (1966).

Leblanc, R. Peripheral nasal field defects. *Docum. Ophthal. Pro. Series* 14: *131-133* (1976).

Matsuo, H. & Endo, N. The visual field. Rinsho-ganka-zensho (Text book of clinical ophthalmology) 1: I-(2) *67-128*, Kanehara, Tokyo (1969).

Matsuo, H., Nakanishi, T., Endo, N., Shinzato, E., Suzuki, R., Furuno, F. & Ikematsu, Y. Glaucomatous visual field. Especially on changes in the central part. *Acta Soc. Ophthalm. Jap.* 79: *1131-1138* (1975).

Shinzato, E., Suzuki, R. & Furuno, F. The central visual field changes in glaucoma using Goldmann Perimeter & Friedmann visual field analyser. *Docum. Ophthal. Pro. Series* 14: *93-101* (1976).

Werner, E.B. & Drance, S.M. Early visual field disturbances in glaucoma. *Arch. Ophthalmol.* 95: *1173-1175* (1977).

Author's address:
Department of Ophthalmology
Tokyo Medical College Hospital
6-7-1 Nishi-shinjuku, Shinjuku-ku
Tokyo, Japan 160

Docum. Ophthal. Proc. Series, Vol. 19

REVERSIBILITY OF GLAUCOMATOUS DEFECTS
OF THE VISUAL FIELD

MANSOUR F. ARMALY

(Washington, U.S.A.)

ABSTRACT

The demonstration of reversibility of glaucomatous defects is complicated by the multiple etiology of field defects; the fact that only ocular pressure level is modifiable by limited mechanisms of pressure reduction, age and technique of perimetry. Nasal step, paracentral scotoma, enlarged blind spot and contraction of the isopter were found to be pressure induced. These defects, when found spontaneously in the ocular hypertensive, were reversible by lowering ocular pressure level in some cases.

I was asked to introduce the subject of reversibility of glaucomatous visual field defects. And to be more specific, the field defects of primary open angle glaucoma. To this end I shall describe my personal experience in this area and highlight some of the difficulties. First, what are glaucomatous field defects? This elementary and basic question proved very difficult to answer; some felt they include all defects that occur in eyes with 'open angle glaucoma'; on the other hand, glaucoma was defined by the presence of damage to the visual field. So, investigators started to look for changes in the visual field in eyes with 'advanced glaucoma' to be sure they were dealing with the unequivocal stage of the disease. But the detection and description of such defects were bound to be greatly dependent upon the method of perimetry and the stage of the disease. This is especially important when we realize that mapping the entire visual field with precision is virtually impossible in any one session or patient because of the time needed, the effort, and the fatigue that may invalidate the test.

Having found defects in glaucomatous eyes, it became clear that they are not unique and may be encountered in other disease conditions. This was the case for nasal step, bjerrum scotoma, enlargement of the blind spot, contraction of the isopter and paracentral scotomas. All these may be encountered in other disease conditions. Other conditions may be ruled out by detailed examination of the fundus or by detailed history. Others cannot be definitively excluded. Thus, it became necessary to narrow the definition of glaucomatous defects to those present in 'glaucomatous' eyes and which cannot be explained by other conditions at that time; a very poor definition and a somewhat circular logic.

In attempting to explain how elevated ocular pressure can produce the

Investigations reported in this study were supported in part by an unrestricted grant from Research to Prevent Blindness, Inc.

types of defects described, Goldmann & Gaffner (1955) proposed a model which explains the greater vulnerability of the circulation of the optic nerve head to elevated ocular pressure and postulated that elevated pressure acts on this vulnerable circulatory bed to produce ischemia which in turn leads to nerve fiber damage and ultimately, fibre death. This model explains not only the mechanism of damage, but also why the same magnitude of pressure elevation may produce, in different individuals, different effects on the visual field: For the effect on the visual field is not that of ocular pressure directly, but of its interaction with the vascular system, and the vulnerability of the nerve fiber to ischemia.

Most importantly, in my view, this model, by accepting the ischemia mechanism, not only explains the mechanism of the effect of increased ocular pressure, but indicates simultaneously that other factors that are capable of producing ischemia of this vascular bed will produce identical field defects. Thus, glaucomatous field defects became a part of a larger domain, namely, ischemic defects. Since this vascular bed is always under the effect of ocular pressure, one may begin to see two extreme situations: The first, where the cause of ischemia is primarily the elevated ocular pressure level and the second, where the primary cause is not the elevated ocular pressure level; in between these extremes are situations in which pressure level and other causes of ischemia exist in varying proportions, Armaly (1962).

The question of reversibility of field defects thus becomes complicated by the following:

1. Reversibility assumes that eliminating the cause at some stage may eliminate the effect. But what is the cause of the defect in a given patient? If ocular pressure level is the modifiable factor, then the effect of lowering it on a given field defect will depend upon how much did the elevated pressure contribute to the production of that field defect. This will be true even in the earliest stages of field defect. Thus, reversibility of a field defect by lowering ocular pressure level even under ideal conditions of earliest detection will not be expected to be demonstrable in each case, but at best in those cases where elevated ocular pressure level was the major, if not the only, factor in the production of ischemia and of the defect.

2. Even if elevated pressure was the primary factor, reversibility will have to depend upon our ability to lower ocular pressure sufficiently to attain reversibility. Just as we are unable to predict in a given patient what magnitude of pressure elevation can produce a field defect, we are equally ignorant of how much should an elevated pressure be reduced so as to become harmless in a given patient. Since lowering ocular pressure level is pharmacologically produced, we may not be able to lower it enough to reach the perfectly safe level. This introduces another complication in demonstrating reversibility of a field defect. Thus, one should produce maximum lowering of ocular pressure before concluding that reversibility is not feasible.

3. The stage of the defect. A defect that results from death of nerve fibers or neurons is not likely to be reversible because the neurons do not

regenerate and the neural organization does not seem to involve expansion of the receptive field of the remaining neurons to cover the area of this absolute defect. Here a question arises as to the nature of the glaucomatous defect. Is it always absolute? Does it always have an absolute nucleus? Do nerve fibers first die before a defect is detected? The answer to this depends upon the stage of the disease with which one deals and the method of testing. If one is dealing with advanced glaucomas referred at the time they become problems of management, then indeed one encounters a high frequency of absolute defects occupying various proportions of the relative defect. Such defects at this stage cannot be expected to be reversible as a rule. I hasten to add that not all absolute defects necessarily represent death of neurons and that one encounters, albeit very infrequently, an absolute defect which is partially or completely reversed when ocular pressure is lowered indicating that the nerve fibers may have lost function but not viability, Armaly (1964). Thus, it would seem clear that if one wishes to reap highest frequency of reversibility, one must deal with the earlier stages of the glaucomatous defect. This is best done, in practice, by following individuals with high ocular pressure but normal visual field at regular intervals such as three to four months and looking, by careful perimetry, for the earliest evidence of field defects. Such defects will typically be relative, not absolute, in nature and will expectedly be the ones with highest frequency of reversibility.

4. Another complication arises from the fact that the effect of ocular pressure on the field when it exists involves an indirect action on two systems: the first, the vascular bed to produce ischemia and consequently, the second, the nerve fibers to produce dysfunction. Reversibility of function requires first that the vacular insult be capable of recovery once ocular pressure is lowered and that the reduced nutrition to the optic nerve be completely reversed. This ability of the vascular system of the optic disc to recover is likely to depend upon a large number of factors that influence the vascular system and especially the small vessels and microcirculations: metabolic, degenerative, and vascular diseases influencing them are indeed numerous. Their frequency increases with age: thus, reversibility of function is more likely to be encountered in the younger age groups and in individuals with otherwise normal circulation and nutritive blood value.

5. Another complicating factor is the method of testing. Faulty techniques may lead to the false impression of reversibility. Kinetic perimetry may fail to detect a previously detected scotoma if the scotoma is smaller than a given size or the speed of movement too fast for the patient. Isopter perimetry may falsely suggest the disappearance of a nasal step; for instance, if the I, 2 target demonstrates a nasal step at 20-25 degrees at one session, and if, in the next session, the I, 2 isopter has expanded to 30 degrees without evidence of nasal step, we should not conclude that the nasal step has reversed to normal until we specifically test the *location* in which it was previously detected. If different individuals are doing these tests, without prior knowledge of the location of the defect, reversibility in such a case may be no more than the unequal attention of technicians towards testing

similar areas of the field. Additionally, if one is dealing with small and shallow defects, their disappearance may be evidence that they did not, in reality, exist, but were to begin with 'artifacts'. Therefore, the design of the experiment and method of testing should take these factors into account to establish true reversibility. These are but some of the factors that complicate the study and demonstration of the reversibility of glaucomatous field defects.

My experience in this area has been limited to the reversibility that follows the lowering of ocular pressure level. I should begin by mentioning that initially I studied the type of defects that follow ocular pressure elevation by topical steroid in the otherwise normal eye and found three identifiable types, Armaly (1964): Paracentral scotoma, nasal step and enlargement of the blind spot with contraction of the isopter. Typically, these are relative defects, not absolute. In the glaucomatous eye with field defects, such pressure elevation produced a bjerrum scotoma, increased the size of the paracentral defect and produced a nasal step. On cessation of dexamethazone and reversal of the ocular hypertension, these defects disappeared. Significant is the fact that their disappearance was not immediate and in some cases took as long as 6-8 weeks during which time ocular pressure was normal and the field defect persisted. These studies identified pressure dependent field defects. I then started to look for these defects in the general population and in those with high ocular pressure and open angles using selective perimetry, Armaly (1972). Their frequency appears in

Table 1. Frequency of field defects

Target	Type	No.
I,2	Nasal step only	5
	Paracentral defects only	73
	Concentric contraction	6
	Nasal step and paracentral	20
I,4	Nasal step only	2
TOTAL		106

Table 2.

	Applanation Pressure (mm Hg.)		Tonographic C-Value (ml./mm Hg./min.)		Field Defect with 1/1,000 white tangent	
Year	OD	OS	OD	OS	OD	OS
1958	28	33	0.04	0.08	Double arcuate	Double arcuate
1959	20	22	0.10	0.11	Seidel's scotoma	Arcuate scotoma
1960	15	15	0.14	0.18	Enlarged blind spot	Enlarged blind spot
1961	15	15	–	–	None	None

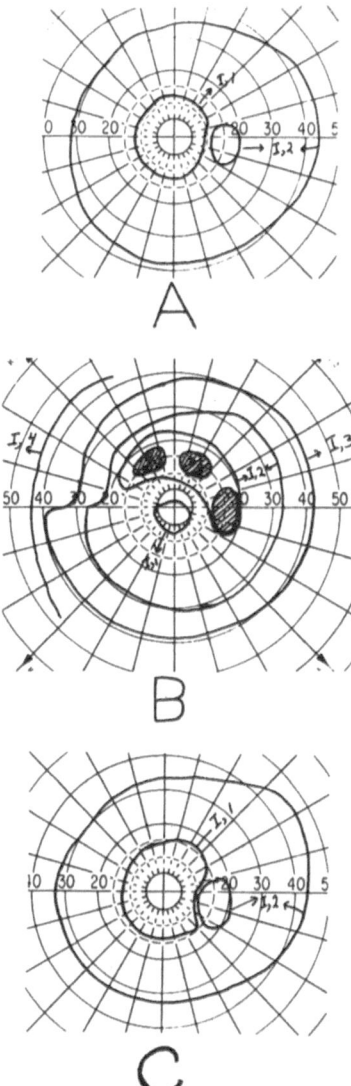

Fig. 1. Visual field of the right eye of a 77-year old lady with visual acuity of 20/20. this patient had been followed for 13 years with ocular pressure renging between 35 and 48 mm Hg., without therapy and with normal visual field.

In notation A — Normal fields and a pressure of 42 mm Hg.

B — The spontaneous appearance of a field defect with an applanation pressure of 37 mm Hg. Note:

I,1,e — contraction of the isopter

I,2,e — nasal step and arcuate scotoma

I,3,e — nasal step and paracentral scotomas (stippled)

I,4,e — normal

This defect was confirmed on several occasions and six months after initial discovery.

C — Field of the same eye one year after the appearance of the defect without any therapy. Ocular pressure is 36 mm Hg., note disappearance of all defects.

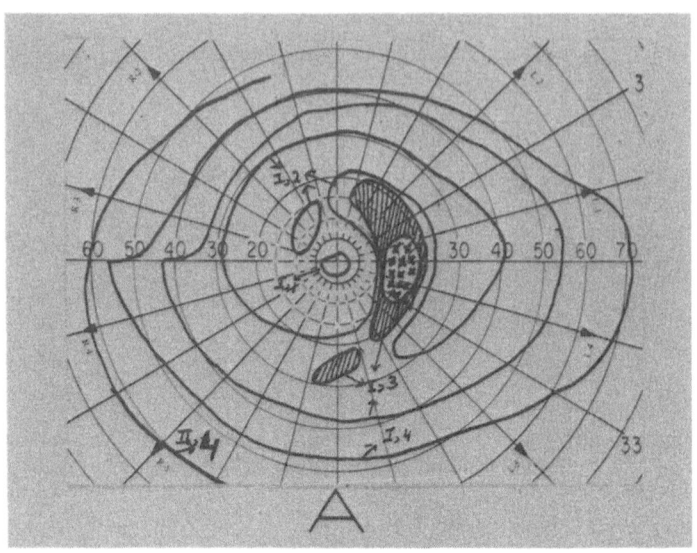

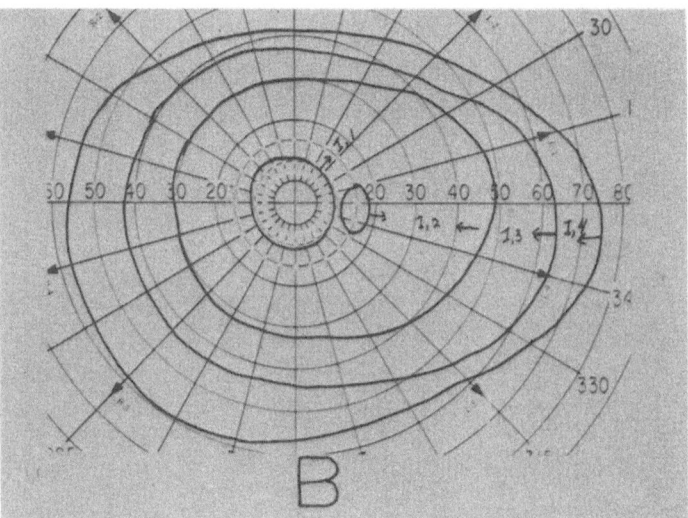

Fig. 2. Visual field of the right eye of a 42-year old man with a pressure of 32 mm Hg.
A – Visual field showing glaucomatous field defects:
I,1,e – contraction of the isopter
I,2,e – arcuate and paracentral scotoma
I,3,e – nasal step and arcuate scotoma (stippled)
I,4,e – nasal step
B – Visual field of the same eye as in A one month after maintaining ocular pressure
level between 15 and 19 mm Hg., by Diamox therapy. Note disappearance of defects.

182

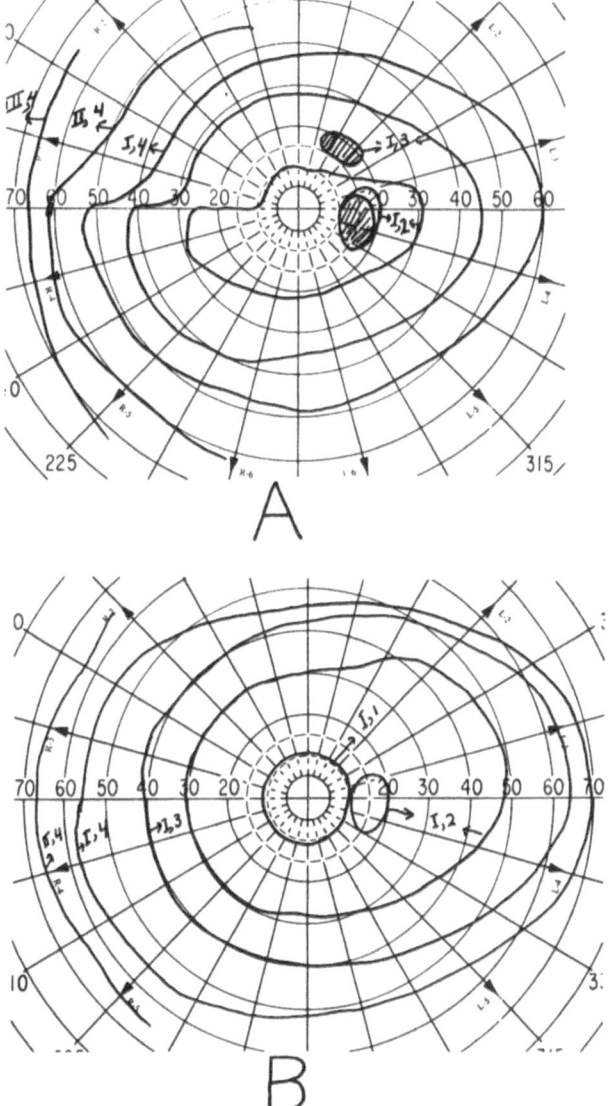

Fig. 3. Visual field of the same right eye in Figure 2.

A – Visual field six weeks after cessation of Diamox therapy, ocular pressure 34 mm Hg. Note the reappeance of the defects:

I,2,e – nasal step

I,3,e – nasal step and paracentral scotoma

I,4,e – nasal step

2,4,e – nasal step

B – Visual field of the same eye following reinstatement of Diamox therapy for six weeks and maintaining ocular pressure level between 14 and 19 mm Hg. Note disappearance of all defects again as ocular pressure is normalized.

Table 1. The same type of defects spontaneously developed in the ocular hypertensive, Armaly (1969).

My experience with reversibility of spontaneously developing defects in open angle glaucoma has three interesting phases: The first, spontaneous reversal over three years with reversal of ocular pressure and fluid dynamics. (Table). The second, spontaneous reversal in spite of the persistence of high ocular pressure (Fig. 1). The third, reversal with pharmacologic lowering of ocular pressure and reappearance when pressure is again elevated. Fortunately, the third is the most frequent (Fig. 2, 3).

The field defects seen in the above cases are large and deep enough defects to preclude artifacts. Each *location* of a previous defect, i.e., paracentral scotoma or nasal step, was tested on follow-up to ascertain reversal was real. The results illustrated above mean at least that a target which previously produced a defect is no more able to outline a defect in that area. This, in most of my cases, meant targets of the Goldmann perimeter with 0.5 log unit increments. It may be argued that the disappearance of the scotoma demonstrable by the same target on a previous occasion does not constitute complete reversibility by these techniques. That may, indeed, be true in some cases where the scotoma is so close to the center that it could conceivably have normally a threshold more than 0.5 log unit below the smallest used target, i.e., I, 1 of the Goldmann perimeter; for each target is supra-threshold within its isopter and the scotoma outlined by it may disappear for it without completely attaining its normal threshold. I have not done routinely static perimetry in these cases and therefore, recovery may not have been thoroughly complete, but recovery and normal threshold nevertheless did occur. This is seen in some of the cases where static perimetry was also performed. In summary, investigations of reversibility of glaucomatous defects are indeed most complex. Numerous factors can operate to produce variation from one case to the next and from one investigator to another. The most important fact is that reversibility does occur albeit not in all cases. This fact presents us with the challenge of seeking and identifying those cases in which reversibility is likely to occur and normalizing their visual function and of protecting them from future glaucomatous damage.

REFERENCES

Armaly, M.F. 'The Vascular Bed of the Retina and Optic Nerve Head,' in A.E. Braley (ed.): *The Retina*, Boston: Little, Brown and Company, 1962, Vol. 2, pp. *133-157*.

Armaly, M.F. 'The Effect of Corticosteroids on Intraocular Pressure and Fluid Dynamics. III. Changes in Visual Function and Pupil Size during Topical Dexamethasone Application,' *Arch. Ophth.*, 71: *636-644* (May 1964).

Armaly, M.F. 'Ocular Pressure and Visual fields, A Ten-Year Follow-Up Study,' *Arch. Ophth.* 81: *25-40* (Jan. 1969).

Armaly, M.F. 'The Visual Field Defect and Ocular Pressure Level in Open Angle Glaucoma,' *Inv. Ophth.*, 8 (No. 1): *105-124* (Feb. 1969).

Armaly, M.F. 'Selective Perimetry for Glaucomatous Defects in Ocular Hypertension,' *Arch. Ophthal.* 87: *518* (1972).

Gaffner, F. & Goldmann, H. 'Experimentelle Untersuchungen über der Tusa wen hang vou augur dweksteigeneug eiud Gesichtsfeld schdigung,' *(Ophthalmologica)* 130: *357* (1955).

Author's address:
George Washington University Medical Center
Washington, D.C. 20037
U.S.A.

VISUAL FIELD DEFECTS IN OPEN-ANGLE GLAUCOMA: PROGRESSION AND REGRESSION

CHARLES D. PHELPS

(Iowa, U.S.A.)

ABSTRACT

How often do glaucomatous visual field defects improve or worsen? What factors pre-dispose a glaucomatous eye to changes in the visual field? Attempting to answer these questions, I reviewed the charts of 130 patients (177 eyes) who met the following criteria: open-angle glaucoma, definite glaucomatous visual field defects, good visual acuity, reliable responses during perimetry, and two perimetric examinations one year apart. Patients were separated into three groups: a surgical group, a group newly started on medical treatment, and a control group continued on previous medication. Visual fields were tested on the Goldmann perimeter, using Armaly's strategy of 'selec-tive perimetry' for detection of defects and quantitative kinetic perimetry for their assessment.

Visual fields improved in 7% and worsened in 15% of the 177 eyes. Improvement occurred more frequently in young patients, in eyes treated surgically, when the reduc-tions of intraocular pressure were large, and when the cup of the optic disc did not extend to its rim. Worsening occurred more often in old patients and in eyes treated medically. Neither systemic blood pressure nor severity or location of visual field defects influenced the prognosis.

INTRODUCTION

Most visual field defects in chronic open-angle glaucoma are permanent and irreversible. With passage of time they either progressively enlarge or remain stable. Occasionally, however, glaucomatous field defects have been ob-served to decrease in size or even disappear altogether (Armaly, 1969; Drance, Bryett & Schulzer 1977; Greve, Dake & Verduin 1977; Heilmann 1978; Janotka & Dubiel 1977; Patterson 1970). The improvement may occur spontaneously but usually follows treatment to lower ocular pressure.

One objective of the present study was to determine how often visual field defects improve or worsen in patients being treated for open-angle glaucoma. An additional objective was to identify factors associated with improvement or worsening of the visual field. The factors investigated in-cluded type of treatment (medical or surgical), age of the patient, pre-treat-ment intraocular pressure, change of intraocular pressure induced by treat-ment, post-treatment intraocular pressure, blood pressure, horizontal cup-to-disc ratio, location of the cup in relation to the neuro-retinal rim of the optic disc, severity of the visual field defect, and location of the visual field defect (upper or lower field).

Charts were reviewed of 232 patients with loss of vision from primary open-angle glaucoma treated at University of Iowa Hospitals between July, 1972, and December, 1977. Each eye of a patient was considered separately and, for purposes of analysis, was assigned an 'age' and 'blood pressure'. This was necessary because in many patients the two eyes either were treated differently or responded differently to treatment. Criteria for inclusion of an eye in the study included (1) at least two visual field examinations separated in time by an interval of about one year (intervals ranged from 9 to 18 months), (2) a glaucomatous visual field defect present during the first examintation, (3) reliable responses during perimetric examination, (4) visual acuity 20/50 or better at time of first examination, and (5) absence of retinal, optic nerve, or neurologic lesions other than glaucoma that might cause a visual field abnormality. Of the charts reviewed, 177 eyes of 130 patients met these criteria. Insufficient follow-up, present in 61 patients, was the major reason for exclusion.

Visual fields were tested with the Goldmann perimeter. To screen for glaucomatous defects, both in the initial and subsequent examinations, we used Armaly's method of 'selective' perimetry as modified by Drance (Armaly 1972; Drance, Brais, Fairclough & Bryett 1972). The size, shape, and density of all detected defects were plotted with kinetic perimetry using multiple test stimuli. We re-examined small or shallow scotomas for refractive cause by altering the near correction in half diopter increments and decrements; refractive scotomas were excluded from the study. If a visual field defect worsened during miotic therapy, the field was re-examined after the pupil had been dilated; field changes due to miosis were excluded from the study.

The following visual field defects were considered glaucomatous: (1) a paracentral scotoma at least 5 degrees wide and 15 degrees in length to the I-2e or brighter stimulus, (2) a nasal step of 10 degrees (if only involving one isopter) or 5 degrees (if involving more than one isopter or when associated with a paracentral scotoma), (3) an arcuate scotoma, (4) a Seidel scotoma (arcuate extension of the blind spot 30° above or 45° below the temporal horizontal meridian), (5) a sector-shaped temporal defect (isopter indentation of 10 degrees or more, often combined with a radial scotomaa pointing towards the blind spot), and (6) advanced defects (loss of most of upper or lower visual field or central or temporal island remnants). Criteria for change in a visual field defect included (1) disappearance of an existing defect, (2) appearance of a new defect, (3) change of 15 degrees in length or 5 degrees in width of an existing scotoma (usually judged from the I-4e stimulus), (4) change in depth of a scotoma by at least two steps in the following sequence of stimuli: I-2e, I-3e, I-4e, II-4e, III-4e, IV-4e, V-4e, and (5) change of 10 degrees in width of a nasal step.

Additional data obtained for each patient included: age at time of initial visual field; visual acuity, refractive error, and pupil size at each visual field examination; and intraocular pressures (measured with a Goldmann applanation tonometer) at time of initial and final visual field examination. Blood pressure measurements were available for 144 of the 177 eyes; if blood pressure was recorded more than once during the year of study, the average reading was used.

Visual field defects were classified according to location (upper field, lower field, or both) and severity (early, moderate, or severe). Early defects included isolated nasal step, paracentral scotoma, and temporal scotoma. Moderate defects included nasal step together with paracentral scotoma, arcuate scotoma, temporal scotoma together with defect in Bjerrum area, and arcuate scotoma in one half the field together with a paracentral scotoma or nasal step in the other half. Advanced defects included double arcuate scotomas, loss of the superior or inferior hemifield, and central or temporal island remnants.

Optic discs, in most instances, were classified from stereophotographs. When photographs were unavailable, the chart description was utilized. The horizontal cup-to-disc ratio was estimated using contour change rather than pallor to define the cup. Information on the cup-to-disc ratio was available in 174 of the 177 eyes. Extension of the cup to the edge of the disc was recorded; this did not necessarily mean a total absence of neuro-retinal rim, but only that the surface of the disc was partially excavated up to the disc margin in at least one sector. Information about the relationship of the cup to the disc margin was available in 169 of the 177 eyes.

Eyes were separated into three groups according to type of treatment:

1. *Surgical:* eyes on which a filtering operation (Scheie thermosclerostomy or trabeculectomy) was performed less than a month after the first visual field exam. Indications for operation were very high intraocular pressures or progressive visual field damage while receiving maximal amounts of tolerated medication.

2. *Medical:* newly diagnosed cases that were receiving no medication at the time of the first examination. Medical treatment (miotics, epinephrine, timolol, and/or carbonic anhydrase inhibitors) was started immediately after the first examination and adjusted throughout the first year with the general goals of lowering ocular pressure to below 20 mm Hg and preventing worsening of the visual field.

3. *Control:* eyes that had been on medical treatment before the start of the study and were maintained on medical treatment for the year of study. The first visual field recorded after July, 1972, was considered as the initial visual field in this study. The control group, whose mean intraocular pressure did not change significantly during the period of study, provided information about how often visual field defects changed or appeared to change in the absence of change in intraocular pressure.

The chi-square test with Yate's correction was used to test the significance of differences in proportions. The t-test for independent means was used to test the significance of differences between mean measurements in separate groups of eyes.

RESULTS

Frequency of visual field change (Table 1): Visual fields improved in 13 (7.3%) and worsened in 27 (15.3%) of the 177 eyes. Field changes were usually slight. However, five early defects (two nasal steps and three paracentral scotomas) disappeared altogether.

Type of treatment (Table 1): Improvement occurred more often (p < 0.5) in the surgically treated eyes (7/52 or 13.5%) than in the control group (1/64 or 1.6%). Visual fields also improved more often in the medically

Table 1. Frequency of visual field changes: relationship to type of treatment.

Visual Field	All	Treatment Group		
Change	Patients	Surgical	Medical	Control
	n (%)	n (%)	n (%)	n (%)
Better	13 (7.3)	7 (13.5)	5 (8.2)	1 (1.6)
Same	137 (77.4)	43 (82.7)	41 (67.2)	53 (82.8)
Worse	27 (15.3)	2 (3.8)	15 (24.6)	10 (15.6)
Total	177 (100)	52 (100)	61 (100)	64 (100)

Table 2. Characteristics of the three treatment groups.

	Surgical	Medical	Control
Number of patients	39	51	52
Number of eyes	52	61	64
Age (mean ± S.D.)	56.0 ± 14.5	67.7 ± 8.6	64.5 ± 13.1
Intraocular pressure (mm Hg)			
Initial	33.2 ± 8.7	27.3 ± 6.5	19.9 ± 5.4
Final	14.6 ± 5.6	18.2 ± 3.6	19.7 ± 5.3
Difference	− 18.6 ± 9.5	−9.1 ± 6.7	− 0.2 ± 4.5
Blood pressure			
Systolic	145.0 ± 17.6	136.2 ± 18.4	145.8 ± 16.7
Diastolic	90.6 ± 11.2	83.9 ± 12.1	88.6 ± 10.7
Optic disc			
Horizontal C/D Ratio	0.82 ± 0.15	0.71 ± 0.15	0.73 ± 0.15
Number with cup to rim	39/49 (79.6%)	38/58 (65.5%)	45/62 (72.6%)
VF defects: severity			
Early	10 (19.2%)	21 (34.4%)	21 (32.8%)
Moderate	22 (42.3%)	30 (49.2%)	34 (53.1%)
Advanced	20 (38.5%)	10 (16.4%)	9 (14.1%)
VF defects: location			
Upper field only	13 (25.0%)	24 (39.3%)	28 (43.8%)
Lower field only	16 (30.8%)	20 (32.8%)	17 (26.6%)
Both	23 (44.2%)	17 (27.9%)	19 (29.7%)

190

treated eyes (5/61 or 8.2%) than in the control group, but this difference was not statistically significant.

Visual fields worsened more often (p < .01) in the medical group (15/61 or 24.6%) than in the surgical group (2/52 or 3.8%). Visual fields also worsened more often in the control group (10/64 or 15.6%) than in the surgical group, but this difference was not quite significant (.10 > p > .05).

Characteristics of the three treatment groups are listed in Table 2. The three groups were roughly comparable in number, average blood pressure, average horizontal cup-to-disc ratio, and location of visual field defects. The surgical group, on the average, had a lower age, higher initial intraocular pressure, greater decrease of intraocular pressure, lower final intraocular pressure, and more advanced visual defects than either of the other groups. The medical group had a similar final intraocular pressure to that of the control group but, of course, a higher initial pressure and a greater decrease in pressure. The control group had no change in mean intraocular pressure between examinations.

Age (Table 3 and 4): Patients whose visual fields improved were, on the average, younger than those whose visual fields did not change (t = 2.07, p < .025). Conversely, patients whose visual fields worsened were, on the average, older than those whose visual field did not change (t = 3.44, p < .005). The percentage of visual field improvement progressively declined and the percentage of worsening progressively increased with advancing age (X^2 = 23.07, 3 × 3 contingency table, p < .005).

Initial intraocular pressure (Tables 5 and 6): Eyes in which the visual fields improved had, on the average, a higher initial intraocular pressure than eyes in which the visual field was stable or worsened (t = 2.74, p < .005). The

Table 3. Changes in visual fields and patient age.

Visual Field Change	n	Age
		(mean ± S.D.)
Better	13	56.0 ± 10.9
Same	137	62.9 ± 11.8
Worse	27	68.3 ± 15.7

Table 4. Frequency of visual field changes: relationship to patient age.

Visual Field Change	Patient Age (years)		
	< 50	50-69	⩾ 70
	n (%)	n (%)	n (%)
Better	6 (28.6)	5 (5.5)	2 (3.1)
Same	15 (71.4)	75 (82.4)	47 (72.3)
Worse	0 (0.0)	11 (12.1)	16 (24.6)
Total	21 (100)	91 (100)	65 (100)

191

frequency of visual field improvement in eyes with initial pressures of 30 mm Hg or higher (9/55 or 16.4%) was significantly higher ($X^2 = 7.71$, p $<$ .01) than the frequency of visual field improvement in eyes with initial pressures less than 30 mm Hg (4/122 or 3.3%). In contrast, the frequency of worsening was not influenced by the initial pressure.

Change of intraocular pressure (Tables 5 and 7): Eyes in which the visual field improved had a somewhat greater reduction of intraocular pressure between examinations than eyes in which the visual field was stable or worsened (t = 1.86, p $<$ .05). Although the frequency of visual field improvement increased progressively with increasing magnitude of intraocular pressure reduction, the trend was not statistically significant. Nor was the frequency of worsening significantly influenced by the amount of pressure reduction.

Final intraocular pressure (Table 5): The final mean intraocular pressure was similar, whether the visual field improved, worsened, or remained stable. Sixty eyes had a post-treatment intraocular pressure of 20 mm Hg or higher: 6 (10.0%) were improved and 11 (18.3%) were worse. One hundred and seventeen eyes had a post-treatment pressure of less than 20 mm Hg: 7 (6.0%) were improved and 16 (13.7%) were worse. The differences were not statistically significant.

Blood pressure (Table 8): The average systolic blood pressures were similar whether the visual fields improved, deteriorated, or remained stable. Diastolic blood pressure tended to be slightly higher in patients whose visual fields improved than in patients whose visual fields worsened, but the difference

Table 5. Changes in visual fields and intraocular pressure.

Visual Field Change	n	Intraocular Pressure (mm Hg)		
		Initial	Change	Final
		(mean ± S.D.)	(mean ± S.D.)	(mean ± S.D.)
Better	13	32.8 ± 8.1	−14.2 ± 10.2	18.7 ± 7.1
Same	137	25.8 ± 8.6	− 8.4 ± 10.3	17.4 ± 5.4
Worse	27	26.1 ± 8.9	− 6.4 ± 10.0	19.7 ± 6.4

Table 6. Frequency of visual field changes: relationship to initial intraocular pressure.

Visual Field Change	Initial Intraocular Pressure (mm Hg)		
	$<$ 20	20-29	$\geqslant$ 30
	n (%)	n (%)	n (%)
Better	0 (0.0)	4 (5.1)	9 (16.4)
Same	36 (83.7)	64 (81.0)	37 (67.3)
Worse	7 (16.3)	11 (13.9)	9 (16.4)
Total	43 (100)	79 (100)	55 (100)

was not quite statistically significant (t = 1.43, .10 > p > .05).

Cupping of the optic disc (Tables 9 and 10): Visual fields improved significantly more often (X^2 = 5.04, p < .025) if the horizontal cup-to-disc ratio was less than 0.8 (10/74 or 13.5%) than if it was 0.8 or greater (3/99 or 3.0%). The cup-to-disc ratio did not influence the frequency of worsening. Visual fields improved much more often (X^2 = 14.37, p < .005) if the cup failed to reach the edge of the disc (10/47 or 21.3%) than if the cup did extend to the edge (3/127 or 2.5%). Whether or not the cup had reached the edge of the disc did not significantly influence the frequency with which the visual field defect worsened.

Severity and location of visual field defect: Early visual field defects underwent change, i.e., either improved or worsened, only slightly more often

Table 7. Frequency of visual field changes: relationship to change of intraocular pressure between field examinations.

Visual Field Change	Change of Intraocular Pressure (mm Hg)			
	Any increase	0 to −9	−10 to −19	⩾ 20
	n (%)	n (%)	n (%)	n (%)
Better	0 (0.0)	4 (6.0)	6 (11.1)	3 (13.6)
Same	28 (82.4)	51 (76.1)	42 (77.8)	16 (72.7)
Worse	6 (17.6)	12 (17.9)	6 (11.1)	3 (13.6)
Total	34 (100)	67 (100)	54 (100)	22 (100)

Table 8. Changes in visual field and systemic blood pressure (data available in 145 of 177 eyes).

Visual Field Change	n	Systolic	Diastolic
		(mean ± S.D.)	(mean ± S.D.)
Better	12	138.8 ± 11.3	91.0 ± 16.8
Same	116	142.4 ± 17.8	87.8 ± 11.3
Worse	17	143.1 ± 22.6	84.0 ± 9.6

Table 9. Frequency of visual field changes: relationship to the horizontal cup: disc ratio (data available for 174 of 177 eyes).

Visual Field Change	Horizontal Cup: Disc Ratio			
	⩽ 0.6	0.7	0.8	⩾ 0.9
	n (%)	n (%)	n (%)	n (%)
Better	6 (13.6)	4 (13.3)	0 (0.0)	3 (5.8)
Same	29 (65.9)	21 (70.0)	43 (91.5)	40 (76.9)
Worse	9 (20.5)	5 (16.7)	4 (8.5)	9 (17.3)
Total	44 (100)	30 (100)	47 (100)	52 (100)

than advanced defects (Table 11). The differences were not statistically significant. Even advanced defects sometimes showed some improvement. Whether the visual field defect was in the upper or lower half of the field did not influence prognosis (Table 12).

DISCUSSION

Visual field changes observed in this study, both for better and worse, were usually minimal. Improvement was in general relative; only five defects, all

Table 10. Frequency of visual field changes: relationship to location of cup in disc (data available for 169 of 177 eyes).

Visual Field Change	Cup of Optic Disc	
	To Rim	Not To Rim
	n (%)	n (%)
Better	3 (2.5)	10 (21.3)
Same	97 (79.5)	32 (68.1)
Worse	22 (18.0)	5 (10.6)
Total	122 (100)	47 (100)

Table 11. Frequency of visual field changes: relationship to severity of visual field defect.

Visual Field Change	Severity of Defect		
	Early	Moderate	Advanced
	n (%)	n (%)	n (%)
Better	6 (11.5)	4 (4.7)	3 (7.7)
Same	36 (69.2)	70 (81.4)	31 (79.5)
Worse	10 (19.2)	12 (14.0)	5 (12.8)
Total	52 (100)	86 (100)	39 (100)

Table 12. Frequency of visual field changes: relationship to location of visual field defect.

Visual Field Change	Location of Defect		
	Upper only	Lower only	Both
	n (%)	n (%)	n (%)
Better	3 (4.6)	4 (7.5)	6 (10.2)
Same	51 (78.5)	39 (73.6)	47 (79.7)
Worse	11 (16.9)	10 (18.9)	6 (10.2)
Total	65 (100)	53 (100)	59 (100)

early, disappeared entirely. However, the improvement, which occurred in seven percent of eyes, was almost certainly real and not artefact. Field defects became smaller only if treatment lowered intraocular pressure. The frequency of visual field improvement was directly related to the magnitude of pressure reduction. This observation underscores the importance of energetic efforts to lower intraocular pressure in patients with glaucoma.

The number of eyes with field improvement was small, and in a disheartening number of eyes (15%) the visual fields worsened in spite of our vigorous attempts to lower intraocular pressure and careful monitoring of treatment. Three factors, in addition to reduction of intraocular pressure, seemed to influence the prognosis: the age of the patient, the type of treatment, and the appearance of the optic disc.

Visual fields improved less often and worsened more frequently in elderly patients. The adverse influence of advanced age on prognosis is probably related to the increased prevalence with aging of certain conditions that predispose an eye to pressure-induced damage. Although much remains to be learned about these conditions, they probably include disorders such as diabetes mellitus, small blood vessel diseases, transient or sustained alterations of blood pressure, cardiac arrhythmias, poor nutrition, and anemia. In the young glaucoma patient, high intraocular pressure is usually the most important factor in the pathogenesis of the visual field defect. In the elderly patient, the other factors may play a more predominant role. Because the other factors are less amenable to treatment than high intraocular pressure, the prognosis in the elderly patient is worse.

Visual fields fared better in eyes treated surgically than in eyes treated medically. This may have resulted from a larger and more sustained reduction of intraocular pressure in surgically treated eyes. In addition, patients using medication often fail to take it as prescribed. It is also possible that medications used for the treatment of glaucoma, which include several vasoactive drugs, might adversely affect the susceptibility of the optic nerve to pressure-induced damage. However, the differences we observed between treatment groups must be interpreted with caution. The study was retrospective and patients were not randomly allocated to one or the other treatment. Our reasons for choosing medical or surgical treatment may have biased the outcome. Analysis of other therapeutic indices, such as effect on visual acuity and complication rates, might be less favorable to surgical treatment. Early results of other investigators have not demonstrated surgery to be decisively better than medical therapy (Demailly, Papoz & Valtot 1974; Smith 1972; Werner & Drance 1977).

When the neuro-retinal rim was obliterated by cupping in one segment of the optic disc, the corresponding portion of the visual field rarely improved. If the cup did not extend to the rim, improvement was frequent. These observations support the concept that pressure-induced damage is initially confined to functional loss, some of which is reversible. Later the damage progresses to structural atrophy with irreversible loss of vision. An analogy may be made to two short-term experiments. In acute pressure amaurosis, elevation of ocular pressure causes a temporary loss of vision that is completely reversible if pressure is promptly lowered. Similarly, elevations of intraocular pressure induced by a few weeks of corticosteroid administration occasionally cause nerve fiber bundle visual field defects that are also reversible, although more slowly, when corticosteroids are stopped and intraocular pressure returns to normal. In neither of these short-term experiments does the optic disc become atrophic. However, if the ocular pressure remains high for a long period of time, structural changes ensue, and visual loss becomes permanent.

REFERENCES

Armaly, M.F. The visual field defect and ocular pressure level in open-angle glaucoma. *Invest. Ophthalmol.* 8: *105-124* (1969).

Armaly, M.F. Selective perimetry for glaucomatous defects in ocular hypertension. *Arch. Ophthalmol.* 87: *518-524* (1972).

Demailly, P.L., Papoz, L. & Valtot, F. Trabeculectomy versus medical treatment in chronic open-angle glaucoma: First results after 16 months follow-up. *International Glaucoma Symposium, Albi, May 20-24, 1974*, ed. by R. Etienne and G.D. Paterson, Diffusion Générale de Librairie Marsaille, *pp 451-460* (1975).

Drance, S.M., Brais, P., Fairclough, M. & Bryett, J. A screening method for temporal visual defects in chronic simple glaucoma. *Canad. J. Ophthalmol.* 7: *428-429* (1972).

Drance, S.M., Bryett, J. & Schulzer, M. The effects of surgical pressure reduction on the glaucomatous field. *Second International Visual Field Symposium, Tübingen, September 19-22, 1976*, ed. by E.L. Greve, Dr. W. Junk bv Publishers, The Hague, *pp 153-157* (1977).

Greve, E.L., Dake, C.L. & Verduin, W.M. Pre- and post-operative results of static perimetry in patients with glaucoma simplex. *Documenta Ophthalmologica* 42: *335-351* (1977).

Heilmann, K. Progression and regression of visual field defects. *Glaucoma: Conceptions of a Disease*, ed. by K. Heilmann, K.T. Richardson, George Thieme Publishers, Stuttgart, *pp 168-175* (1978).

Janotka, H. & Dubiel, J. Ergebnisse der operativen Behandlung bei chronischem Glaukom mit grösseren Gesichtsfeldausfällen. *Klin. Mbl. Augenheilk.* 170: *105-108* (1977).

Patterson, G. Effects of intravenous acetazolamide on relative scotomas and visual field in glaucoma simplex. *Proc. Roy. Soc. Med.* 63: *865-869* (1970).

Smith, R-J.H. Medical versus surgical therapy in glaucoma simplex. *Brit. J. Ophthalmol.* 56: *277-283* (1972).

Werner, E.B. & Drance, S.M. The effect of trabeculotomy on the progression of glaucomatous visual field defects. *Second International Visual Field Symposium, Tübingen, September 19-22, 1976*, ed. by E.F. Greve, Dr. W. Junk bv Publishers, The Hague, *pp 67-73* (1977).

Author's address:
C.D. Phelps, M.D.
Department of Ophthalmology
University Hospitals
Iowa City, Iowa 52242
U.S.A.

Docum. Ophthal. Proc. Series, Vol. 19

THE CLINICAL SIGNIFICANCE OF REVERSIBILITY OF GLAUCOMATOUS VISUAL FIELD DEFECTS

E.L. GREVE, F. FURUNO & W.M. VERDUIN

(Amsterdam, The Netherlands)

ABSTRACT

This paper decribes some aspects of the normal and pathological variation of perimetric measurements. It stresses the difference between the two. A significant change of a glaucomatous visual field defect (GVFD) has to be larger than the pathological variation. Reversibility of GVFD is not a frequent phenomenon. It is found mainly in the early stages of the development of GVFD, notably in the stage of the wedge shaped defect (w.s.d.). It is difficult to induce substantial amounts of reversibility by short-term reduction of IOP. Short-term large elevations of IOP however can produce substantial deterioration.

The study of reversibility or improvement of glaucomatous visual field defects (GVFD) has a theoretical and practical interest. If reversibility exists this implicates that any theory of the cause of glaucomatous damage has to include the possibility of recovery of function.

If a reversible stage exists than this may have practical implications for the management of the glaucoma patient and specially for the decision to treat or not to treat. Reversibility can be defined as the total or partial recovery of a significant GVFD.

Reversibility is well known from, e.g., optic neuritis or chiasmal lesions. Some vascular disorders may show reversible VFD. Reversibility of GVFD has not received much attention, probably because it is not as frequent as deterioration and certainly not an easy measurable phenomenon. We are used to thinking in terms of deterioration and glaucoma would not be an important cause of blindness if substantial improvement of serious GVFD would regularly occur.

Large improvements of GVFD are very rare. It might be, however, that subtile improvements have escaped attention. Before any statement on improvement of GVFD can be made a few facts should be known:
1. Variation of measurements in normal areas of the VF;
2. Variation of measurements in VF defects.

In other words: what is the *reproducibility* of measurements in normal areas and in GVFD?

We have examined 5 patients repeatedly over a period of seven to ten days. During this period the IOP and blood pressure did not vary extensively. At least two meridians were examined by static perimetry. The examiner did not have preceeding results available during each examination.

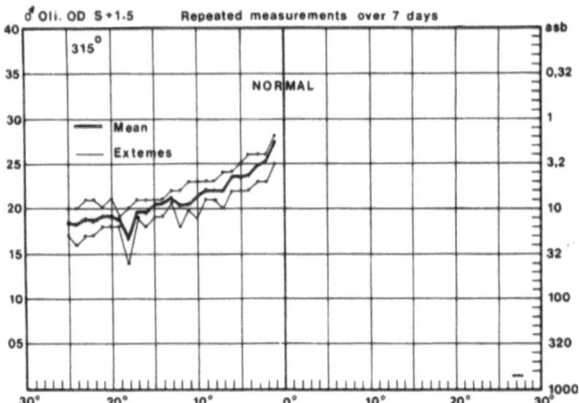

Fig. 1. Day-to-day variation of S.P. measurements in one meridian of a normal subject.

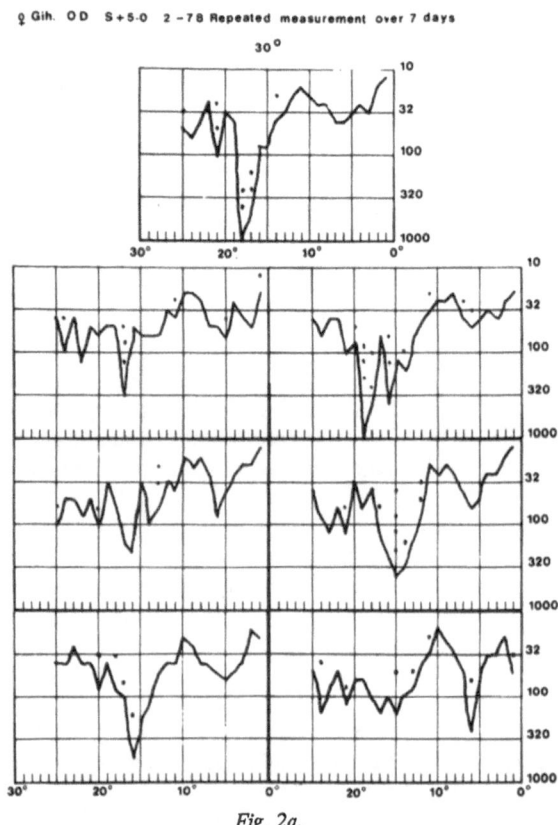

Fig. 2a.

The results of this investigation expressed as the range of measurements, are as follows: In a normal area the variation is 0.3 - 0.4 log. unit (fig. 1). In a defect area a variation of 0.5 log. unit regularly occurs (fig. 2). On separate points variations between two measurements of 0.6 - 0.9 log. unit may occur. It is rare that this size of variation occurs over a larger area. At the edge of defects for max. L. large variations (up to 1.5 log. unit) may occur.

The mean of all measurements of one meridian with a VFD (30 points) does not vary more than 0.3 log. unit indicating that plus-variation occurs next to minus-variation. This is where pathological variation differs from improvement or deterioration. In the latter case most changes are in one direction, either plus or minus.

It is of practical importance to differentiate between change in the sense of pathological variation and change that exceeds pathological variation. The first change indicates a malfunction of one or more nerve fibers, the second indicates deterioration or improvement of the disease. Variations of measurements in static perimetry is typical for pathological areas in the visual field. Significant changes of the VF have to exceed this pathological variation in one direction (plus or minus). Significant changes should take place over a number of positions. Ideal would be if change could be established after a number of measurements of successive examinations, unless of course the change is so great that no confusion with pathological variation is possible.

Reversibility of GVFD due to changes of IOP has to be a change that is significantly more than the pathological variation.

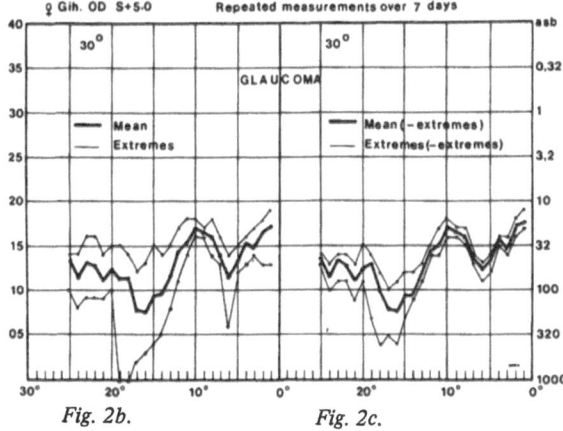

Fig. 2b.   *Fig. 2c.*

Fig. 2. Variation of S.P. measurements over 7 days in one meridian of a patient with glaucoma.
a) results of individual days.
b) mean and extreme values.
c) mean and extreme values minus one i.e. only the most extreme values of fig. 2b were omitted.

199

Unless one can prove that pathological variation itself is influenced by changes of IOP.

It is clear that observations on reversibility require accurate perimetric measurements. In our hands the best results are obtained with single stimulus static perimetry (SSSP).

With the above mentioned considerations in mind we want to report on two studies: a retrospective study of our visual field records and a short term study of the effect of variations of IOP on GVFD.

I. We studied our records of GVFD and extracted those cases where a significant improvement of the VF occured. We found the following types of improvement:

1. wedge-shaped defects (w.s.d.) to normal; (see Greve et al: A Critical phase etc in this vol).
2. small paracentral defects for max. L. (usually with some variation) to either w.s.d. or normal.;
3. the edges of larger defects for max. L. may show improvement and also relative areas adjacent to a defect for max. L.;
4. large defects for max. L. may show some recovery in the form of isolated peaks of decreased sensitivity.

We have seen no total recovery of complete glaucomatous nerve fibre bundle defects (NFBD) for max. L.

In this list changes that may occur outside the 20° parallel are not included.

The type of change of group 1 is frequent. The type of improvement of group 2 is less frequent. The improvement of group 3 is comparable with that of group 1 in so far as relative defects are concerned. However, the rest of the eye is in a worse state than group 1.

Group 4 shows that our max. L. (mistakenly called 'absolute') only indicates that we cannot measure the total intensity of the defect. Were stronger luminance available a remaining sensitivity might have been found. In this last group it is hard to differentiate from pathological variation. Clinically in our opinion only groups 1 and 2 are interesting.

A fluctuating w.s.d. is a typical example of pathological variation. It is certainly not the consequence of the examination procedure. It possibly indicates that the level of functioning of the nerve fibre serving that area of the VF is changing. The fiber may function adequately one day but may fail on another day. Of course we would like to see a correlation between IOP and VF change. For the w.s.d. this has not yet been established. It may vary independently from IOP.

In a study of the results of filtrating surgery a GVFD improvement of GVFD occured in 4 of 42 eyes. Two of these improvements were still evident after 4 years postoperative (Greve et al. 1977).

II. In this second investigation it was aked whether short-term variations in IOP could influence visual field defects. We also wanted to compare the effect of increase and decrease of IOP. 12 patients, of which 10 had GVFD, were planned for the following examinations:

200

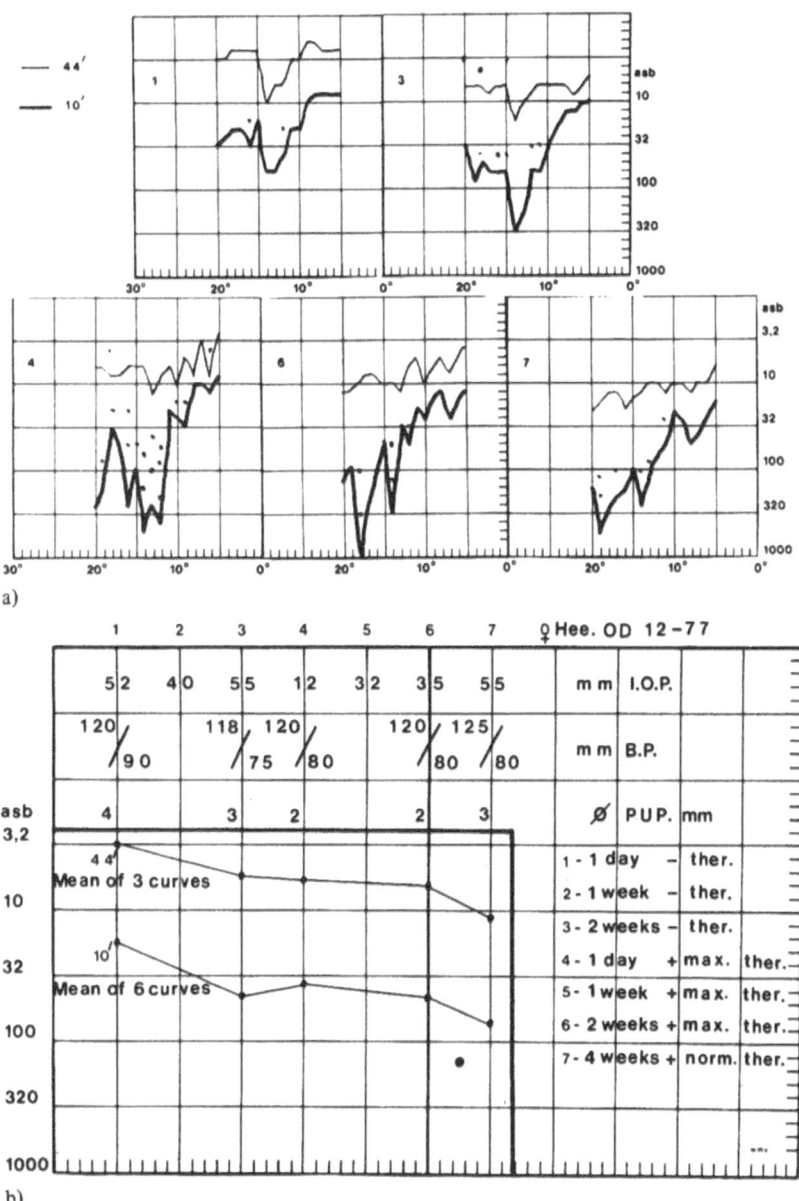

a)

b)

Fig. 3. Deterioration of the visual field after withdrawal of therapy; IOP went up to 55 mm; see curves 1 and 3. After reduction of IOP to 12 mm ($\Delta p = 43$ mm) the new defect did not improve; see curve 4. Nor was there any improvement after 2 weeks.

a) results of individual curves.

b) mean values of all measurements in 6 meridians (10′ object) and 3 meridians (44′ object).

1. VFE + TM + BP under present medical therapy.
2. Stop medical therapy for 2 weeks.
3. VFE + TM + BP under highest untreated IOP.
4. Max. decrease of IOP with medical therapy including diamox and glycerine.
5. VFE + TM + BP under lowest possible IOP.
6. Maintenance of lowest possible IOP level with medical therapy.
7. VFE + TM + BP after 2 weeks.

(TM = Tonometry / BP = Blood Pressure / VFE = Visual Field Examimation.

This means that 4 times VFE was performed under different circumstances. All VFE were done by means of static perimetry in at least 4 meridians.

RESULTS

In 2 patients without a defect no defect could be induced during the high IOP stage.

In 3 patients the VF deteriorated significantly in the high IOP stage without any tendency towards recovery even under low IOP (fig. 3).

In these patients a w.s.d. developed into a defect of greater intensity, and in a normal area a w.s.d. developed. All three patients had high IOP without therapy.

In 2 patients some improvement of the VF occured after reduction of IOP; the same 2 patients were examined in the reproducibility-study. Their changes, although minor, did exceed the pathological variation.

In 2 patients a w.s.d. disappeared without any evident'relation to the IOP level. Both patients never had an IOP over 30 mm. Their IOP was reduced from 28 mm to 12 mm.

One patient developed a w.s.d. when his IOP rose to 38 mm; he could not be examined after reduction of the IOP. 2 patients did not respond to therapy and neither did their visual fields.

DISCUSSION

The first conclusion from this investigation is that the deterioration of the VF was much more impressive than the improvement. The group that deteriorated is a bad-risc group without any tendency towards improvement. In the other group improvement was slight and occured mainly in early VFD related or unrelated to IOP level.

It seems that some patients are in a marginal stage of functioning and others have some reserve that enables them to tolerate periods of high IOP without deterioration.

OVER-ALL CONCLUSIONS

Some degree of reversibility exists but it is by no means as frequent and as extensive as deterioration.

Most frequently we have found reversibility in the early stages of the development of GVFD, notably the stage of the fluctuating w.s.d. For practical purposes we feel that this is the only interesting aspect of reversibility.

It is important to differentiate between pathological variation and true changes of GVFD. This differentiation may be difficult. It is unknown what mechanism causes the early stages of GVFD; it is unknown which mechanism is responsible for reversibility.

REFERENCES

Greve, E.L., Dake, C.L. & Verduin, W.M. Pre- and postoperative results of static perimetry in patients with glaucoma simplex. *Docum. Ophthal.* 42,2: *335-351* (1977).

Authors' address:
Eye Clinic of the University of Amsterdam
Wilhelmina Gasthuis
1e Helmerstraat 104
Amsterdam
The Netherlands

RECOVERY OF VISUAL FUNCTION DURING
ELEVATION OF THE INTRAOCULAR PRESSURE

J. TERRY ERNEST

(Madison, Wisconsin, U.S.A.)

ABSTRACT

Acute glaucoma was induced in a normal subject by the application of a suction cup ophthalmodynamometer. Static perimetry was carried out with a $\frac{1}{4}$ degree white test target in the Bjerrum area adjacent to the blind spot on the 135 degree axis 15 degrees from fixation. Rapid elevation of the intraocular pressure resulted in an elevation of the visual threshold but a slow elevation of the intraocular pressure had little effect on visual function. It is concluded that the eye is capable of adapting to acute elevations in the intraocular pressure and it is hypothesized that the mechanism of this compensation is circulatory.

INTRODUCTION

The effects of acute elevations of the intraocular pressure on visual function are controversial because it is difficult to obtain reliable measurements and thus there have been only a few studies reported. Artificial elevation of the intraocular pressure by ophthalmodynamometry results in decreased visual function but the design of previous studies prohibited both the detailed measurement of the visual loss and the study of its time course (Jaeger, et al., 1964; Vanderburg & Drance, 1966). Moreover, Douglas et al. (1975) found nerve fiber bundle field defects in only 7 of 18 acute closed angle eyes and a recent study of twenty-four patients with acute elevation in intraocular pressure due to angle closure glaucoma, mydriasis, and following cataract extraction, failed to demonstrate any glaucomatous visual field defects (Radius & Maumenee, 1977). To explain both the visual loss with ophthalmodynamometry and the lack of a consistent change in function in patients with acute glaucoma, we hypothesized that the eye is initially compromised but then is capable of compensating with a return to normal vision even though the intraocular pressure remains elevated. The following study was carried out to test this hypothesis.

MATERIALS AND METHODS

One subject, the author, a 39-year-old white man in excellent general health with no ocular disease, was used. Static perimetry was performed on the left

This study was supported in part by United States Public Health Service Research Grant EY 02526 and a Research to Prevent Blindness, Inc., Eye Research Professorship.

eye with a modified Goldmann-Weekers adaptometer. Background illumination was adjusted to the same order of magnitude as that of the Goldmann perimeter. The fixation target was a projected circular white light that subtended one-third degree on the retina. The fixation light was adjusted so that a $\frac{1}{4}$ degree white test target was in the Bjerrum area adjacent to the blind spot on the 135 degree axis 15 degrees from fixation. The target was presented continuously and the method of limits was used. The test target light intensity that was just not visible was started with and its intensity increased until it was just seen. The intensity of the light was then decreased until it was no longer visible. Approximately three ascending and three descending thresholds were obtained every 30 seconds and the measurements were continued for 90 seconds and then the intraocular pressure was changed. The threshold intensities were mechanically recorded on a logarithmic (log.) scale. The threshold for each 30 second segment was measured as the arithmetic mean of the upper and lower log. values. The self-recording, semi-automatic scleral suction cup modeled after Kukan was used (Galin, et al., 1969). The suction cup, because of its relatively large volume, maintains the intraocular pressure at a constant level as long as the negative pressure remains constant and calibration was carried out as previously described (Ernest, et al., 1972).

The suction cup was applied to the temporal scleral area of the globe and the negative pressure decreased to -50 mm Hg. The negative pressure was maintained at this level for 90 seconds and the difference thresholds measured. The negative pressure was then decreased in 25 mm Hg increments, pausing for 90 seconds at each level and testing. The intraocular pressure was thus raised until the visual threshold was grossly elevated. The suction cup pressure was then slowly brought back to 1 atmosphere and removed.

One hour after the first testing sequence, the suction cup was again applied to the same eye and the intraocular pressure elevated in approximately 3 seconds to the maximum level reached during the first session. The pressure was held at this level for 90 seconds.

RESULTS

The experiment was performed three times one week apart. In the Table the results from the first session are shown. The data from the three sessions were not averaged because slightly different testing conditions were employed but the results were similar. Elevation of the intraocular pressure had little effect on the visual threshold in the Bjerrum area until approximately 50 mm Hg was reached. The thresholds decreased toward the control value over the course of each of the 90 second testing periods. It is important to point out that the subject's blood pressure, 135/85, did not change between the first testing session and the second, one hour later.

During the second testing session, the threshold obtained during the first 30 seconds after the intraocular pressure had been quickly elevated to 72 mm Hg was 1 log. higher than the control level. It was also double the threshold obtained during the first session when the intraocular pressure had been gradually elevated. After 30 seconds, however, the visual threshold increased 3 logs, over the control level. The threshold then returned toward the original level.

DISCUSSION

The visual threshold in the Bjerrum area was elevated to a maximum of approximately 0.5 log. at an intraocular pressure of 72 mm Hg providing the pressure was elevated slowly over a period of 10 minutes. The fact that the visual threshold increased 3 logs. when the intraocular pressure was elevated rapidly to the same level means that the intraocular visual apparatus is able to compensate given time. Moreover, each of the 90 second testing sequences obtained during the first session show a gradual lowering of the visual thresholds toward normal following the initial elevation. This compensation is a form of autoregulation wherein local changes take place to restore homeostasis and normal function following intraocular pressure elevation. This is most evident from the fact that the visual threshold had returned toward control levels by 90 seconds even after it had been acutely elevated. One to two minutes are required for blood flow and tissue oxygen to return to normal following a decrease in perfusion pressure. It is important to note that axoplasmic flow blockage would be expected to take longer.

The observation that the visual threshold remained low and then increased steeply after 30 seconds of increased intraocular pressure in the second testing session is evidence that the reduced function was due to ischemia rather than direct pressure on the optic nerve. Direct pressure effects would be expected to act instantly while the effects of vascular compromise require time since oxygen and metabolites must be exhausted before there can be decrease in function.

It is evident that the eye is capable of adapting to acute glaucoma. There is evidence that the conduction of nerve impulses can be compromised by pressure but the levels are inordinately high and have not been shown to recover during the exposure to high pressure (Meek & Leaper, 1911). The

Table: Intraocular pressure versus Bjerrum area thresholds. Increase in visual threshold with elevation of the IOP (log. micromicrolamberts)

| IOP mm Hg | 90 seconds at each IOP level | | | 90 seconds at maximum IOP level | | |
	1st 30″	2nd 30″	3rd 30″	1st 30″	2nd 30″	3rd 30″
35	control			control		
41	0.00	0.05	0.06			
47	0.16	0.08	0.01			
53	0.22	0.20	0.08			
60	0.38	0.35	0.19			
66	0.36	0.28	0.22			
72	0.51	0.44	0.28	1.01	3.01	1.38

flow of axoplasm in the optic nerve may be blocked by acute glaucoma but there is no evidence to suggest this mechanical process is restored during the time the intraocular pressure is elevated (Anderson & Hendrickson, 1974; Minckler, et al., 1977).

The ocular vasculature, however, could be the site of compensatory mechanisms operating during ocular hypertension. The choroidal circulation appears to decrease when the intraocular pressure is elevated (Weiter, et al., 1973). The choroidal blood flow, however, is many times greater than required for normal nutrition of the outer retina and moreover the receptors have not been implicated in the pathology of a least early glaucoma. The retinal circulation has been suggested as a possible site of pathology in glaucoma (Henkind, 1967). The retinal circulation has been shown capable of compensation for acute elevations in the intraocular pressure. The blood cells traversing the retinal vessels in the macular region may be seen entoptically (flying corpuscles). If the intraocular pressure is then experimentally elevated, the cell movement slows but it requires a continual increase in the pressure applied to the eye to maintain the slowed cell circulation (Loebl & Riva, 1977). It is thus evident that the retinal circulation, while initially compromised by acute ocular hypertension, does compensate and return towards normal levels of retinal perfusion. This autoregulation of the retinal circulation has been demonstrated in experimental animals (Ffytche, et al., 1974; Alm & Bill, 1972). A decrease in perfusion pressure caused an initial decrease in the retinal circulation but it then returned to normal even though the perfusion pressure remained low.

The circulation of the optic disk has been implicated by many authors as the primary site affected by elevations in the intraocular pressure in glaucoma. It is difficult to assess the optic disk circulation in man, even with fluorescein angiography, because the superficial vessels disappear early in the course of the disease and the deep vessels within the optic disk are difficult to resolve. In subhuman primates, however, blood flow in the optic disk has been measured by a variety of means. Probes measuring temperature changes, oxygen tensions, and hydrogen wash-out, have been inserted into the optic disk to measure blood flow (Ernest & Potts, 1971; Armaly & Araki, 1975; Ernest, 1976; Ernest, 1977). Recently microsphere impaction in the optic disk blood vessels of experimental animals has been used to quantitate blood flow (Bill & Geijer, 1977). All of these studies have shown that the blood flow of the optic disk can compensate for elevations in the intraocular pressure by the process of autoregulation and it seems reasonable to extrapolate the animal studies to humans.

There is no question that visual function can be compromised by induced ocular hypertension, at least for the first minute. The normal eye then recovers and the time course of the recovery is similar to the recovery of blood flow following elevation of the intraocular pressure in experimental animals. It is persuasive that patients with acute glaucoma need not have visual field defects because the ocular vasculature has been able to adjust to the increased intraocular pressure. This does not necessarily mean, however, that the glaucomatous optic atrophy and visual field loss of chronic open angle glaucoma are due to mechanisms other than circulatory compromise. It could well be that while the circulation can initially compensate for elevations in the intraocular pressure, over the course of months and years, the autoregulatory mechanisms breakdown with resultant loss of optic nerve substance and visual function.

ACKNOWLEDGEMENT

Part of this material was used in a Thesis for membership in the American Ophthalmological Society accepted by the Committee on Theses.

REFERENCES

Alm, A. & Bill, A. The oxygen supply to the retina. II. Effects of high intraocular pressure and of increased arterial carbon dioxide tension on ureal and retinal blood flow in cats. *Acta Physiol. Scand.* 84: *306-319* (1972).

Anderson, D.R. & Hendrickson, A. Effect of intraocular pressure on rapid axoplasmic transport in monkey optic nerve. *Invest. Ophthal.* 13: *771-783* (1974).

Armaly, M.F. & Araki, M. Optic nerve circulation and ocular pressure. *Invest. Ophthal.* 14: *724-731* (1975).

Bill, A. & Geijer, C. Effect of intraocular pressure on regional blood flow in the retina and optic nerve. Association for Research in Vision and Ophthalmology. Spring 1977 Meeting, Sarasota, Florida.

Douglas, G.R., Drance, S.M. & Schulzer, M. The visual field and nerve head in angle closure glaucoma: A comparison of the effects of acute and chronic angle closure. *Arch. Ophthal.* 93: *409-411* (1975).

Ernest, J.T. Optic disc blood flow. *Trans. Ophthal. Soc. U.K.* 96: *348-351* (1976).

Ernest, J.T. Optic disk oxygen tension. *Exp. Eye Res.* 24: *271-278* (1977).

Ernest, J.T., Archer, D. & Krill, A.E. Ocular hypertension induced by scleral suction cup. *Invest. Ophthal.* 11: *29-34* (1972).

Ernest, J.T. & Potts, A.M. Pathophysiology of the distal portion of the optic nerve. IV. Local temperature as a measure of blood flow. *Am. J. Ophthal.* 72: *435-444* (1971).

Ffytche, T.J., Bulpitt, C.J., Kohner, E.M., Archer, D. & Dollery, C.T. Effect of changes in intraocular pressure on the retinal microcirculation. *Brit. J. Ophthal.* 58: *514-522* (1974).

Galin, M.A., Baras, I. & Best, M. Suction Ophthalmodynamometry. *Trans. Am. Acad. Ophthal. Otol.* 73: *335-336* (1969).

Henkind, P. New observations on the radial peripapillary capillaries. *Invest. Ophthal.* 6: *103-108* (1967).

Jaeger, E.A., Weeks, S.D. & Duane, T.D. Perimetric and visual acuity changes during ophthalmodynamometry. *Arch. ophthal.* 71: *484-488* (1964).

Loebl, M. & Riva, C.E. Macular circulation and the flying corpuscles. *Am. Acad. Ophthal. Otol. Eighty-second annual meeting,* October, 1977, Dallas, Texas.

Meek, W.J. & Leaper, W.E. Effects of pressure on conductivity in nerve and muscle. *Am. J. Physiol.* 27: *308-322* (1910-1911).

Minckler, D.S., Bunt, A.H. & Johanson, G. Orthograde and retrograde axoplasmic transport during acute ocular hypertension in the monkey. *Invest. Ophthal. Visual Sci.* 16: *426-441* (1977).

Radius, R.L. & Maumenee, A.E. Visual field changes following acute elevation of intraocular pressure. *Trans. Am. Acad. Ophthal. Otol.* 83: *61-68* (1977).

Vanderburg, D. & Drance, S.M. Studies of the effect of artificially raised intraocular pressure on retinal differential thresholds of the Bjerrum area. *Am. J. Ophthal.* 62: *1049-1063* (1966).

Weiter, J.J., Schachar, R.A. & Ernest, J.T. Control of intraocular blood flow. I. Intraocular pressure. *Invest. Ophthal.* 12: *327-331* (1973).

Author's address:
Dept. of Ophthalmology
Clinical Sciences Center
1300 University Avenue
Madison, Wisconsin 53792 600 Highland Avenue
U.S.A.

Docum. Ophthal. Proc. Series, Vol. 19

THE MODE OF DEVELOPMENT AND PROGRESSION OF FIELD DEFECTS IN EARLY GLAUCOMA — A FOLLOW-UP STUDY

YOSHIAKI KITAZAWA, OSAMU TAKAHASHI & YOHKO OHIWA

(Tokyo, Chiba, Japan)

ABSTRACT

One hundred twenty ocular hypertensive patients without demonstrable field defects and twenty primary open-angle glaucoma patients with unilateral field defects were followed up for 2 to 14 years (average: 5.4 years) without medical therapy. Visual field was examined with kinetic and static methods. Quantitative, kinetic and static, selective perimetry (Armaly's method) were performed with a Goldmann perimeter. Multiple stimulus static campimetry was done with a Friedmann Visual Field Analyser. Eleven eyes (ten cases) of ocular hypertensives and four eyes (four cases) of primary open-angle glaucoma patients developed field defects during the period of observation. the defects was detected by means of kinetic Goldmann perimetry initially. While kept untreated the relative defects increased in size and severity without further elevation of parafoveal region in association with the changes in the upper Bjerrum area. None of the defects was detected by means of kinetic Goldmann perimetry. While kept untreated the relative defects increased in size and severity without further elevation of IOP. The relative defects in the upper Bjerrum area extended toward the blind spot rather than to nasal periphery. Multiple stimulus static campimetry is of great value in the detection of early field change in primary open-angle glaucoma.

INTRODUCTION

The results of recent prospective follow-up studies support the prevailing trend toward observing rather than medically treating the patient with moderately increased intraocular pressure (IOP) until the field defect is detected (Kitazawa, Horie, Aoki, Suzuki & Nishioka 1977; Linnér & Stromberg 1967, Perkins 1973; Wilensky, podos & Becker 1974). The presence of the charactiristic glaucomatous field defects is considered to be one of the most important criteria for the diagnosis of primary open-angle glaucoma (POAG) along with the elevated IOP and the changes in the optic disc. Therefore, the detection of early glaucomatous field defect is of cardinal importance for the early diagnosis of primary open-angle glaucoma. The knowledge of form and location of early defects is indispensable for the detection of the field defects while they are still imperceptible to the patient and hopefully reversible. Although there are many reports on the 'early' field defects in glaucoma there is much left to be known about the mode of development of the field defect in the individual patient (Aulhorn & Harms 1967; Lobstein & Gerhard 1975; Suzuki, Furuno, Shinzato, Tomonaga, Endo & Matsuo 1976). We initiated a prospective study at the Glaucoma Service of Chiba University Hospital 15 years ago in an attempt to determine the fate of the patients with elevated IOP but without demonstrable field defects. The purpose of the present paper is to report the various characteristics and the temporal course of the field defects in the same individuals which took place during the period of observation.

SUBJECTS AND METHODS

A total of 120 patients with ocular hypertension and 20 POAG patients with unilateral field loss were enrolled in this study between 1963 and

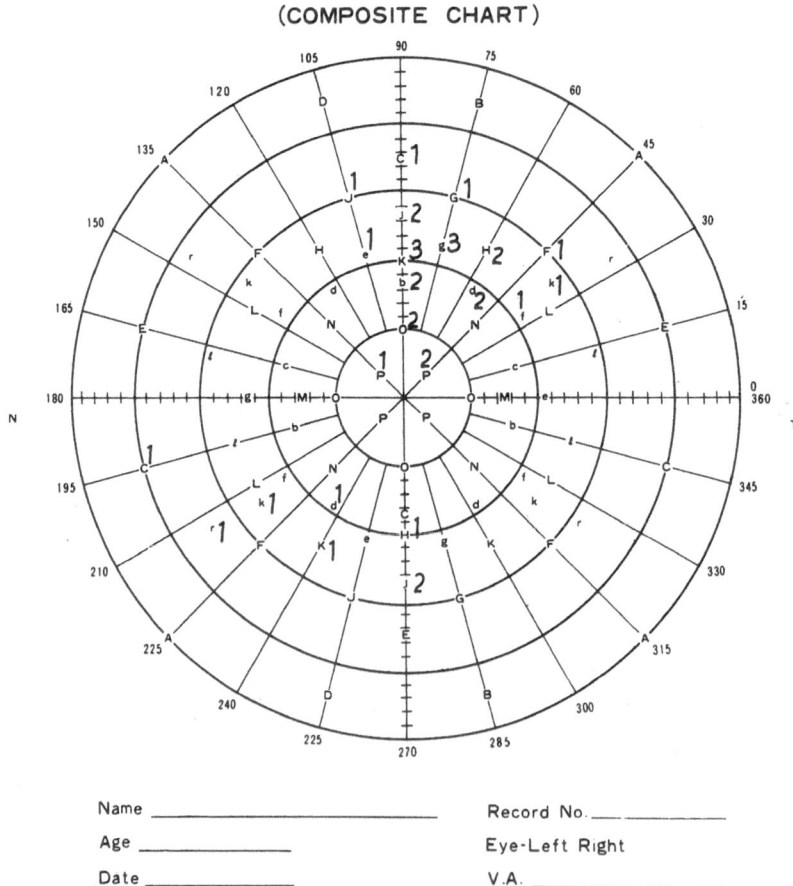

Fig. 1. Distribution of relative defects when first detected (15 eyes), a: right eye, b: left eye.

1975. Each had IOP greater than 21 mm Hg, an unoccludable normal open-angle (grade 3 to 4), and no demonstrable field defect. Prior to enrollment in the study the following data were recorded: age, sex, applanation IOP, facility of outflow, Po/C ratio, horizontal cup/disk ratio. The IOP was measured with a Goldmann applanation tonometer. Visual field examination was done by means of kinetic perimetry with a Goldmann perimeter and multiple stimulus static campimetry using a Friedmann Visual Field Analyser (Friedmann 1966). The latter examination was included in 1974. The cup/disc-ratio was determined by comparing the horizontal diameter of the cup to that of the disc on ophthalmoscopic examination. All patients were asked to return to the Glaucoma Service at least every 3 to 6 months for follow-

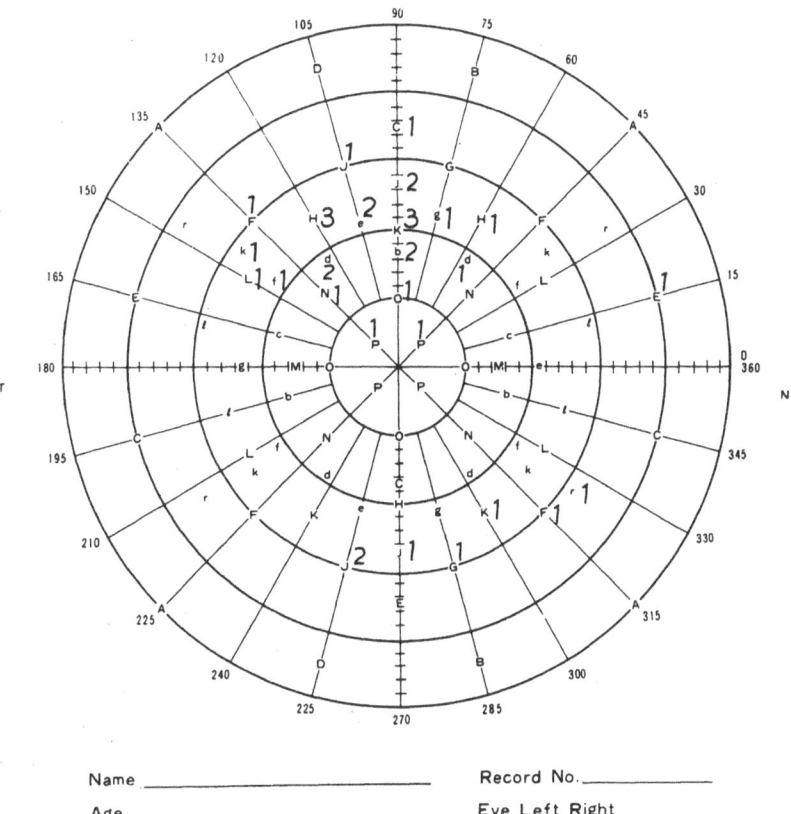

Fig. 1b.

up examinations. All the eyes without field changes were kept untreated and no systemic, ocular hypotensive drugs were administered. Examinations included tonometry, perimetry, direct ophthalmoscopy, gonioscopy, and tonography. Quantitative, kinetic perimetry with a Goldmann perimeter was performed through the period of follow-up. Static, selectice perimetry was performed with a Goldmann perimeter according to Armaly's method after 1971 (Armaly 1969). Multiple stimulus static campimetry was done in the following manner: Two different front plates, the standard one and the one divised for the examination of glaucoma patients, were used, i.e. 80 stimuli were presented in 25 phases in the 25 degree (radius) visual field. The The threshold was defined by the denset filter compatible with the perception of the two paracentral spots located at 2 degrees from the center (spots P). Failure to perceive the stimulus with a luminance of 0.4 log unit above the threshold level was suspected to be pathological and the examination was repeated to confirm the finding. Multiple stimulus static campimetry was also performed in the separate series of 81 ocular hypertensive patients in which quantitative, kinetic Goldmann perimetry failed to reveal abnormality.

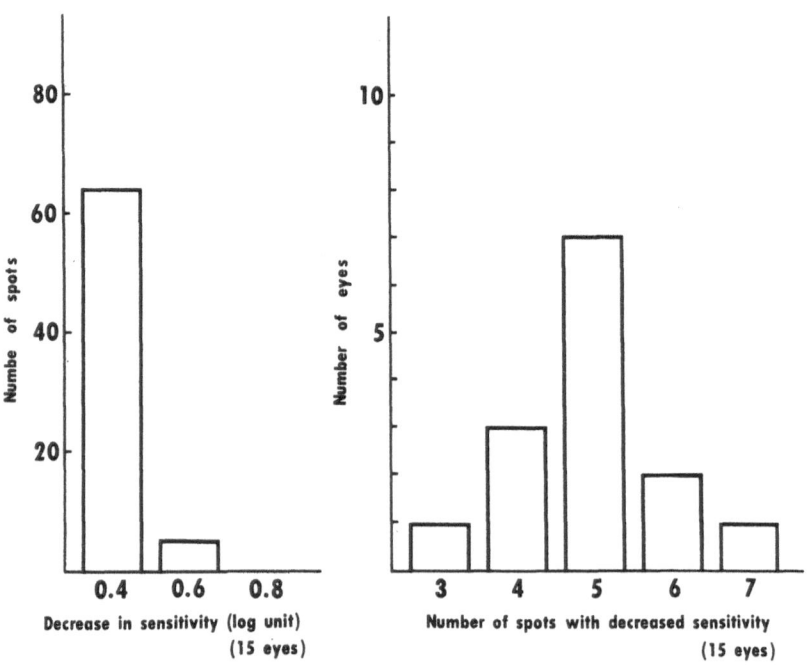

Fig. 2. a: Number of spots with the different degree of decrease in sensitivity when first detected (15 eyes), b: Number of eyes with the variable number of spots with decreased sensitivity (15 eyes).

214

The average duration of follow-up of 120 ocular hypertensives and 20 primary open-angle glaucoma was 5.4 years. During the period of observation, eleven eyes of ten ocular hypertensives and four eyes (four cases) of primary open-angle glaucoma with unilaterial field loss developed field changes which were revealed by Friedmann Visual Field Analyser. When the defects were first detected and confirmed to be reproducible by multiple stimulus static campimetry, kinetic quantitative perimetry failed to disclose any abnormality in all cases. The distribution of the spots with decreased sensitivity is shown in Figure 1. The majority of the spots with decreased sensitivity,

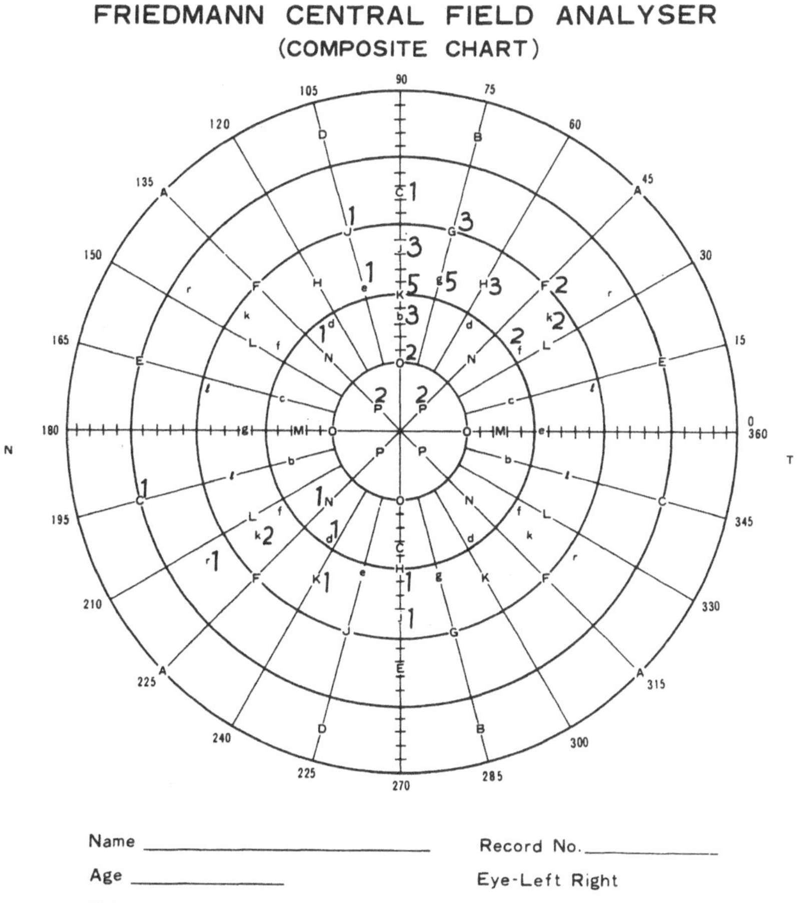

FRIEDMANN CENTRAL FIELD ANALYSER
(COMPOSITE CHART)

Name _____   Record No._____
Age _____   Eye-Left Right
Date _____   *Fig. 3a.*   V.A. _____

Fig. 3. Distribution of relative defects at the end of follow-up without therapy (average period of follow-up: 1.6 years) in 11 ocular hypertensive eyes, a: right eye, b: left eye.

41 among 69 (59%), were located in the upper Bjerrum area and the decrease in sensitivity in the parafoveal region was associated with that in the upper Bjerrum area in all cases but one. In the majority of cases the spots with decreased sensitivity took place in a cluster either in upper or lower Bjerrum area. The severity of the sensitivity decrease was 0.4 log units in the vast majority of spots (93%) when first detected (Fig. 2). Four eyes of primary open-angle glaucoma with unilateral field defect were placed on glaucoma medications when the field defects were confirmed. In these eyes the field defects remained essentially unchanged for the following two years in spite of the normalization of IOP. The eleven eyes of the ocular hypertensives were kept under close observation without therapy after they devel-

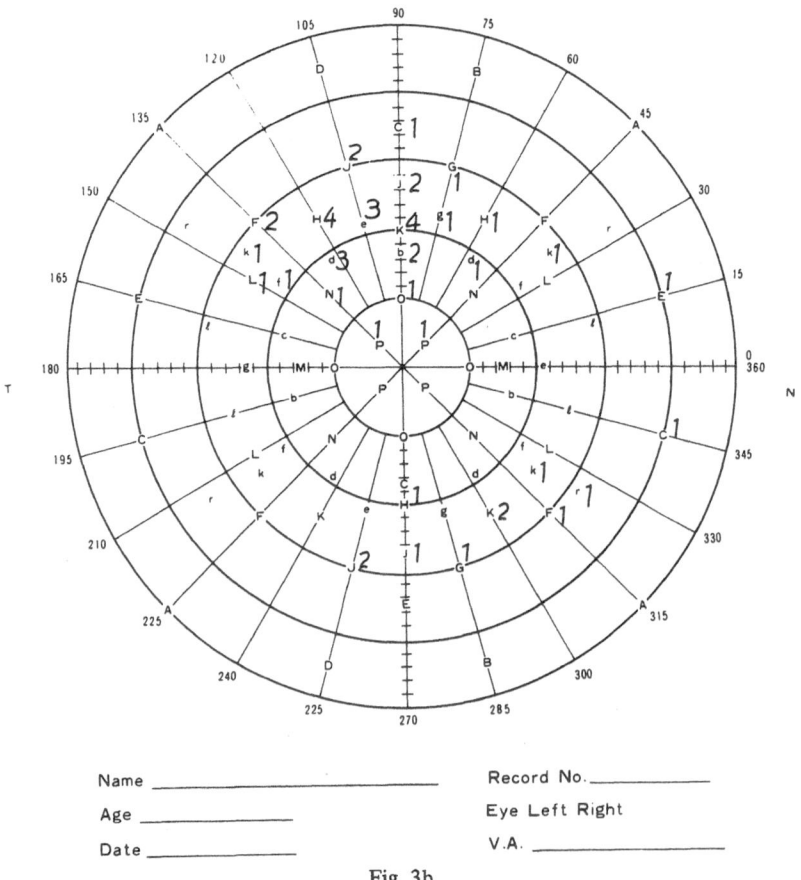

FRIEDMANN CENTRAL FIELD ANALYSER
(COMPOSITE CHART)

Name _____   Record No. _____

Age _____   Eye Left Right

Date _____   V.A. _____

Fig. 3b.

216

Table 1. IOP (mm Hg) before and after detection of field defects

Case	Eye	before the detection mean ± S.D.	peak pressure	after the detection mean ± S.D.	peak pressure
1	OD	20.3 ± 2.8 (24)	24	20.8 ± 2.8 (12)	26
2	OS	22.1 ± 5.3 (27)	30	22.9 ± 3.1 (34)	28
3	OD	22.4 ± 2.2 (70)	26	22.7 ± 2.5 (20)	24
4	OD	22.7 ± 2.1 (11)	25	21.4 ± 1.8 (15)	23
5	OS	22.8 ± 2.5 (6)	26	21.8 ± 2.2 (20)	23
6	OS	23.0 ± 2.2 (19)	27	22.0 ± 2.2 (24)	22
7	OD	21.8 ± 2.8 (20)	25	24.1 ± 2.0 (20)*	22
8	. OD	24.7 ± 2.7 (20)	29	23.5 ± 2.8 (17)	28
9	OD	21.3 ± 3.5 (13)	28	20.0 ± 2.4 (23)	26
	OS	21.5 ± 3.5 (13)	26	20.8 ± 2.0 (23)	24
10	OD	20.7 ± 2.6 (43)	24	20.1 ± 1.5 (9)	22
Total		22.1 ± 1.2		24.4 ± 2.2	

*: difference between before and after the detection is statistically significant ($p < 0.05$). Parenthesis denotes number of measurements.

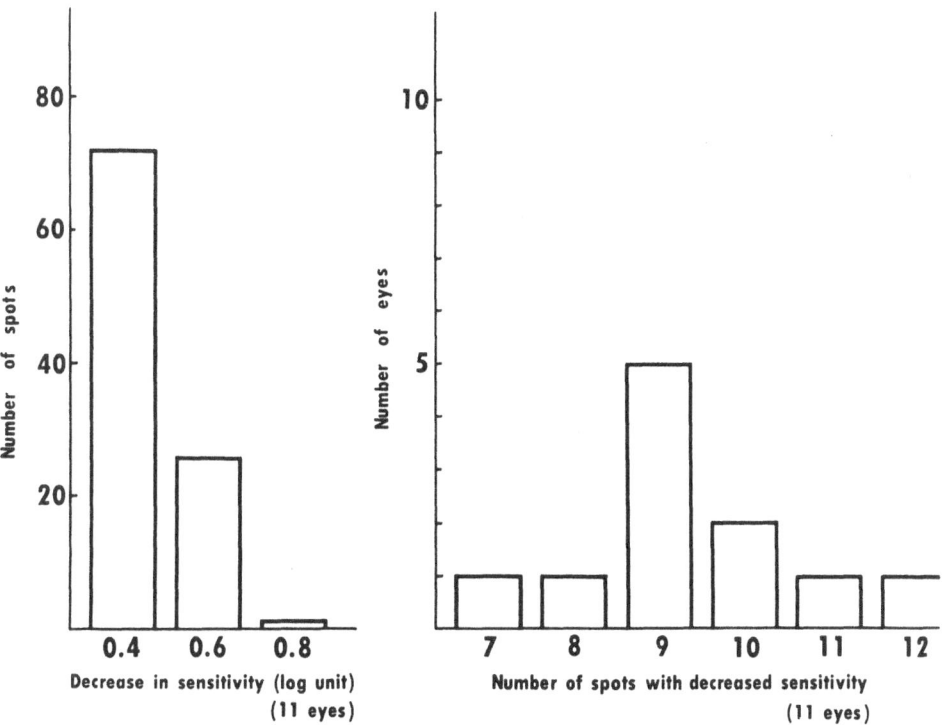

Fig. 4. a: Number of spots with the different degree of decrease in sensitivity at the end of follow-up without therapy in 11 ocular hypertensive eyes, b: Number of eyes with the variable number of spots with decreased sensitivity (11 eyes).

oped relative field defects. In the following two to three years the relative defects increased in size and severity (Fig. 3 & 4). The comparison of the distribution of the relative defects noted on the different occasions in the same individual suggested that the defects take place first in the upper half of the field in 10 to 15 degrees eccentricity on or close to 90 degree meridian and extends toward the blind spot. The changes in the lower half of the field appeared always later. In no case of the present series initial changes occurred exclusively in the lower half without accompanying changes in the upper Bjerrum area. Although the defects became more and more conspicuous while kept untreated IOP failed to show any significant change between before and after the field defects were detected in all but one eye (Table 1). In the separate series of 81 ocular hypertensives (162

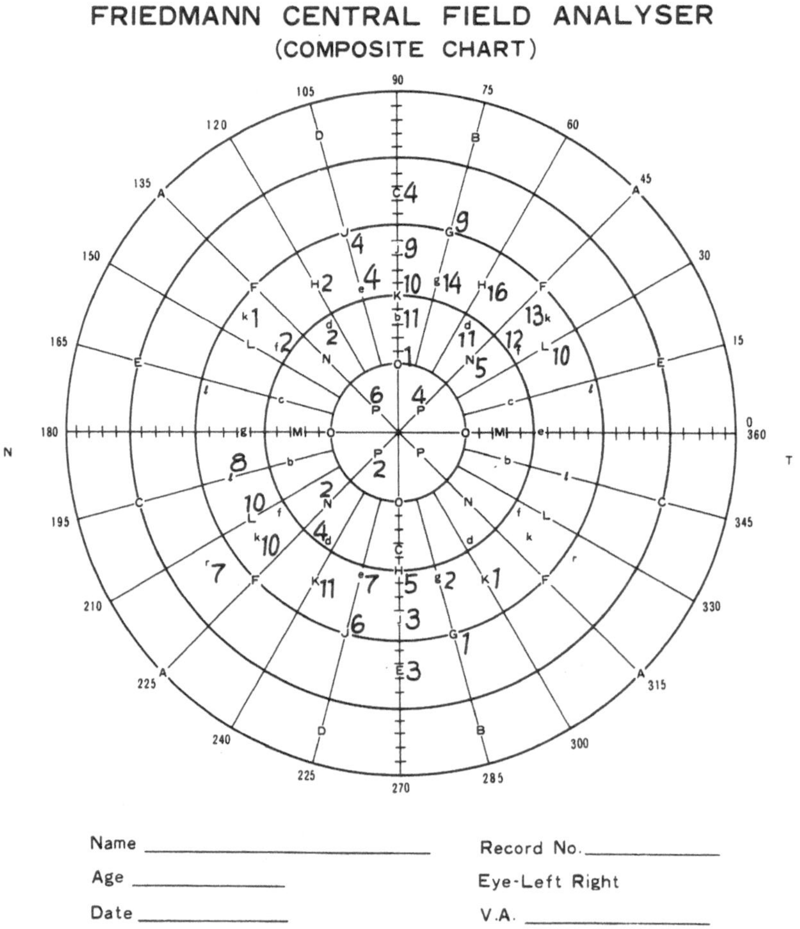
FRIEDMANN CENTRAL FIELD ANALYSER
(COMPOSITE CHART)
N
T
Name
Record No.
Age
Eye-Left Right
Date
V.A.

Fig. 5. Distribution of relative defects in 17 consecutive ocular hypertensions (24 eyes), a: right eye, b: left eye.

eyes) without demonstrable field loss by kinetic perimetry with a Goldmann perimeter the multiple stimulus static campimetry disclosed relative defects in 24 eyes (14.8%) of 17 patients. The severity of the decrease in sensitivity ranged from 0.4 to 0.8. The distribution of the spots with decreased sensitivity is almost identical to that in ocular hypertensives who developed field changes during the follow-up period without therapy. IOP ranged from 22 to 29 mm Hg and was 24.0 ± 1.3 mm Hg (mean $\pm$ S.D., n = 162).

DISCUSSION

The morphological and topographical characteristics of early glaucomatous field loss have been elucidated considerably by the recent investigations

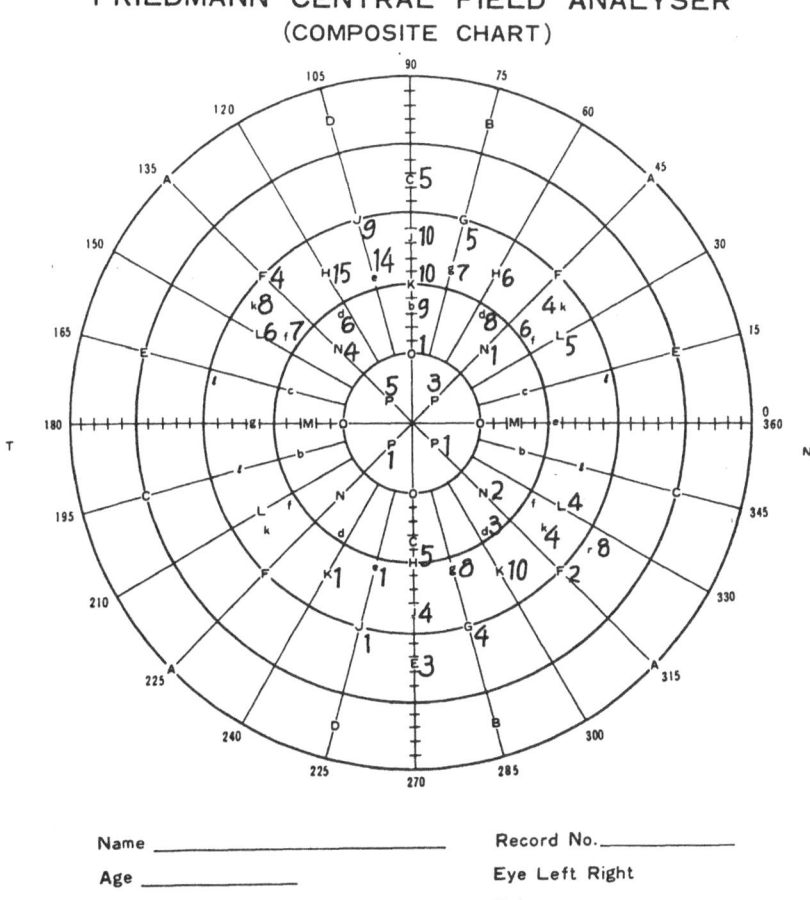

Fig. 5b.

219

utilizing the static method of perimetry. The wedge-shaped, relative defects in Bjerrum area and possibly, isolated, paracentral scotoma are considered to be representative changes of early primary open-angle glaucoma (Aulhorn & Harms 1967; Greve 1973). Most of the investigators, however, studied consecutive cases with elevated IOP and their studies are essentially 'horizontal' studies in chronological terms. Although the horizontal studies add to the knowledge of the pathological changes in various stages of the disease, prospective (longitudinal) studies provide a more solid ground for understanding the mode of evolution of the disease process. Many reports of the prospective studies on ocular hypertensives are now available. Although all the reports indicate the incidence of field loss which took place during the period of observation, neither the characteristics or the temporal changes of the detected field loss are described in detail in most of the studies (Kitazawa, Horie, Aoki, Suzuki & Nishioka 1977; Linner & Stromberg 1967; Perkins 1973; Wilensky, Podos & Becker 1974). The periodic monitoring of the visual field with a Friedmann Visual Field Analyser disclosed that the decrease in sensitivity in the upper Bjerrum area is the commonest and earliest change in primary open-angle glaucoma. This finding confirms the results of previous horizontal studies (Aulhorn & Harms 1967; Suzuki, Furuno, Shinzato, Tomonaga, Endo & Matsuo 1976). The sensitivity decrease in parafoveal region can be regarded as a common finding but is almost always associated with the relative defects in upper Bjerrum area. By following-up the field without therapy we could confirm that relative defects extend toward the blind spot and that similar relative defects take place in the lower Bjerrum area.

It is interesting to note that the field changes did progress although IOP remained unchanged in all ocular hypertensive cases but one. This seems to indicate that chronic and moderate elevation of IOP is that all necessary for the evolution of field loss in primary open-angle glaucoma and a further rise of IOP is not always needed for the further progression of the field defects once they are established. It should be noted, however, that the peak IOP found during the period of observation was considerably higher than the average IOP throughout the observation period. This suggests that the fluctuation of IOP or the transient elevation of IOP can threaten the integrity of visual function and seems to stress the importance of meticulous monitoring of IOP along with perimetric examination and the determination of diurnal variation of IOP during the follow-up period.

In the present study the normalization of IOP failed to reverse the relative field defects while the patients were followed-up for at least two years with reduced IOP. This finding is in contrast to the previous papers reporting the prompt regression of early field changes following the reduction of IOP and warns against undue optimism about the prognosis of ocular hypertension without field loss (Lobstein & Gerhard 1975).

It must be emphasized that when one defers treatment on the ocular hypertensives the visual field has to be monitored regularly. As demonstrated by the present study the static campimetry is definitely more useful in detecting the early glaucomatous field defects as compared with kinetic perimetry with a Goldmann perimeter. Multiple stimulus static campimetry was found to be quite useful for the detection of early defects and should be included in the examinations of the ocular hypertensive patients.

REFERENCES

Armaly, M.F. Ocular pressure and visual fields. *Arch. Ophthalmol.* 81: *25-40* (1969).

Aulhorn, E. & Harms, H. Early visual field defects in glaucoma. Tutzing Symposium, ed. by Leydhecker, W., Karger, Basel (1967), pp. 151-186.

Friedmann, A.I. Serial analysis of change in visual field defects, employing a new instrument, to determine the activity of disease involving the visual pathways. *Ophthalmologica* 152: *1-12* (1966).

Greve, E.L. Single and multiple stimulus static perimetry in glaucoma: The two phases of visual field examination. *Doc. Ophthalmol.* 136: *1-346* (1973).

Kitazawa, Y., Horie, T., Aoki, S., Suzuki, M. & Nishioka K. Untreated ocular hypertension, A long-term prospective study. *Arch. Ophthalmol.* 95: *1180-1184* (1977).

Linnér, E. & Stromberg, U. Ocular hypertension. Tutzing Symposium, ed. by Leydhecker, W., Karger, Basel (1967), pp. 187-214.

Lobstein, A. & Gerhard, J.P. Prognostic value of the visual field response to corticosteroid provocative testing in ocular hypertension: A follow up study, Glaucoma, Albi Symposium 1974, Diffusion Generale de Librairie, Marseille, (1975), pp. 205-210.

Perkins, E.S. The Bedford glaucoma survey: 1. Long-term follow-up of borderline cases. *Brit. J. Ophthalmol.* 57: *179-187* (1973).

Suzuki, R., Furuno, F., Shinzato, E., Tomonaga, M., Endo, N. & Matsuo, H.: The glaucomatous visual field changes using Friedmann Visual Field Analyser. *Acta Soc. Ophthalmol. Jpn.* 80: *345-352* (1976).

Wilensky, J.T., Podos, S.M. & Becker, B.: Prognostic indicators in ocular hypertension. *Arch. Ophthalmol.* 91: *200-202* (1974).

Authors' address:
Department of Ophthalmology
University of Tokyo
School of Medicine
7-3-1 Hongo
Tokyo 113
Japan

Docum. Ophthal. Proc. Series, Vol. 19

PERIPHERAL NASAL FIELD DEFECTS
IN GLAUCOMA

ELLIOT B. WERNER

(Montreal, Canada)

ABSTRACT

One hundred fifty one eyes of 101 consecutive patients with chronic open angle and low tension glaucoma showed typical visual field changes. Sixty of the eyes had a nasal step, either alone or in combination with other defects. In 17 of these eyes, it was possible to demonstrate an isolated scotoma in the nasal periphery. It was concluded that the peripheral nasal step is a nerve fiber bundle defect, and in its earliest phase produces a scotoma. In this sense, it behaves similar to the more central defects, rather than simply as a depression of isopters nasally. Photographs of the optic discs were obtained, and the appearance of the disc and field was correlated.

INTRODUCTION

The visual field defects of glaucoma result from damage to the retinal ganglion cell axons at the optic disc. The anatomy of the nerve fibers in the retina and optic nerve explains the characteristic shape and location of the field defects seen in glaucoma (Lynn, 1975).

When the nerve fibers are first damaged, the most common field defect is the paracentral scotoma (Aulhorn & Harms, 1966, Armaly, 1971). The nasal step is also a well known field defect in glaucoma, although its incidence as an isolated early glaucomatous field defect is a matter of some controversy. (Leblanc & Becker, 1971).

Like the paracentral defect, the nasal step is also caused by damage to nerve fiber bundles at the optic disc. These types of defects are known collectively as 'nerve fiber bundle' defects. (Drance, 1975).

When peripheral nasal steps are carefully evaluated, an isolated peripheral nasal scotoma is often found. Although this phenomenon has previously been described, (Armaly, 1972, Scott, 1957) it receives little attention in the standard texts on glaucoma and perimetry. Reed & Drance (1972) mention it in passing. Kolker and Hetherington (1976) Gorin (1977) and Harrington (1976) all fail to mention it. Leblanc (1976) did not describe isolated peripheral nasal scotomas in his series of nasal steps.

MATERIALS AND METHODS

The visual fields of 101 consecutive, unselected open angle and low tension glaucoma patients were reviewed. All patients were tested on the Goldmann perimeter using static and kinetic techniques. In each case, field defects were confirmed on repeat testing. Peripheral fundus examination showed no other lesion to account for the field defects.

RESULTS

One hundred fifty one eyes demonstrated typical nerve fiber bundle defects. Of this number, 64 had advanced field loss, that is a central defect breaking through to the periphery. Of the 87 eyes with earlier defects, a nasal step of 10° width or more was present in 60, either alone or associated with paracentral or arcuate defects. In 17 of the 60 nasal steps, a separate scotoma was present near the horizontal meridian in association with the nasal step.

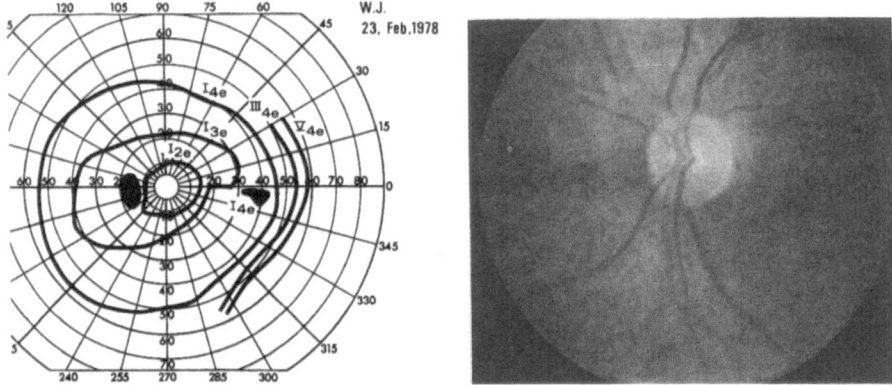

Fig. 1. Case number one; left visual field; left optic disc

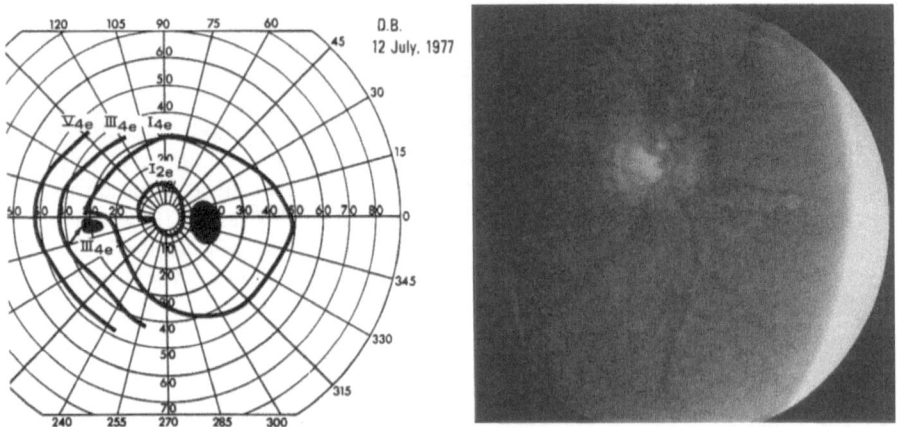

Fig. 2. Case number two; right visual field; right optic disc

224

CASE PRESENTATIONS

For the first two cases both the visual field and the optic disc are shown. For case number two to six only the visual field is shown.

Case number one: a 67 year old man with open angle glaucoma in the left eye shows a nasal step in the I/3e isopter (Figure 1). With the I/4e test object, no nasal step is detected, but a rather dense isolated scotoma is present near the horizontal meridian. The optic nerve head shows a small, round central cup with an intact neuro-retinal rim.

Case number two: a 70 year old man with open angle glaucoma. In the

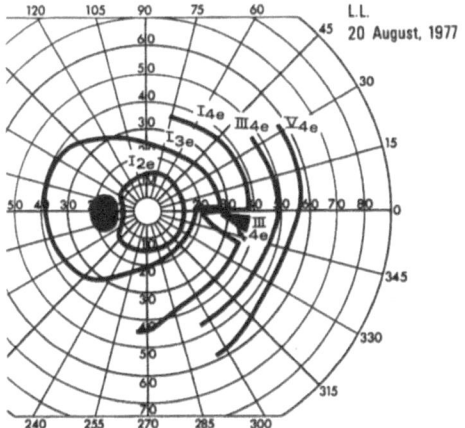

Fig. 3. Case number three; left visual field.

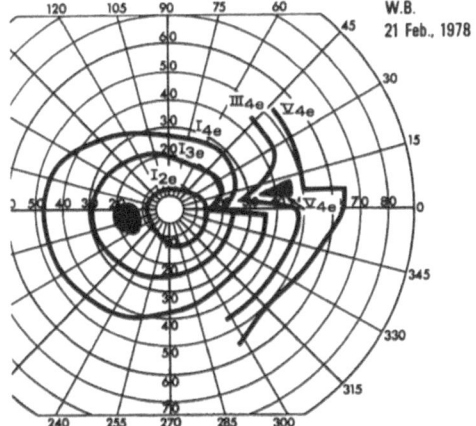

Fig. 4. Case number four; left visual field

225

right eye (Figure 2) nasal steps are present in the central but not peripheral isopters. With the III4e test object, a scotoma is found near the horizontal meridian. The optic nerve head shows an intact neuroretinal rim which is somewhat thinned superotemporally.

Case number three: a 67 year old woman with open angle glaucoma. The left eye (Figure 3) shows an isolated peripheral nasal scotoma with the III4e test object. In the disc the neuroretinal rim was intact, but more markedly thinned superiorly.

Case number four: a 64 year old man with open angle glaucoma. The left eye (Figure 4) demonstrates that even with a nasal step present to the V4e, the largest test object, an isolated nasal scotoma can still sometimes be demonstrated. The optic nerve head was more clearly pathologic and showed a large cup with a notch in the inferior neuroretinal rim.

Case number five: a 75 year old man with open angle glaucoma. Here, the peripheral nasal scotoma in the right eye is associated with a dense central arcuate defect (Figure 5). The optic nerve head showed, as one would predict, extensive loss of the inferior neuroretinal rim with the notch extending to the disc margin.

Case number six: a 65 year old man with open angle glaucoma. Despite treatment, intraocular pressures in the right eye range between 24 and 30 mm Hg. In November, 1977 (Figure 6) an isolated peripheral nasal scotoma is found to the V4e test object associated with nasal steps in the more central isopters. The field of February, 1978 (Figure 7) demonstrates progression. A dense paracentral scotoma has now appeared and the peripheral nasal scotoma has broken through to the periphery completing the nasal step with the V4e. The optic nerve head showed an inferior notch in the neuroretinal rim. The appearance of the disc did not change despite the progression in the field.

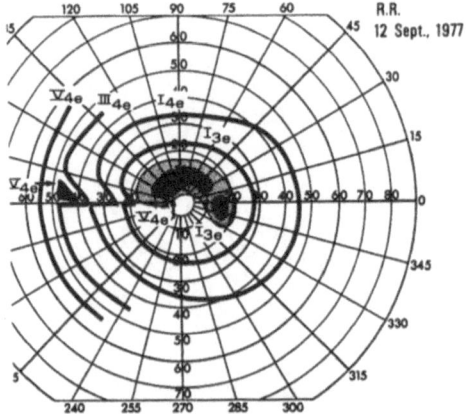

Fig. 5. Case number five; right visual field.

DISCUSSION

As a bundle of nerve fibers is damaged by the glaucomatous process, the ganglion cells from which the bundle arose in a particular area of the retina cease to function. A defect will then appear in the corresponding area of the visual field. In the central field, this defect is almost always a scotoma. Depressions of certain isopters will also occur, depending on the test object used and the location of the scotoma, but the scotoma is the basic defect.

We now can see that exactly the same process occurs when peripheral nerve fiber bundles are involved. A scotoma in the peripheral field appears,

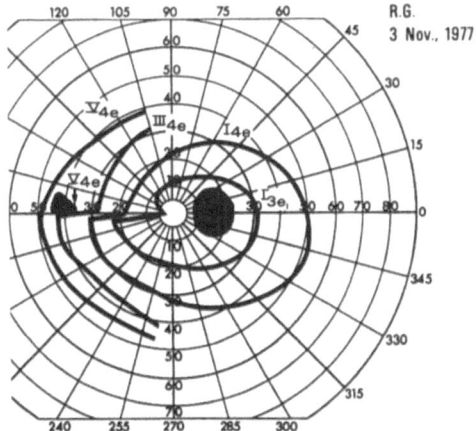

Fig. 6. Case number six; right visual field, 3 November, 1977

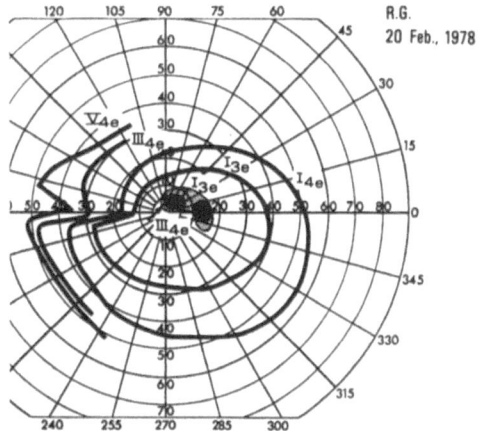

Fig. 7. Case number six; right visual field, 20 February, 1978

227

usually near the horizontal nasal meridian. This scotoma will be associated with depressions of certain isopters producing the classic nasal step. As the scotoma enlarges, it will break through to the periphery, and a nasal step will be present in all isopters.

We might, therefore, think of the nasal step not as a depression which begins peripherally and progresses inward, but as a discrete scotoma which progresses outward as well. We should also consider the possibility that most, if not all, peripheral nasal steps begin as an isolated peripheral nasal scotoma.

REFERENCES

Armaly, M.F. Visual field defects in early open angle glaucoma. *Trans. Amer. Ophthal. Soc.* 69: *147-162* (1971).

Armaly, M.F. Selective perimetry for glaucomatous defects in ocular hypertension. *Arch. Ophthal.* 87: *518-524* (1972).

Aulhorn, E. & Harms, H. Early visual field defects in glaucoma. Glaucoma Symposium Tutzig Castle 1966, pp. 151-186, Karger/Basel, New York (1967).

Drance, S.M. Visual field defects in glaucoma, Symposium on Glaucoma. Transactions of the New Orleans Academy of Ophthalmology, pp. 190-209, C.V. Mosby Co./ St. Louis (1975).

Gorin, G. Clinical Glaucoma, Marcel Dekker/ New York, Basel (1977).

Harrington, D.O. The Visual Fields Fourth Edition. C.V. Mosby/ St. Louis (1976).

Kolker, A.E. & Hetherington, J. Becker-Shaffer's Diagnosis and Therapy of the Glaucomas Fourth Edition. C.V. Mosby/ St. Louis (1976).

Leblanc, R.P. Peripheral nasal defects. Second International Visual Field Symposium Tübingen 1976, pp. 131-133, Dr. W. Junk/ the Hague (1977).

Leblanc, R.P. &Becker, B. Peripheral nasal field defects. *Amer. J. Ophthal.* 72: *415-419* (1971).

Lynn, J.R. Correlation of pathogenesis, anatomy and patterns of visual fields loss in glaucoma, Symposium on Glaucoma. Transactions of the New Orleans Academy of Ophthalmology, pp. 151-186, C.V. Mosby Co./ St. Louis (1975).

Reed, H. & Drance, S.M. The Essentials of Perimetry: Static and (1972).

Scott, G.L. Traquair's Clinical Perimetry Seventh Edition, p. 132, Henry Kimpton, London (1957).

Author's address:
Royal Victoria Hospital
Department of Ophthalmology
687 Pine Ave.West.
Montreal, Quebec H 3A 1A1
Canada

REVERSIBILITY OF VISUAL FIELD
DEFECTS IN SIMPLE GLAUCOMA

IWAO IINUMA

(Wakayama, Japan)

ABSTRACT

Considering that simple glaucoma may be a disease of a generalized metabolic disorder because of its genetic, geriatric and progressive nature, the present author has prescribed anthranilic acids and vitamin B_{12}, when necessary also with other anti-glaucomatous treatments, in 15 simple glaucoma patients for over 10 years and gets a good result in about half of the patients without apparent progress especially in visual fields. The discontinuance of these medications contributed to the progression of visual field defects while re-establishment of their use reversed the process.

INTRODUCTION

Broadly viewing the etiology of simple glaucoma, it may be presumed that progressive loss of visual field is caused not only by elevated intraocular pressure (IOP) or reduced blood supply to the optic disc but also by some noxious agents suspected to be present in the patient's body as an abnormal metabolite. It is because simple glaucoma is defined as a disease of genetic, geriatric and progressive nature with reduced glucose tolerance and other constitutional characteristics. Based on this hypothesis, short-term studies on the treatment of simple glaucoma with anthranilic acids (A.A.) (1, 2) and vitamin B_{12} (V.B_{12}) (5) were initiated. This paper reports the results of a long-term study with these medications.

MATERIALS AND METHODS

A.A. (anthranilic acid in dosis of 1o-60 mg/day or 5-hydroxyanthranilic acid in dosis of 1-6 mg/day) and V.B_{12} (in dosis of 2-3 mg/week) were used singly or in combination. During last 1 year, 47 simple glaucoma patients were treated with A.A. and V.B_{12} and when necessary with miotics, carbonic anhydrase inhibitors or operations. During the previous 10 years period, however, only 15 patients received the treatment involving an extensive course of therapy.

RESULTS AND CASE REPORTS

The effects of A.A. and V.B_{12} on visual fields of 15 cases of simple glaucoma receiving treatment for over 10 years are considered to be beneficial

229

under present conditions of glaucoma treatment. The results can be divided into following 4 groups;

I. In 7 cases (14 eyes) there was no apparent progress, but reversible depressions occurred when the medication was discontinued (Case 2).

II. One case (2 eyes) had a good course for 13 years in our clinic, then went other ophthalmologist who operated her both eyes and treated only with miotics for 18 months, and consequently gradual field loss occurred, but recovered moderately by re-administration of A.A. and V.B$_{12}$ in our clinic.

III. One case (2 eyes) h-a a good course for 8 years in spite of moderately elevated IOP in winter seasons, but when medication tended to be terminated, progressive field defects occurred.

IV. In 6 cases (12 eyes) with almost normally controlled IOP by use of miotics, carbonic anhydrase inhibitors or operations progressive field loss occurred in spite of administration of A.A. and V.B$_{12}$.

DISCUSSION

It is reported that anthranilic acid or 5-hydroxyanthranilic acid is a metabolite of tryptophan and has following physiological functions, 1) promotion of liver functions, 2) promotion of glucose metabolism, 3) diuretic action, 4) recovery from anemia, 5) compensatory function of the adrenal cortex, and 6) partial compensatory function of vitamin C (Kotake 1949, Kotake & Inoue 1955).

Following studies by the present author and his co-laborators (Ando 1958, Iinuma 1975, Iinuma, Ando Murazi & Kawasaki 1956) or other authors (Matsui 1956, Shimizu 1957, Soh, Yanagisawa & Sugawara 1965, Sugawara & Hamada 1957) confirmed the beneficial effects of A.A. in a short-term treatment of simple glaucoma, especially in recovery of defected visual fields and promotion of reduced glucose tolerance.

On the other hand, it is known that V.B$_{12}$ has following physiological functions, 1) aids in recovery from anemia, 2) aids in recovery from lesions of the nervous system, 3) function for transmethylation, 4) formation of nucleic acid, 5) accelating functions for metabolism of amino acids, proteins, carbohydrates or fats (Wakizaka 1961).

Effectiveness of V.B$_{12}$ on defected visual fields of glaucoma was already known by Russian authors (Martynovskaya 1961, Shlopak & Kushnir 1963). Our results of administration of V.B$_{12}$ 2-3 mg/week to simple glaucoma were good and appeared to be especially effective for recovery of defected visual fields and reduced facility of outflow (Iinuma, Ohmi & Toda 1965). Similar reports on the effectiveness of V.B$_{12}$ have also been published (Kishimoto & Nakamori 1965, Okayama, Inoue & Toyofuku 1965).

Although our results of the experience in treating simple glaucoma with both A.A. and V.B$_{12}$ for short period of time have been very good (Kotake & Inoue 1949), it is still too early to make any conclusion about long-term therapy.

As 10 year course may be too short to discuss the prognosis of simple glaucoma with use of some agents but in using A.A. and V.B$_{12}$ over a period of time, better results have been obtained than if used a short-term period. Long-term treatment has proved to be the better course in 7 patients out of 15.

According to Goldmann (1959) or Laydhecker (1959), there is a period of 13 or 18-20 years between the onset of elevated IOP and earliest evidence of field defects. As seen in the description of the most representative cases (Case 1-3), the discontinuance of A.A. and V.B$_{12}$ contributed to the progression of visual field defects while re-establishment of their use reversed the process. These findings support the hypothesis under this study is being conducted.

REFERENCES

Ando, J. Treatment of primary glaucoma by international administration of anthranilic acid. *Folia Ophth. Jap.* 9: *264-271; 274-280; 338-347; 347-353; 405-415; 415-420* (1958) (in Japanese).

Goldmann, H. Some basic problems of simple glaucoma. The Proctor Medal Lecture. *Amer. J. Ophth.* 48: *213-220* (1959).

Iinuma, I. Whole bodily treatment of glaucoma. *Ganka Rinsho Iho* 69: *615-625* (1975) (in Japanese).

Iinuma, I., Ando, J., Murazi, K. & Kawasaki, Y. Use of anthranilic acid, a metabolite of tryptophan, in simple glaucoma. *Acta Soc. Ophth. Jap.* 60: *953-962* (1956) (in Japanese).

Iinuma, I., Ohmi, E. & Toda, M. Preserving treatment from visual dysfunction in glaucoma without ocular hypertension. *Ophthalmology* (Tokyo) 7: *166-173* (1965) (in Japanese).

Kishimoto, M. & Nakamori, F. Effects of vitamin B$_{12}$ on reduced visual function due to glaucoma. *Folia Ophth. Jap.* 16: *291-297* (1965) (in Japanese).

Kotake, Y. Biochemistry of kynurenin. *Biochemistry* (Tokyo) 21: *155* (1949) (in Japanese).

Kotake, Y. & Inoue, K. Studies on xanthurenic acid. *Proc. Jap. Academy* 31: *100-105* (1955).

Leydhecker, W. Zur Verbreitung des Glaucoma simplex in der scheinbar gesunden, augenärztlich nicht behandelten Bevölkerung. *Docum. Ophth.* 13: *357-388* (1959).

Martynovskaya, V.I. Vitamin B$_{12}$ in certain eye disease. *Vest. Oftal.* 74 (3): *31-33* (1961) (in Russian).

Matsui, M. On the effects of 5-oxyanthranilic acid administration on simple glaucoma. *Gamka Rinsho Iho* 50: *867-871* (1956) (in Japanese).

Okayama, T., Inoue, Y. & Toyofuku, H. A therapeutic experience of V.B$_{12}$ (Redisol) in glaucoma. *Ganka Rinsho Iho* 59: *518-522* (1965) (in Japanese).

Shimizu, S. Administration of anthranilic acid tablets, 5-oxyanthranilic acid tablets and 5-oxin tablets for glaucoma. *Clin. Ophth.* 11: *57-62* (1957) (in Japanese).

Shlopak, T.V., Kushnir, P.K. The use of cobalt-containing preparations in a complex treatment of primary glaucoma. *Vest. Oftal.* 76 (1): *15-20* (1963) (in Russian).

Soh, Y., Yanagisawa, K. & Sugawara, H. On the long-term administration of 5-hydroxyanthranilic acid to asthenopia or simple glaucoma patients. *J. Jap. Med. Ass.* 45: *1225-1260* (1965) (in Japanese).

Suda, K. Diagnosis and therapy of primary glaucoma. *Acta Soc. Ophth. Jap.* 69: *595-632* (1965) (in Japanese).

Sugawara, A. & Hamada, M. Effects of 5-oxin tablets on several ocular diseases. *Clin. Ophth.* 11: *683-687* (1957) (in Japanese).

Wakizaka, K. Physiological functions of vitamin B_{12} and its clinical application. *Advances in Vitaminology* III; pp. 243-323, *Jap. Vitam. Soc., Tokyo* (1961) (in Japanese).

Author's address:
Department of Ophthalmology
Wakayama Rosai Hospital
435 Koya Wakayama 640
Japan

REVERSIBLE CUPPING AND REVERSIBLE FIELD DEFECT IN GLAUCOMA

KAZUO IWATA

(Niigata, Japan)

ABSTRACT

For the early diagnosis and the treatment of open-angle glaucoma it is very important to reveal the nature of the reversibility of field defect. The correlation between fundus and visual field change during 5 years in 42 cases of open-angle glaucoma was studied retrospectively and was analyzed stereoscopically and stereometrically. Reversible cupping showed no observable retinal nerve fiber layer defect and left no permanent field defect. Well defined wedge-shaped retinal nerve fiber bundle defect demonstrated permanent arcuate scotoma and large nasal step which showed no significant recovery. Narrow slit-like retinal nerve fiber layer defect showed small nasal step or small scotomata, however, they were unstable and intermittently disappeared. It should be recognized·that the loss of optic nerve fibers can never recover, and leaves corresponding permanent field loss.

INTRODUCTION

As generally accepted, reversible cupping in glaucoma can be observed in younger patients, and leaves no permanent field defect (Iwata et al. 1977; Shaffer & Hetherington 1969). On the other hand, in eyes with enlarged cupping by structural destruction, the retinal nerve fiber bundle (RNFB) defect (Hoyt et al. 1973), arcuate scotoma and nasal step were always proved.

To decide on the right time of treatment of early open-angle glaucoma, it is very important to reveal the nature of the reversibility of field defect. The purpose of this study is to reveal such nature.

MATERIAL AND METHOD

From our glaucoma clinic well documented open-angle glaucoma patients who have been well controlled during the past 5 years 42 patients were selected. In this series 2 patients showing reversible cupping, 22 patients showing clearly defined retinal nerve fiber bundle (RNFB) defect, and 18 patients showing narrow slit-like RNF layer defect were retrospectively studied. Each patient was followed by stereophotography in color of large size and·by Goldmann perimeter and Friedman's visual field analyzer.

For the stereophotogrammetry of optic cupping the previously reported method (Iwata et al. 1974) was employed. To eliminate the factors affecting the visual field cases with cataracta, retinal vascular disease and inflammation were not included in this series.

RESULTS

Reversible cupping and defect
of visual field

Case 1. A 21-year-old man, who was referred to us for bilateral steroid glaucoma. As showed in Fig. 1, one month after the reduction of the IOP to normal level C/D became 0.62 from the initial 0.80 (Fig. 1). The stereophotogrammetry revealed that the excavated cup wall was put back to the original place, and any irregular recovery was not observed (Fig. 2).

Any RNFB defect or any slit-like RNF layer defect before and after the recovery was not found by stereophotography. By Goldmann perimeter no isopter change and no field defect were demonstrated before and after the recovery, however, paracentral spot-like slight depressions were proved at the initial examination. But 4 weeks after the normalization of IOP the depressions disappeared completely.

Case 2. An 11-year-old boy, who was referred to us for the management of steroid glaucoma which was induced by application of 6 months steroid eye drops on the left eye.

IOP: r = 19 mmHg,   l = 35 mmHg
C/D: r = 0.42,   l = 0.82 $\longrightarrow$ 0.54 (one month after normalisation of IOP)

Stereophotogrammetry revealed the same pattern of recovery as seen in Case 1. No irregularity of cup and no RNF layer defect were identified before and after recovery. Goldmann isopter was normal. Friedman's ana-

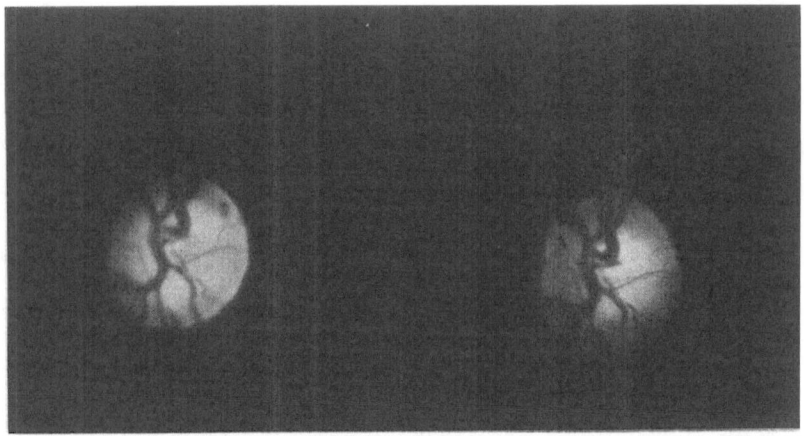

Fig. 1. 21 year-old man, steroidglaucoma. Remarkable recovery of cupping.
C/D: 0.80 $\longrightarrow$ 0.62

lyzer showed paracentral slight spot-like depression, which disappeared completely after 2 weeks of normalization of IOP. The findings of these two cases indicate that reversible cupping occurs without any observable optic nerve fiber loss, and proved that paracentral scotomata due to high IOP can occur without any demonstrable loss of optic nerve fibers. Therefore, such scotomata may be attributable to transient pressure dependent impairment of optic nerve fiber function.

Retinal nerve fiber bundle
defect and visual field

As Hoyt already demonstrated, well defined RNFB defect with connecting localized elongation of cup means without doubt loss of neural elements. Observed cases were divided into 2 types according to the RNF layer defect on the correlation to visual field defects.

1. WELL DEFINED WEDGE SHAPED RNFB
DEFECT AND FIELD DEFECT

The findings of 30 eyes of 22 patient of open-angle glaucoma showing well defined wedge shaped RNFB defect with connecting localized disc tissue loss were analyzed. All these patients were well controlled under 20 mm Hg of IOP during the past 5 years (Fig. 3).

As showed in Table 1, sharply defined RNFB defect demonstrated permanent arcuate scotoma, and relatively well defined RNFB defect demonstrated nasal step and paracentral small scotomata. During 5 years the nasal step and the arcuate scotoma demonstrated no significant improvement and

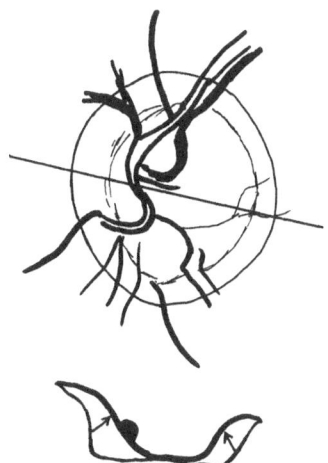

Fig. 2. Stereophtogrammetry of cupping recovery

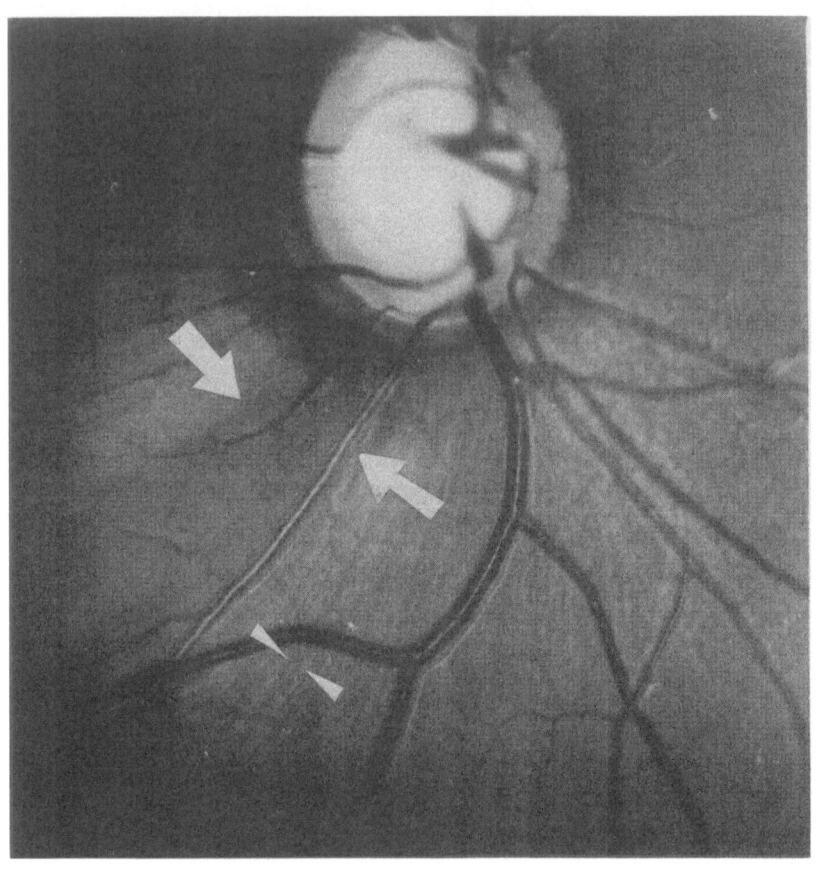

Fig. 3. Well defined wedge shaped RNFB defect and slit-like RNF layer defect

Table 1. Five years course of visual field defects accompanied by RNFB defect on 30 eyes of open-angle glaucoma

	No. of eyes	Increase	Non significant change	unstable	Dis- appearance
Nasal step	26	4	22	none	none
Arcuate scotoma	15	2	13	none	none
Additional Paracentral scotomata	22	3	16	3	none

no disappearance. In 9 eyes progressive visual field impairment was observed. Paracentral spot-like scotomata were, however, unstable in 3 eyes. The rest of the eyes showed no significant variation of field changes.

From the results it may be concluded that well developed RNFB defects cannot cause any reversible visual field defect and any significant improvement, except for paracentral spot-like scotomata.

2. SLIT-LIKE RNF LAYER DEFECT AND VISUAL FIELD

In the earliest stage of open-angle glaucoma one or two slit-like RNF layer defect with ca 200μ width can be identified by stereoscopic observation as a slit-like gap in RNF layer (Fig. 3). The 5 years variations of 20 eyes of 18 patients with such slit-like defect were followed. As showed in Table 2, slit-like RNF layer defect caused small nasal step, vertical step and paracentral small spot-like scotomata in I-2-c level of Goldmann's perimeter (Table 2). These small visual field defects disappeared intermittently in some cases. No arcuate scotoma was proved. Therefore, this slit-like RNF layer defect may be evaluated as the earliest sign of structural destruction of optic nerve fiber.

DISCUSSION

It is well experienced that induced constriction of isopter and Bjerrum scotoma by artificially elevated or by spontaneously raised IOP disappear completely after reduction of IOP (Radius & Maumenee 1977, Vanderburg

Table 2. Five years course of visual field defect accompanied by slit-like RNF layer defect on 20 eyes of open-angle glaucoma

	No. of Eyes	No significant change	Intermittent disappearance	Complete disappearance
Small Nasal step	16	11	5	none
Small Vertical step	4	2	2	none
Small Spot-like scotomata	8	5	3	none
Arcuate scotoma	none	none	none	none

237

& Drance 1966). In open-angle glaucoma in which the IOP does not reach to high a level, the change of the visual field is different from acute angle-closure glaucoma, even if it can be reversible within a reversible lesion.

In open-angle glaucoma it is correct without doubt that when relatively high IOP accompanies paracentral visual field defect, then the diagnosis of glaucoma is established. Therefore, the earliest detection of field defect is indispensable for the early diagnosis. If the earliest defect of visual field can be completely reversible, it is still early enough to begin to treat at the moment when the earliest defect is detected. Armaly (1969) reported reversible visual field defect and concluded that the field defect in glaucoma may be completely reversible and its recovery is related to reduction in ocular pressure level. Reversibility of the glaucomatous defect underlines the need for its early detection by careful examination of the visual field.

According to my observations the early visual field defect, however, is not always completely reversible. Therefore, it should be clarified which type of field defect is reversible. To solve such problem I attempted to search a morphological fundus change for an index of reversibility of field defect. The reversible cupping could occur without any optic nerve fiber loss, and the caused paracentral spot-like scotomata disappeared completely in the course. This recovery of visual field means that there was no organic structural damage in optic nerve fibers.

In the earliest open-angle glaucoma with narrow slit-like RNF layer defect the proved small nasal step and small spot-like scotomata disappeared intermittently. This unstable scotoma means that the destruction of optic nerve fiber is on a borderline of organic and functional destruction. Recently Sommer et al. (1977) reported that each eye that lost visual field demonstrated consistent abnormalities of the nerve fiber layer, beginning as early as 5 years before it developed glaucomatous visual field defects on routine Goldmann perimetry. They applied as routine isoptometry I-2-e. However, according to my analysis, I-2-e level is not enough to catch the earliest change of visual field. Therefore, I applied I-2-c or I-2-b. The result, which differs from the result of Sommer et al., was that with the identification of narrow slit-like RNF layer defect, the corresponding nasal step, vertical step and spot-like scotomata on Bjerrum area could be surely demonstrated. Therefore, in open-angle glaucoma the narrow slit-like RNF layer defect should be estimated as the earliest sign of organic destruction of optic nerve fiber. On the contrary, well defined RNFB defect demonstrates permanent arcuate scotoma and nasal step and proves never significant recovery of field defect, under well controlled IOP.

Finally, it is most important to recognize that loss of optic nerve fiber can never recover and leaves permanent field loss.

SUMMARY

The development of 42 patients with early open-angle glaucoma over a period of 5 years was retrospectively studied by stereophotography, stereo-photogrammetry and campi- and perimetry. Different from acute angle-closure glaucoma, in early stage identified RNFB defect showed permanent stable field defect or nasal step, and in the earliest stage identifiable narrow slit-like RNF layer defect demonstrated occasionally unstable small nasal step or spot-like scotomata. This narrow slit-like RNF layer defect should be, therefore, estimated as the earliest sign of organic destruction of open-angle glaucoma.

REFERENCES

Armaly, M.F. The visual field defect and ocular pressure level in open-angle glaucoma. *Invest. Ophthalm.* 8: *105* (1969).

Hoyt, W.F. et al. Fundoscopy of nerve fiber layer defects in Glaucoma. *Invest. Ophthalm.* 13: *815* (1973).

Iwata, K. et al. On the correlation between Glaucomatous Disc and Visual field. *Acta. Soc. Ophthalm.* Jap. 78: *148* (1974).

Iwata, K. et al. On the reversibility of the Glaucomatous Disc Cupping and the Visual Field. *Jap. J. Clini. Ophthalmol.* 31: *759* (1977).

Radius, R.L. & Maumenee, A.E. visual field changes following acute elevation of IOP. *Trans. Amer. Acad. Ophthal. Otol.* 83: *op-61* (1977).

Shaffer, R.N. & Hetherington, J.Jr. The glaucomatous disc in infants. *Trans. Amer. Acad. Ophthal. Otol.* 73: *929* (1969).

Sommer, A. et al. The nerve fiber layer in the diagnosis of glaucoma. *Arch. Ophthalm.* 95: *2149* (1977).

Vanderburg, D. & Drance, S.M. Studies of the effects of artificially raised IOP on retinal defferential thresholds of the Bjerrum area. *Am. J. Ophthal.* 62: *1049* (1966).

Author's address:
Dept. of Ophthalmology
Niigata University
School of Medicine
Niigata-shi, Asachicho – 1
Japan

Docum. Ophthal. Proc. Series, Vol. 19

THE REVERSIBILITY OF VISUAL FIELD
DEFECTS IN THE JUVENILE GLAUCOMA CASES

KUNIYOSHI MIZOKAMI, YUSAKU TAGAMI
& YOSHIMASA ISAYAMA

(Kobe, Japan)

ABSTRACT

In the early stage of juvenile glaucoma cases, we followed up the changes of the spot-like scotomas in the Bjerrum area with newly developed our Quantitative Maculometry with direct fundus examination and the other perimetries. In the present study, we analysed the relationship between the appearance of scotomas and the defects of the arcuate nerve fiber bundles which were photographed through red-free filters, in other words, we marked the scotomas on the fundus photographs and determined their accurate position in the fundus. In some cases with no nerve fiber bundle defects, the scotomas diminished or disappeared after the intraocular pressure was controlled. However, if the nerve fiber bundle defects had already appeared, the scotomas did not diminish under the control of the ocular pressure. In the cases of the juvenile glaucoma, the scotomas without nerve fiber bundle defects were considered that they have the possibility of a transient loss of the nerve fiber function.

INTRODUCTION

In the recent studies, it has been documented that the glaucomatous visual field defects sometimes improve after the control of the ocular pressure (Armaly, 1969; Heilmann, 1972; Greve, 1975). However, the mechanism of their reversibility in field changes still remains an enigma inspite of extensive studies. On the other hand, atrophic changes of retinal nerve fiber bundles corresponding to the glaucomatous visual field defects could be observed by exact red-free fundus photography (Hoyt, 1973; Sommer, 1977). In this paper, we studied the correlation between the reversibility of the early glaucomatous visual field defects and the atrophic changes of retinal nerve fiber bundles in juvenile glaucoma cases.

MATERIALS & METHODS

The materials include 5 early stages of juvenile glaucoma cases with clear optical media, which is the most important factor aiding the visualization of the nerve fiber bundles. In every case several spot-like scotomas were detected by the campimeter (Auto-plot tangent screen) and the quantitative perimeter (Tübinger's static perimeter) with high ocular pressure (over 20 mm Hg) at the time of the first consultation. The spot-like scotomas were re-examined by Quantitative Maculometry with direct fundus examination

(Isayama & Tagami, 1977) in order to obtain the exact position of the scotomas in the fundus. The retinal nerve fiber bundles were also examined by red-free fundus photography using a Topcon TRC-FB fundus camera with its 2x magnification attachment. A Fuji BPB 53 filter with a transmission peak of 530 nm was used for the red-free filters. Controlling the ocular pressure (under 20mmHg), these spot-like scotomas were followed up using the same perimeter and Quantitative Maculometry. The atrophic changes of the retinal nerve fiber bundles were also followed up through red-free fundus photography.

RESULTS

In our follow-up cases, the scotomas in two cases clearly diminished (Case 1, Case 2 in Table 1), while in the other cases the scotomas did not improve (Case 3, 4, 5).

A. Recovered Cases

Case 1 (Fig. 1, 2); 23 year-old-male. He was admitted to our glaucoma clinic on December, 9, 1976. At that time, his ocular pressure was 24 mmHg (C-value, 0.08), and a spot-like scotoma on the Bjerrum area could be detected using the campimeter and the quantitative static perimeter. The scotoma was re-examined through Quantitative Maculometry for locating the accurate position in the fundus. In red-free fundus photography, the nerve

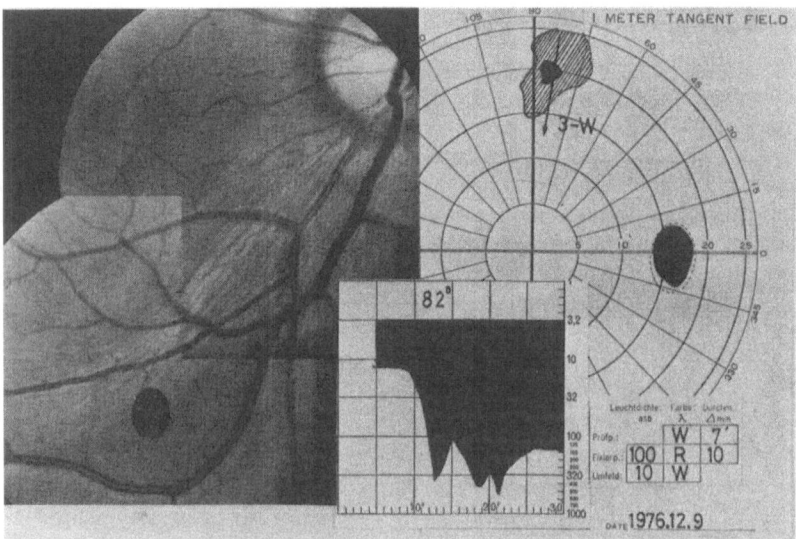

Fig. 1. Case 1, the spot-like scotoma under high ocular pressure and the red-free photograph.

242

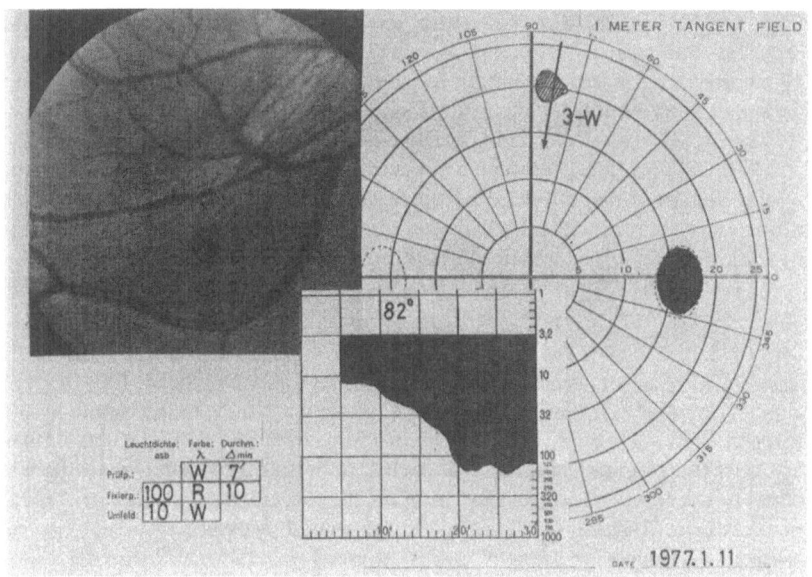

Fig. 2. Case 1, the diminished scotoma after controled ocular pressure.

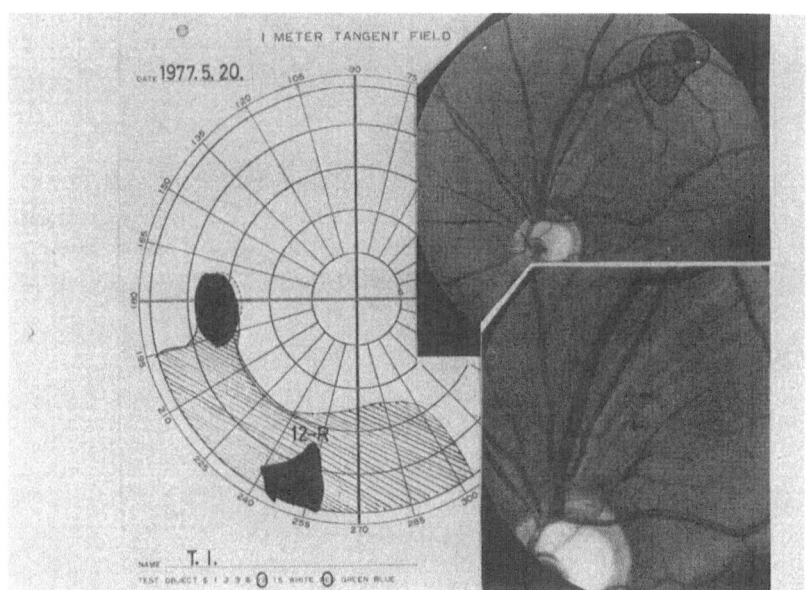

Fig. 3. the scotoma in Case 3 and the red-free fundus photography, (slit-like nerve fiber defects corresponding to the scotoma are seen arrows).

fiber bundle defects did not correspond to the position of the scotoma (Fig. 1). One month following the control of the ocular pressure (below 17 mmHg) by 1% pilocarpine, the scotoma was significantly diminished and the nerve fiber bundles unchanged (Fig. 2).

Case 2: 34 year-old-female. She was admitted to our clinic on February, 3, 1976. At that time, her ocular pressure was 25 mmHg (C-value, 0.10) and a spot-like scotoma on the Bjerrum area could be found. There were no nerve fiber bundle defects corresponding to the scotoma. Following the control of the ocular pressure, the scotoma gradually diminished (Fig. 3).

B. Not Recovered Cases

Case 3: 33 year-old-male. At the time of his first admission, the pressure was 22 mmHg (C-value, 0.08) and a scotoma could be detected in the Bjerrum area. Through red-free fundus photography slit-like nerve fiber bundle defects could be observed, corresponding to the scotoma, which was then re-examined through Quantitative Maculometry with direct fundus examination. Despite the control of the ocular pressure, the scotoma remained unchanged.

Case 4 and 5: 35 year-old-male, 25 year-old-male. At the time of their first consultation, high ocular pressure and scotomas were found. And the nerve fiber bundle defects corresponded to the presence of the scotomas. Despite the control of the ocular pressure, their scotomas remained unchanged.

Therefore, in our cases with no nerve fiber bundle defects, the scotomas diminished or disappeared after the ocular pressure was controled. However, if the nerve fiber bundle defects corresponding to the scotoma had already appeared, the scotomas did not change even under the control of the ocular pressure.

DISCUSSION

In recent studies, it has been documented that the glaucomatous visual field defects sometimes diminish after control of the ocular pressure. However the mechanisms of their reversibility still remains an enigma inspite of ex-

Table 1. The subjects and the results.

	Ocular pressure	C-value	Visual acuity	Changes of scotoma after controlled O.P.	Nerve fiber bundle Defect corresponded to the scotoma
Case 1 23-y M Right	24	0.08	20/20	significantly improved	No-bundle defect
Case 2 34-y F Right	25	0.10	20/20	improved	No-bundle defect
Case 3 33-y M Right	22	0.08	20/20	no-change	Slit-like defect
Case 4 35-y M Right	27	0.11	20/20	no-change	Slit-like defect
Case 5 25-y M Right	28 mmHg	0.13	20/20	no-change	Wedge-like defect

tensive studies. Greve, E.L. and co-workers (1975, 1977) reported that the glaucomatous visual field defects sometimes improve after a filtering operation. There were no dramatic changes in the extent and the intensity of the defects. One case showed no significant improvement of visual field defects and it seemed that the nerve fibers were dead. According to Armaly, M.F. (1969), the field defects in glaucoma may be completely reversible and their recovery related to the reduction of the ocular pressure level.

However, marked indivisual variabilities exist, indicating the operation of other factors. One of these factors is aging. With increasing age a smaller magnitude of pressure rise is required to produce changes in the visual field. Thus an increase of the pressure level can indeed produce field defects identical to those of open angle glaucoma and increase with advancing age. Equally significant is the course of recovery of those defects.

In this study, juvenile glaucoma cases were examined because factors aiding reliable visualization of nerve fiber layers are dilated pupils and clear optical media. In our cases, significant and dramatic improvement of visual field defects were seen after the control of the ocular pressure. Therefore, it seems that a more detailed study of the relationship between these improvements and aging have to be undertaken.

On the other hand, glaucomatous nerve fiber bundle defects such as slit-like defects in arcuate fibers can be observed at a stage of this desease when abnormality of the optic disc and the visual field would be regarded as marginal (Hoyt, 1973). Sommer, A. and co-workers (1977) reported that nerve fiber bundle defects appeared several years before the visual field defects were detected in routine Goldmann's perimetry. But, Iwata, K. and co-workers (1975) demonstrated that the nerve fiber bundle defects can not be observed photographically in many open angle glaucoma cases with visual field defects. In this study, we found glaucomatous visual field defects with or without nerve fiber bundle defects in the early stages of juvenile glaucoma. We believe that the visual field defects attributed to the functional nerve fiber bundle damage occur at first and later the nerve fiber degeneration increases the nerve fiber bundle defects which can be observed photographically and correspond to the visual field defects.

In this study, it is demonstrated that in cases with no nerve fiber bundle defects the scotomas diminish after the ocular pressure is controlled, while cases with nerve fiber bundle defects corresponding to the scotomas the scotomas remain unchanged even after the control of the pressure.

In recent studies, the axoplasmic transport of material from the nerve cell down its axon has caught the interest of researchers (Anderson, 1974; Minckler, 1977). Alteration in the axoplasmic transport may play a significant role in the pathogenesis of visual damage in glaucoma. This concept is supported by experimental studies demonstrating that orthograde transport in ganglion cell axons is blocked in the nerve head in experimental ocular hypertension. Therefore it can be speculated that the early stage of ocular elevation may be associated with the interference of the axoplasmic flow in normal appearaning nerve fiber bundles. The changes interfere in the function of the nerve fibers and cause result visual field defects.

However, after the ocular pressure is controlled, the axoplasmic flow may be recovered and the result visual field defects improved.

Therefore, visual field improvement related to the ocular pressure can be expected in the early stages of the defects as in the subjects of this study.

REFERENCES

Anderson, D.R. & Hendrickson, A.E. Effect of intraocular pressure on rapid axoplasmic transport in monkey optic nerve. *Invest. Ophthalmol.* 13: *771-783* (1974).

Armaly, M.F. The visual field defect and ocular pressure level in open angle glaucoma. *Invest. Ophthalmol.* 8: *105-124* (1969).

Greve, E.L., Dake, C.L. & Verduin, W.M. Pre- and postoperative results of static perimetry in patients with glaucoma simplex. *Ophthalmologica* 175: *1* (1977).

Greve, E.L., Dake, C.L. & Verduin, W.M. Reversibility of visual field defects in glaucoma. *Exp. Eye Rec.* 20: *183* (1975).

Heilmann, K. Intraocular Druck und Gesichtsfeldschädigung. In: Augendruck, Blutdruck und Glaukomschaden, Bücherei des Augenarztes, 61: *29-46* (1972).

Hoyt, W.F., Frisén, L. & Newman, N.M. Fundoscopy of nerve fiber layer defects in glaucoma. *Invest. Ophthalmol.* 12: *814-829* (1973).

Isayama, Y. & Tagami, Y. Quantitative Maculometry using a new instrument in cases of optic neuropathies. *Docum. Ophthal. Proc. Series* 14: *237-242* (1977).

Iwata, K., Yaoeda, H. & Sofue, K. Changes of nerve fiber layer in glaucoma. Report 2. Clinical Observation. *Acta Soc. Ophthalm. Jap.* 79: *1110-1118* (1975).

Minckler, D.S., Bunt, A.H. & Johanson, G.W. Orthograde and retrograde axoplasmic transport during acute ocular hypertension in the monkey. *Invest. Ophthalmol. Visual Sci.* 16: *426-441* (1977).

Author's address:
Department of Ophthalmology
School of Medicine
Kobe University
Kusunoki-cho, 7-chome
Ikuta-ku
Kobe, Japan

EARLY STAGE PROGRESSION IN
GLAUCOMATOUS VISUAL FIELD CHANGES

FUMIO FURUNO & HARUTAKE MATSUO

(Tokyo, Japan)

ABSTRACT

A group of visual fields of 39 eyes of glaucoma patients which progressed from normal te defective was investigated to find the frequency of early glaucomatous changes based on the results of quantitative examination with an FVFA. The frequency distribution was discussed.

Fourteen selected glaucomatous eyes were investigated to see the progression of the early stages of glaucomatous visual field changes. Three patterns of progression were found.

The spot-like scotoma on the Bjerrum's Area (BA) and the peripheral nasal defect have been considered to be the most important early visual field changes in glaucoma. We have already reported in 1976 the frequency distribution of the early glaucomatous changes on central visual field (within 30°) as measured by Kinetic Perimetry (KP) using the Goldmann Perimeter (GP) and Multiple Stimulus Static Perimetry (MSSP) using the Friedmann Visual Field Analyser (FVFA) (Shinzato et al., 1976). Also, every one can well remember the report of Aulhorn's frequency distribution which was analysed from a great number of kinetic visual fields (Aulhorn & Karmeyer, 1976).

In KP, the results of the examinations are variable using different techniques depending on how careful the technician is, how the target was moved and how fast the target was moved in each examination. Therefore, if successive visual fields showed different results, this different result might be caused by a technical mistake. On the other hand, MSSP measures at fixed examination points and hardly uses any meticulous technique. Hence the results can be more stable than KP and Single stimulus static perimetry which requires a high degree of technical skill. Therefore MSSP has an advantage to evaluate progression of the visual field changes and also the frequency distribution.

In this study we have analysed the early glaucomatous visual field changes and their progression based on the results of the FVFA.

MATERIALS AND METHODS

This study was done in Amsterdam and Tokyo. In the eye clinic of Amsterdam, 39 FVFA visual fields with early glaucomatous defects that developed

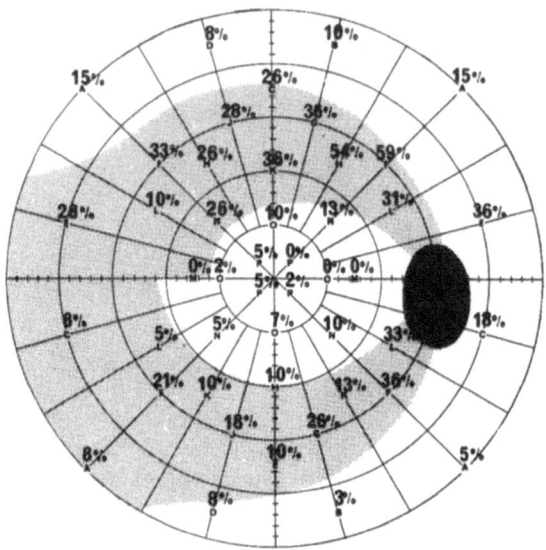

Fig. 1. The frequency of early glaucomatous visual field changes in a group of Amsterdam patients (39 eyes). The shadowed area indicates the presumed nerve fiber pathway including the higher frequency stimulus points.

Table 1. Number of eyes in the 3 types of progression pattern (14 eyes).

Types	Temp. BA to Nasal BA	Middle BA	Nasal BA to Temp. BA	TOTAL
Upper half	4	3	2	9
Lower half	3	1	1	5
TOTAL	7	4	3	14

after documented normal fields were analysed to determine the frequency of finding an early glaucomatous defects on each stimulus point. For that purpose, each result of the left eye was converted to the right eye. The value of the neutral density filter indicating the intensity of the defect at each stimulus point was converted into the value of depression as a difference from the normal level of each visual field. This normal level was defined as the highest value of filter in each visual field (excluding the value of fovae). More than 0.6 log U depression was regarded as a pathological depression. The frequency of finding a pathological depression was analysed on each stimulus point of the FVFA.

In Tokyo, early glaucomatous visual field were selected from the results of FVFA which had been examined for the past two years in our clinic. Finally, 14 eyes which had a good follow-up study from a normal field to an early glaucomatous visual field or from very early visual field changes to significant changes in the progression, were selected for studying the pro-

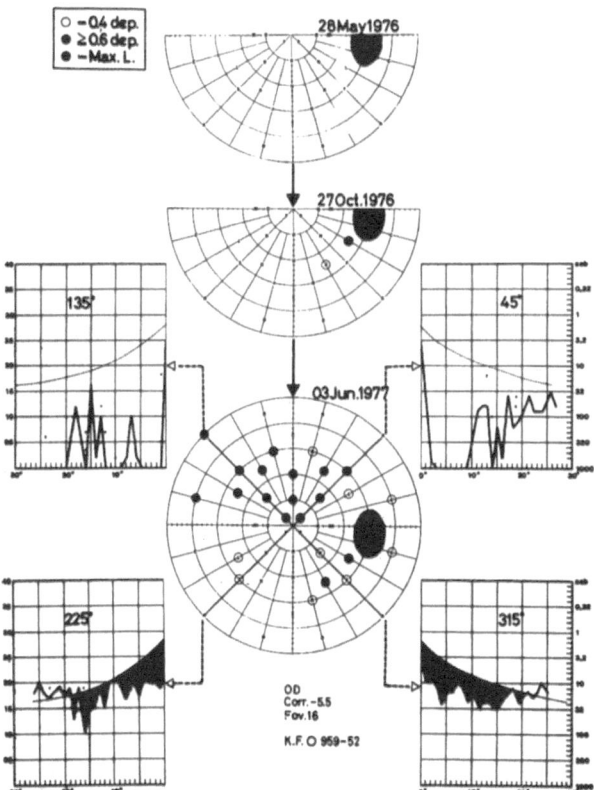

Fig. 2. An example of the type of temporal BA to nasal BA. The upper half field had absolute arcuate defect and no defect in the lower half at first. Then, 0.8 log.U and 0.4 log.U of depressions were observed in the lower half close to the blind spot.

gression. Each visual field was divided into upper and lower half fields, because the stage of progression in the each half was different in the glaucomatous visual field.

RESULTS

I) The frequency of finding early glaucomatous visual field changes in a group of Amsterdam patients (Fig. 1), resulted in following 3 tendencies.
1) Higher frequency was found in the upper half field (67%) than the lower half (33%).
2) In each half field, the highest frequency was located on the temporal side on the BA close to the blind spot.
3) An area of nerve fiber pathway corresponding to the higher frequency stimulus points was indicated in each half field as in figure 1. The upper half defects are situated closer to the fixation point than in the lower half.
II) The following three patterns of progression were seen in the study of 14 eyes in Tokyo (Table 1).

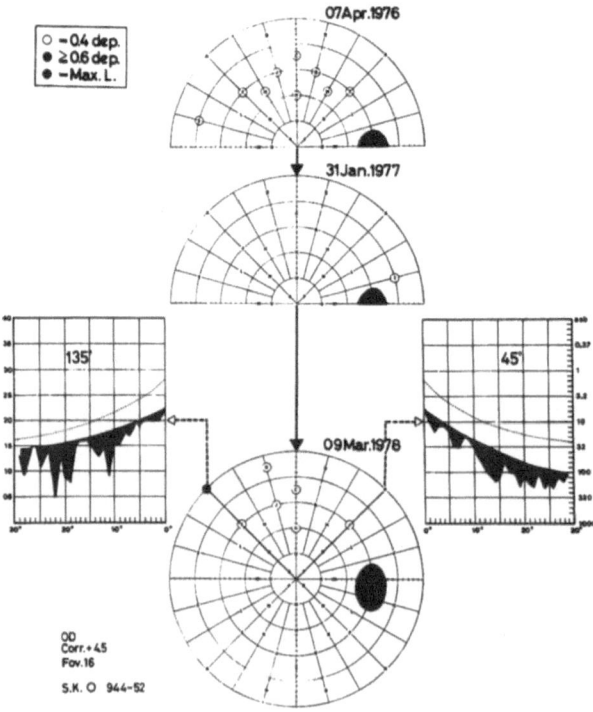

Fig. 3. An example of the type of middle BA. In this case, the visual field had no defect at the beginning of the follow-up study. Then, the 0.4 log.U of depressions were detected on the BA of the upper half. Afterwards, these depressions first improved and became deeper than at their first appearance later on.

250

1) A type of temporal BA to nasal BA. This means, relative depressions appear in the temporal of BA first, then in the nasal side. 7 eyes of the 14 had this type of progression and it was most common in the cases study (Fig. 2).

2) A type of middle BA which stretches over the vertical meridian. In this type, the depression area developed to either one or both sides along the presumed nerve fiber pathway. This type was observed in 4 eyes of the 14 (Fig. 3).

3) A type of nasal BA to temporal BA. 3 eyes of the 14 had this type of progression (Fig. 4).

In this early stage progression, the location and depth of depression were variable in the individual visual field. However, the location of the depression seems to follow the presumed nerve fiber pathway in each eye.

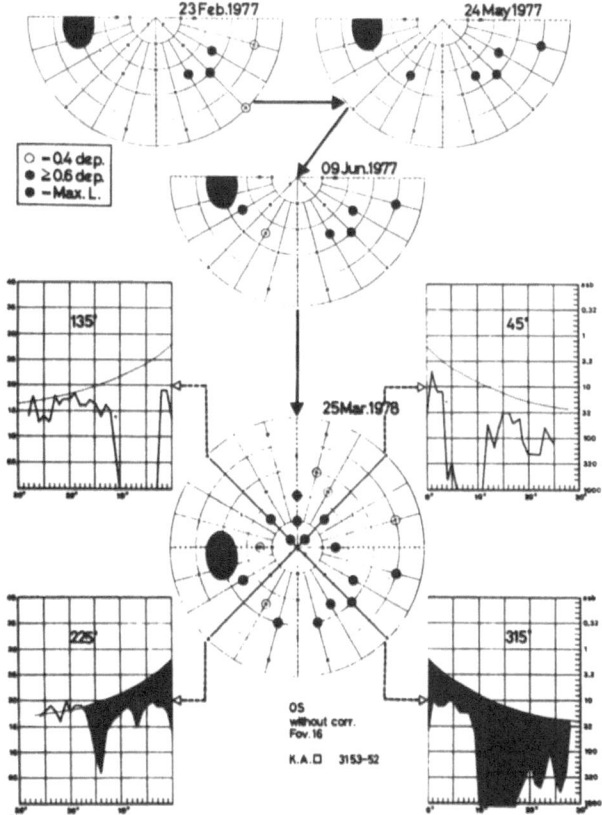

Fig. 4. An example of the type of nasal BA to temporal BA. The upper half field had an absolute arcuate defect already when the lower half had a relative defect. This relative defect was observed in the nasal side on the BA first then temporal side.

Aulhorn devided the progression of glaucomatous visual field into 5 stages. A stage of 'spot-like, stroke-like or arcuated absolute defect, still without connection to the blind spot' was considered as an important stage and a stage of relative defects was omitted from the study. For that reason, the stage of relative defects has not yet been established. Nevertheless, in my opinion, this stage of relative defects is the most important stage for keeping the visual field and for getting some information for management. The highest incidence of early defects found in the temporal BA close to the blind spot. This result is similar to our earlier result (Shinzato et al., 1976), and is little different from Aulhorn's (Fig. 5) (Aulhorn & Karmeyer, 1976). This small difference could occur due to different stages analysed in these studies. However, the most interesting thing is that in the upper half of the VF the defects are more close to the fixation point than in the lower one regardless of the different stages. Presumably, this indicates a small morphological difference of nerve fiber pathway in the upper and lower halves of the disc and retina.

The anatomy of the nerve fiber layer of the retina has long attracted the attention of researchers. Most papers were based on red-free light examination. There are a few interesting studies by Vrabec (1966), Laties (1970) of nerve fiber pathway using microscope and by Ogden using auto-radiography (1974) (Ogden, 1974). However, the correlation between the so-called nerve fiber bundle defect and nerve fiber pathway is not yet proven to be valid.

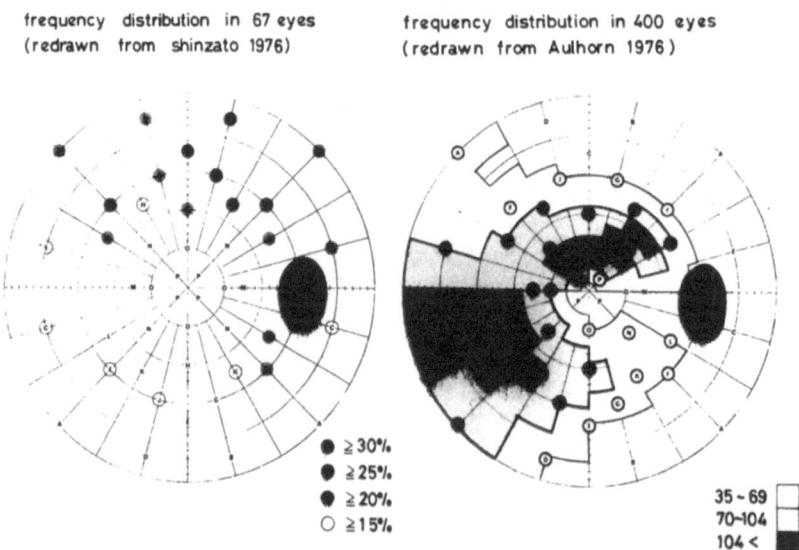

frequency distribution in 67 eyes (redrawn from shinzato 1976)

frequency distribution in 400 eyes (redrawn from Aulhorn 1976)

● ≧30%
● ≧25%
● ≧20%
○ ≧15%

35~69
70~104
104<

Fig. 5 Frequency distributions of early glaucomatous defects according to our result in 1976 and to Aulhorn's in that same year.

Hence, more physiological and morphological studies of nerve fiber bundles would be welcomed. The pattern of progression was divided into 3 types from this study in Tokyo. Half of our 14 eyes had a type of temporal BA to the nasal side and this result will support the frequency of early glaucomatous changes found in Amsterdam.

In early stage progressions, the location and depth of depression changed in the individual visual fields. However, the location of the depression seems to wander along the presumed nerve fiber pathway in each eye. Then, if the early depression deteriorated to an absolute defect, the location did not undergo further change. This stage indicates not only the functional damage of the nerve fiber bundle but the beginning of atrophy.

A reduction of sensitivity of 0.6 log.U was defined as the critical value for a pathological depression, although sometimes 0.4 log.U of depression suggested the early glaucomatous change. In my opinion most 0.4 log.U of depressions are part of the spontaneous normal variations.

However, if a few 0.4 log.U depressions are distributed along the nerve fiber pathway, these will suggest a glaucomatous change. Also, if a pathological depression was related to 0.4 log.U depressions along the nerve fiber pathway, these 0.4 log.U depressions should be regarded as pathological. On the other hand, if an isolated 0.6 log.U of depression was observed in the temporal BA this depression has a high possibility of an angioscotomata and a re-examination with eccentric fixation target will be necessary.

REFERENCES

Aulhorn, E. & Karmeyer, H. Frequency Distribution in Glaucomatous Visual Field Defect. *Doc. Ophthal. Proc. Series* 14: *75-83* (1976).
Laties, A.M. Method for Permanent in Situ Display of Retinal Nerve Fiber Layer Anatomy. *Amer. J. Ophthal.* 70: *284-287* (1970).
Ogden, T.E. The Nerve-Fiber Layer of the Primate Retina: An Autoradiographic study. *Invest. Ophthal.* 13: *95-100* (1974).
Shinzato, E., Suzuki, R. & Furuno, F. The Central Visual Field Changes in Glaucoma using Goldmann Perimeter and Friedmann Visual Field Analyser. *Doc. Ophthal. Proc. Series* 14: *93-101* (1976).
Vrabec, F. The Temporal Raphe of the Human Retina. *Amer. J. Ophthal.* 62: *926-938* (1966).

Author's address:
Department of Ophthalmology
Tokyo Medical College Hospital
6-7-1 Nishishinjuku, Shinjuku-ku
Tokyo, 160, Japan

THE EARLIEST VISUAL FIELD DEFECT (IIa STAGE) IN GLAUCOMA BY KINETIC PERIMETRY

HIROSHI KOSAKI

(Osaka, Japan)

ABSTRACT

Using two groups of patients with early glaucoma, the location of scotomas and whether or not these scotomas are characteristic of early glaucoma were studied by kinetic Goldmann perimetry.

It was revealed that scotomas were most frequently found in the above the blind spot area, precisely 45 degrees direction and 15 degrees away from the fixation point and that these scotomas were characteristic of early glaucomas.

In 1966 Aulhorn & Harms concluded that the characteristic first visual field disturbances in glaucoma are spot-like scotomata in the Bjerrum area, which enlarge and only later join with the blind spot. Aulhorn also showed in the last symposium of the I.P.S. in 1976 that the defects in the upper half of the visual field were placed closer to the center than those in the lower half of the visual field. On the other hand, in 1969 Drance revealed that the earliest changes in eyes with open angle glaucoma that could be discovered with the use of static perimetry were paracentral scotomas in the Bjerrum area separated from the blind spot, coalescing into an arcuate scotoma joining the blind spot.

It is the purpose of this report to study the clinical usefulness of kinetic Goldmann perimetry which has been most widely used in ophthalmological practice, in the diagnosis and follow-up studies of early glaucoma. Using two groups of patients with early glaucoma, we studied the location of scotomas (Study 1) and we also studied whether or not these scotomas are characteristic of early glaucoma (Study 2).

MATERIALS AND METHOD (STUDY 1)

The location of scotomas in the early stage of glaucoma was studied in 56 eyes of 47 cases of early glaucoma, by the kinetic method using Goldmann perimeter. Twelve cases were male and 35 cases were female. Their ages ranged from 15 to 85, with the average of 64.4 years of age. We used 5 isopters, including at least one isopter in the Bjerrum area. All field changes were expressed as those of the right eyes. Glaucoma cases with only one scotoma were chosen for the present investigation.

RESULT

Figure 1 is the actual plot of isolated scotomas of 56 eyes of 47 cases of early glaucoma. Scotomas were most frequently found in the 'above the blind spot' area. If the number of the above cases was plotted against direction and distance, scotomas were found most frequently in the 45 degrees direction and 15 degrees away from the fixation point (Figure 2). Figure 3 is a typical case of early glaucoma. A scotoma was found above the blind spot. We called this scotoma 'above the blind spot' scotoma or 'A.B.S.' scotoma.

MATERIALS AND METHOD (STUDY 2)

An attempt was thus made as a next step to ascertain whether or not this 'above the blind spot' scotoma was characteristic of early glaucoma in a new series of cases. Provocative tests such as tonography after drinking water were performed on cases with only 'above the blind spot' scotoma but without any increase in intraocular pressure and retinal diseases. Our new series of cases consisted of 54 eyes of 47 cases, ranging from 20 to 78 years of age. The average age was 66.6 years. Five cases were male and 42 cases were female.

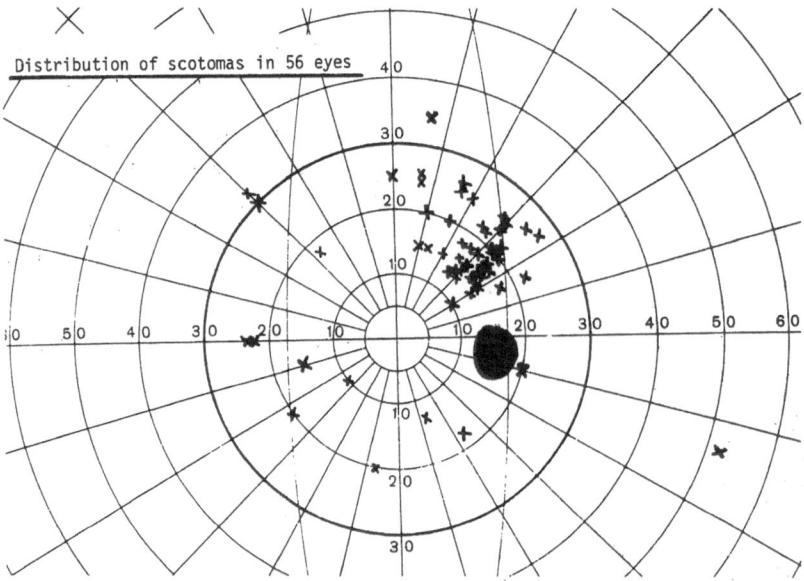

Fig. 1. Distribution of new position of early isolated scotomas in 56 eyes of 47 patients all converted to a right visual field.

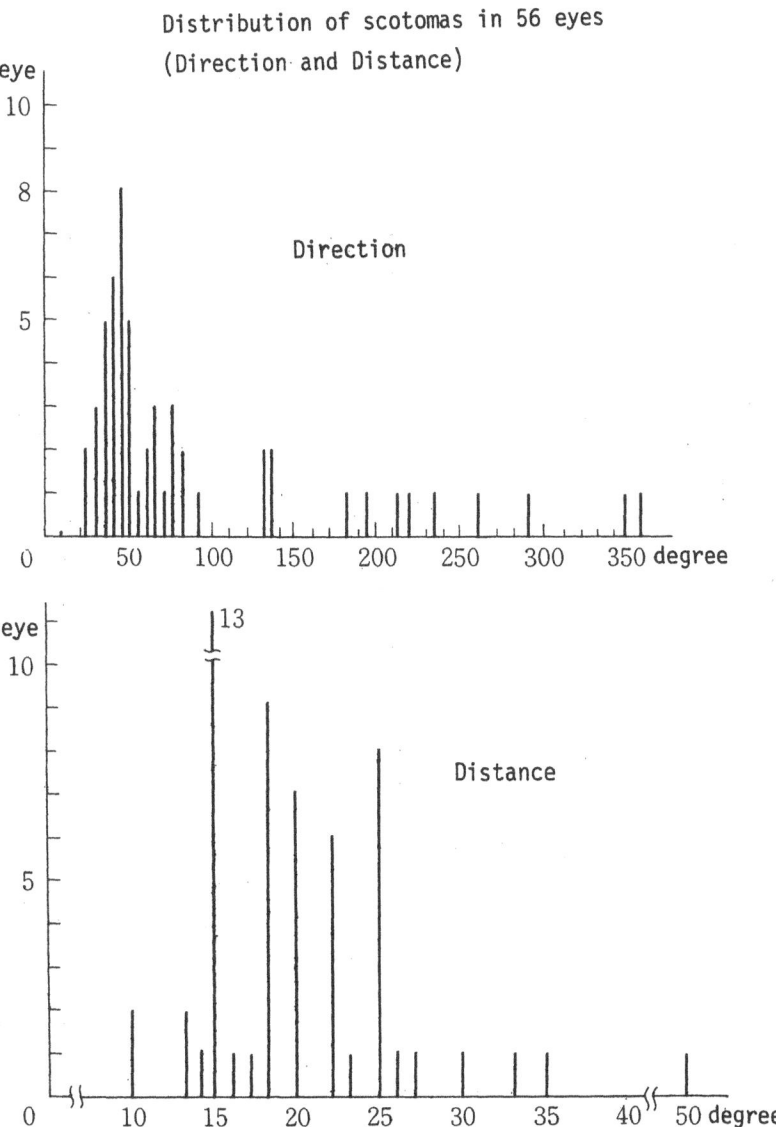

Fig. 2. Distribution of Scotomas according to direction and distance. The number of eyes is indicated along the ordinate. In the upper part is indicated along the abscissa and in the lower part the distance from the center in degrees.

RESULT

Analyses of provocative tests on these patients revealed that 23 eyes of 19 cases were positive and 31 eyes of 25 cases were negative. Follow-up studies of the above patients with negative provocative test disclosed that 16 eyes showed either increased intraocular pressure or lowering of C-value in tonography in two years. If these cases suspected of glaucoma were added to the above mentioned cases with positive provocative tests, 39 eyes, i.e. *72% of the new* series of cases were diagnosed as *glaucoma or glaucoma-suspect.*

SUMMARY

Field studies of 56 eyes of 47 cases of early glaucoma revealed that scotomas were most frequently found in the 'above the blind spot' area, precisely 45 degrees direction and 15 degrees away from the fixation point. A new series of patients (54 eyes of 47 cases) with only one scotoma 'above the blind spot' area was chosen to confirm that the 'above the blind spot' scotoma (A.B.S. scotoma) was characteristic of glaucoma. Follow-up studies demonstrated that the 'above the blind spot' scotoma is pathognomonic of glaucoma in 39 eyes (72%) of the examined cases. It is therefore suggested to conclude that kinetic Goldmann perimetry is quite useful in the diagnosis and follow-up studies of early glaucoma.

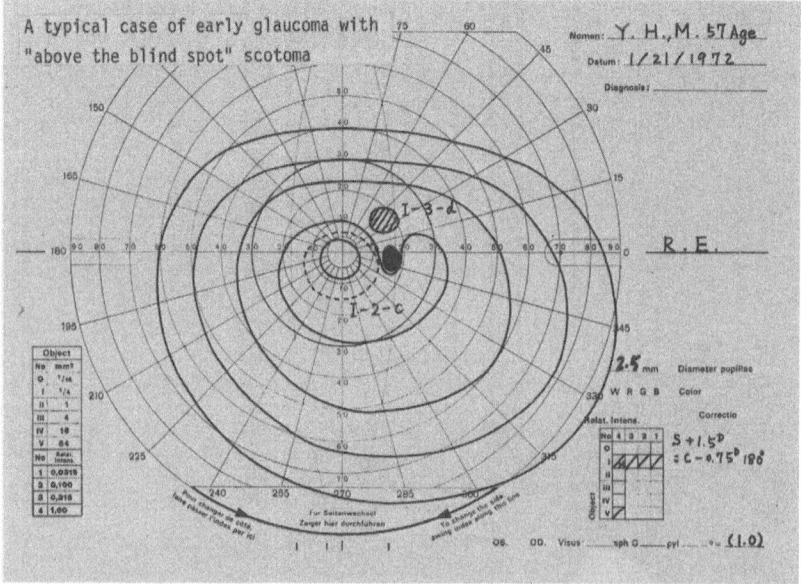

Fig. 3. See text.

REFERENCES

Aulhorn, E. & Harms, H. Early visual field defects in glaucoma, Glaucoma, 151-186 Karger, Basel/New York (1967).

Aulhorn, E. & Karmeyer, H. Frequency distribution in early glaucomatous visual field defects. *Docum. Ophthal. Proc. Series* 14: *75-83* (1977).

Drance, S.M. The early field defects in glaucoma. *Invest. Ophthal.* 8: *84-91* (1969).

Author's address:
1-51-10 Hannan-cho
Abenoku
Osaka 545
Japan

Docum. Ophthal. Proc. Series, Vol. 19

RELATIONSHIP BETWEEN IOP LEVEL AND VISUAL FIELD IN OPEN ANGLE GLAUCOMA (STUDY FOR CRITICAL PRESSURE IN GLAUCOMA)

S. YAMAZI, K. YAMASOWA & I. AZUMA

(Osaka, Japan)

ABSTRACT*

Measurements of the visual sensitivity at various IOP levels in primary open angle glaucoma by using diurnal variation of IOP were carried out.

The visual sensitivity was examined at 5 points including central fixation point by using white and white flickering light spot with Tübinger static perimetry.

A decrease of visual sensitivity was observed following an increase of IOP.

It was possible to estimate the critical in the ocular pressure (Pc), which produces a damage of visual function in each case, from the relationship between IOP level and visual sensitivity.

The numerical values of estimated Pc with this method were similar to those of other methods.

* The original paper will be published elsewhere.

Docum. Ophthal. Proc. Series, Vol. 19

THE RELATIONSHIP BETWEEN VISUAL FIELD CHANGES AND INTRA-OCULAR PRESSURE

A Preliminary Report*

A.I.FRIEDMAN

(London, England)

To assess to what degree progression and regression of visual field defects may occur in the clinical environment, it was decided to analyse the records of patients with open angle glaucoma attending the glaucoma clinic at the Royal Eye Hospital, and to relate visual field changes to the intra-ocular pressures found at routine visits. It is felt that these 'routine' intra-ocular pressures will have the most significance for the clinician.

Generally most cases had either controlled intra-ocular pressures and unchanging visual fields or not such well-controlled pressures, but still unchanging visual fields. These cases were simply kept on medical treatment. Other cases showed uncontrolled intra-ocular pressures on treatment and increasing visual field defects. These cases were advised to have surgery.

Between these two types of cases there are a varied group in which clinical decisions are much more difficult, and this paper describes some such patients who like all patients attending this clinic have their visual fields monitored on the visual field analyser at almost every visit. All cases described in this paper had good visual acuity and the visual field examinations were done by experienced technicians.

METHOD

The charting of analyser visual fields allows the findings to be converted into a number which will be called the visual field function. The conversion is simple. The filter densities with which each stimulus was seen are added together and multiplied by 10. Where any stimulus could not been seen without any filters, an arbitrary value of -0.4 log. unit was given it.

A normal subject who sees all 46 stimuli with a 1.6 log. unit filter will have a visual field function of $46 \times 1.6 \times 10 = 736$. Whilst the same subject on the 100 stimuli plate would have a function of $1.6 \times 100 \times 10 = 1600$.

It is felt that in order to gain more understanding of visual field changes, a numerical conversion is almost essential.

---

* Due to the absence of figures this report had to be reduced to an abstract. In the complete report 7 cases were presented.

Although the intra-ocular pressures recorded at routine visits can in no way be assumed to reflect accurately either 'damaging' or 'relieving' pressures in the months preceding or succeeding such a reading, it is just on such readings that decisions may be made and it was therefore decided that correlating these 'routine' intra-ocular pressures graphically with progression or regression of visual field defects might be instructive.

CONCLUSIONS

No conclusions can be drawn at this stage in a retrospective study of this kind. It is fairly clear from the cases shown in this paper (and other) that the recorded intra-ocular pressure at routine visits may give no indication as to whether the visual field defects in a case of open angle glaucoma will get worse or improve.

There is no doubt that considerable recovery can take place. One of the many questions unanswered is that perhaps where the field defect has fairly rapidly deteriorated and then equally rapidly recovered, should not a filtration operation be performed to prevent a later serious and possibly permanent reduction in visual function.

The correlation of a number of other facets of glaucoma will be required before a greater understanding of the vulnerability of the 'visual field' is reached.

I wish to thank Mrs. J. Claringbold and Miss. P. Glock for technical and secretarial assistance.

Author's address
Courage Laboratory
Royal Eye Hospital
St. George's Circus
London S.E. 1
England

Docum. Ophthal. Proc. Series, Vol. 19

VISUAL FIELD CHANGE EXAMINED BY PUPILLOGRAPHY IN GLAUCOMA

TATSUYA AOYAMA

(Hyogo-ken, Japan)

INTRODUCTION

Early visual field change in glaucoma have been considered as a spot-like scotoma in the Bjerrum area since the report of Aulhorn & Harms (1967). The author performed 'Pupillographic Perimetry' on very early glaucoma cases where no abnormalities were found in kinetic visual field or static visual field measurements and obtained findings which matched spot-like scotoma as was reported previously (Aoyama, 1977).

In this work, diurnal variation of the pupillographic perimetry and the water drinking test was performed and investigations were conducted concerning the correlation between the pupillary threshold (Hereafter abbreviated as P-th) and changes in the subjective static visual threshold (hereafter abbreviated as V-th) and the intraocular pressure. The results are reported here.

METHODS AND SUBJECTS

The apparatus and measuring methods were the same as reported previously except for the 10asb. photopic adaptation for background luminosity.

The subjects included four normal controls and seven patients with glaucoma or suspected glaucoma showing an almost normal visual field in kinetic visual field measurements. Prior to these measurements the intraocular pressure was measured. There were four measurement times: 6.00a.m., 0.00p.m., 6.00p.m. and 10.00p.m.. The water drinking test was performed 30 minutes after the subjects drank 1,000 ml of water for five minutes after the 0.00p.m. measurement. To obtain correct data just after the subjects got up the time of the 6.00a.m. measurement, the subject slept in examination room from the night before. The measurement range was from the central part of the 45° and 135° meridians to 30° nasal and temporal.

RESULTS

Fig. 1 shows the changes in the average values of intraocular pressure in the normal controls (group A) and the glaucomatous cases (group B). The average diurnal variation of the intraocular pressure was 4.4 mmHg in group A and 5.1 mmHg in group B with a maximum of 8.0 mmHg. The difference after the water drinking test was 1.2 mmHg in group A and 3.0 mmHg in group B (max. of 6.0 mmHg).

Fig. 2 shows the pupillographic perimetries of groups A and B respectively. In group A, P-th (·O–O·) was about 0.6 log unit in the center and about 1.0 log unit higher than the V-th (□-□), but the parallerism was good. In group B, V-th (■-■) showed almost the same threshold as group A. However, P-th values (●-●) were 0.9 log unit in the center and the threshold increases were not very large, but at 15°, there was a very great increase to 2.3 log unit.

Fig. 3 and 4 show the pupillographic perimetries before and after the water drinking test for group A (case a, left eye, 135° meridian) and group B (case b, right eye, 45° meridian) respectively. In case a, there was

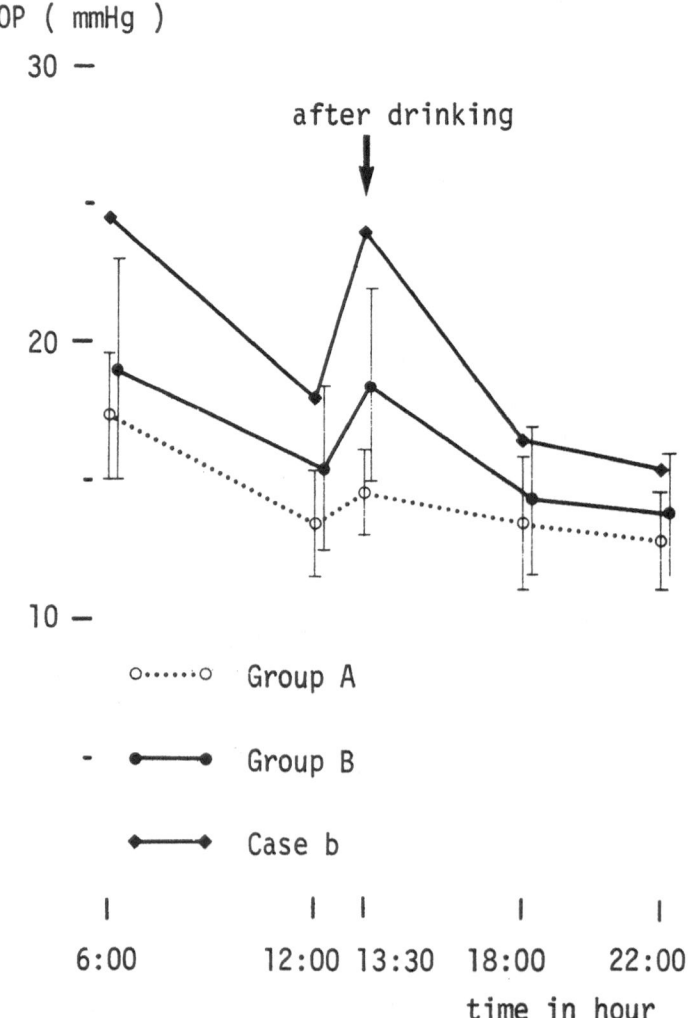

Fig. 1. Diurnal variation of intraocular pressure.

no major effect of the water drinking test on either V-th and P-th. In case b, there were threshold increases of 0.1 log unit for V-th and 0.3 log unit − 0.5 log unit for P-th at 15°.

Table 1 shows the diurnal changes of V-th and P-th in the center and at each 15° nasal and temporal of group A. Table 2 shows that of group B. In group A, the difference of V-th in the center and at 15° of each hour was

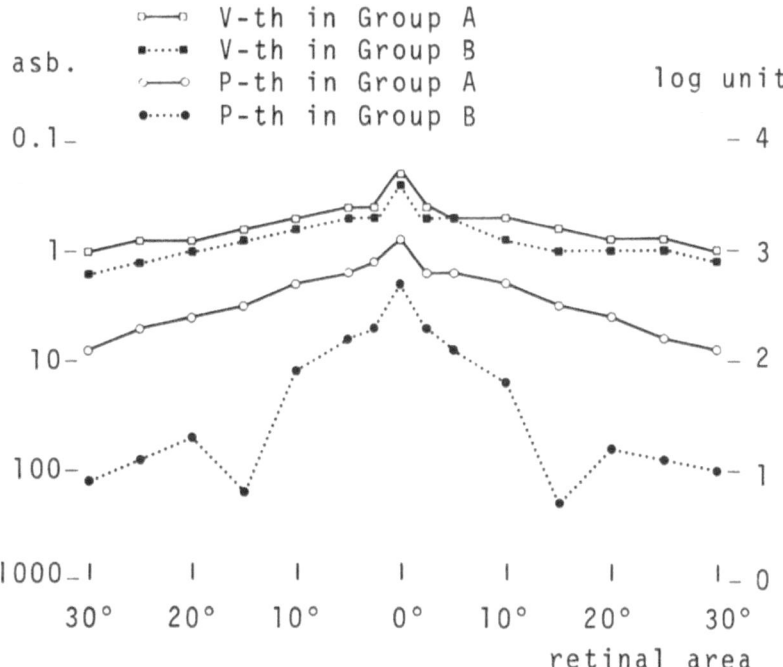

Fig. 2. Pupillographic perimetry in groups A & B.

Table 1. V-th and P-th measured at a certain hour (Group A).

<table>
<tr><th></th><th colspan="3">retinal area</th><th></th></tr>
<tr><th>hour</th><th>nasal 15°</th><th>0°</th><th>temporal 15°</th><th></th></tr>
<tr><td rowspan="2">6:00</td><td>3.2 ± 0.2</td><td>3.7 ± 0.1</td><td>3.2 ± 0.2</td><td>V-th</td></tr>
<tr><td>2.5 ± 0.2</td><td>3.1 ± 0.2</td><td>2.5 ± 0.2</td><td>P-th</td></tr>
<tr><td rowspan="2">12:00</td><td>3.1 ± 0.1</td><td>3.6 ± 0.1</td><td>3.1 ± 0.1</td><td>V-th</td></tr>
<tr><td>2.5 ± 0.1</td><td>3.1 ± 0.2</td><td>2.5 ± 0.1</td><td>P-th</td></tr>
<tr><td rowspan="2">18:00</td><td>3.2 ± 0.1</td><td>3.6 ± 0.2</td><td>3.2 ± 0.2</td><td>V-th</td></tr>
<tr><td>2.6 ± 0.1</td><td>3.1 ± 0.2</td><td>2.6 ± 0.1</td><td>P-th</td></tr>
<tr><td rowspan="2">22:00</td><td>3.2 ± 0.2</td><td>3.7 ± 0.1</td><td>3.1 ± 0.1</td><td>V-th</td></tr>
<tr><td>2.5 ± 0.1</td><td>3.1 ± 0.2</td><td>2.5 ± 0.1</td><td>P-th</td></tr>
</table>

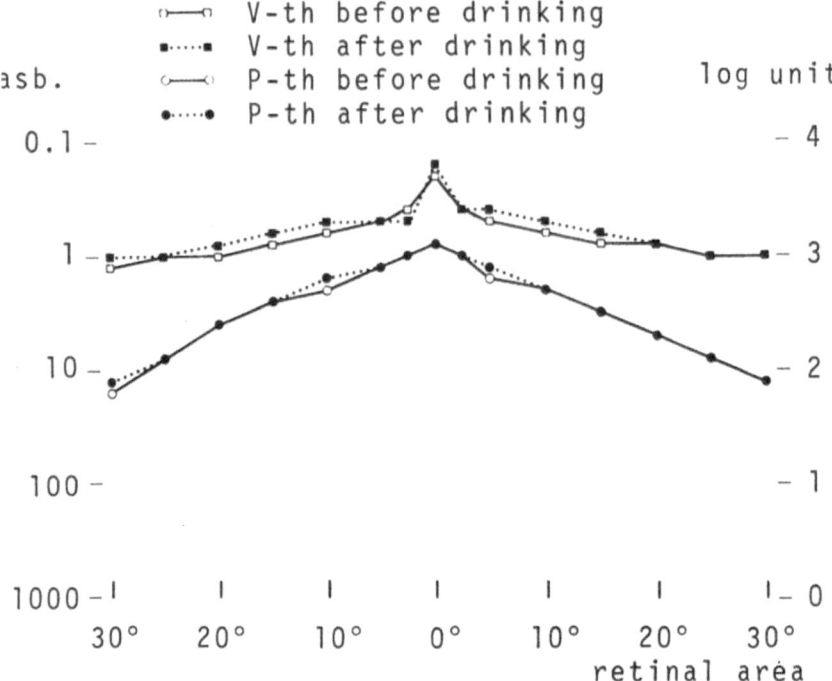

Fig. 3. Water drinking test in Group A (case a, left eye, 135° meridian).

Table 2. V-th and P-th measured at a certain hour (Group B).

hour	nasal 15°	retinal area 0°	temporal 15°	
6:00	3.0 ± 0.1	3.5 ± 0.1	3.0 ± 0.1	V-th
	0.8 ± 0.5	2.6 ± 0.5	0.6 ± 0.3	P-th
12:00	3.1 ± 0.2	3.5 ± 0.2	3.0 ± 0.1	V-th
	0.9 ± 0.5	2.7 ± 0.3	0.7 ± 0.3	P-th
18:00	3.1 ± 0.1	3.6 ± 0.2	3.0 ± 0.2	V-th
	0.8 ± 0.3	2.8 ± 0.3	0.7 ± 0.3	P-th
22:00	3.0 ± 0.2	3.6 ± 0.1	3.0 ± 0.1	V-th
	0.8 ± 0.4	2.7 ± 0.3	0.7 ± 0.3	P-th

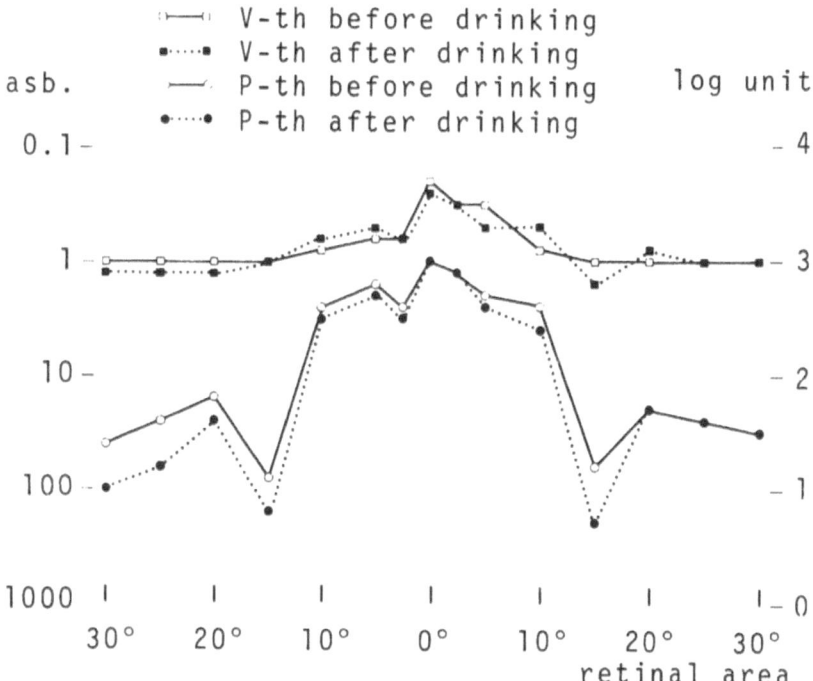

Case b, right eye, 45° meridian

<table>
<tr><td>:—∙</td><td>V-th before drinking</td></tr>
<tr><td>∙····∙</td><td>V-th after drinking</td></tr>
<tr><td>—.</td><td>P-th before drinking</td></tr>
<tr><td>∙····∙</td><td>P-th after drinking</td></tr>
</table>

Fig. 4. Water drinking test in Group B (case b, right eye, 45° meridian).

Table 3. Comparison with water drinking test (Groups A & B).

| | | retinal area | | | |
		nasal 15°	0°	temporal 15°	
Group A	before drinking	3.1 ± 0.1	3.6 ± 0.1	3.1 ± 0.1	V.th
		2.5 ± 0.1	3.1 ± 0.2	2.5 ± 0.1	P-th
	after drinking	3.1 ± 0.1	3.6 ± 0.1	3.1 ± 0.1	V-th
		2.5 ± 0.1	3.1 ± 0.1	2.5 ± 0.1	P-th
Group B	before drinking	3.1 ± 0.2	3.5 ± 0.2	3.0 ± 0.1	V-th
		0.9 ± 0.5	2.7 ± 0.3	0.7 ± 0.3	P-th
	after drinking	3.0 ± 0.1	3.5 ± 0.2	3.0 ± 0.1	V-th
		0.6 ± 0.4	2.6 ± 0.4	0.5 ± 0.3	P-th

269

not so large as 0.4 - 0.5 log unit for V-th and 0.5 - 0.6 log unit for P-th. In group B, V-th shows the same pattern as that of group A. On the other hand, P-th was somewhat low in the center as compared with group A, however, no difference was seen at each hour. At 15°, the difference in the center increased remarkably as 1.8 - 2.1 log unit at each hour. By the V-th and P-th ratio, no difference was seen in the center and at 15° as 0.5 - 0.6 log unit and 0.6 - 0.7 log unit in group A. In group B, therefore, while no special difference was seen in the center as 0.8 - 0.9 log unit, it became extremely larger at 15° as 2.2 - 2.4 log unit. No differences were seen either in groups A and B at each hour.

Table 3 shows the comparison with both P-th and V-th before and after the water drinking test of both groups A and B. V-th was invariable either in groups A and B. P-th was invariable in group A but it showed increase as 0.2 - 0.3 log unit in group B.

DISCUSSION

There have been several reports on early visual field changes in glaucoma, but they have all concerned subjective perimetry of the kinetic and static visual fields. There have been no reports of objective perimetry. The author performed pupillographic perimetry in subjects in which no abnormalities in subjective perimetry and found the so-called Bjerrum scotoma. As was mentioned in the previous report, the P-th and V-th ratio in the Bjerrum area was much higher in the patients than in the normal controls with no relation to the level of the intraocular pressure. This should be a very effective method for screening and the early discovery of glaucoma.

In the case of diurnal variations, the variation in the P-th and V-th ratio was a maximum of 0.2 log unit and this result reconfirmed that pupillographic perimetry has excellent reproducibility. After the water drinking test, there were no changes in group A and only a 0.3 log unit increase in group B. The maximum variation was 0.5 log unit as shown in Fig. 4. These results indicate that water drinking tests have no meaning in pupillographic perimetry and pupillographic perimetry itself is of diagnostic value in the detection of glaucoma.

CONCLUSIONS

1) Pupillographic perimetry is effective method for glaucoma diagnosis since it can detect early visual field changes in glaucoma which can not be detected in subjective perimetry.
2) Pupillographic perimetry shows no diurnal variations and reproducibility is excellent.
3) The water drinking test has no significance in pupillographic perimetry.

REFERENCES

Aoyama, T. Pupillographic Perimetry – The Application to Clinical Cases – *Acta Soc. Ophthalm. Jpn.* 81: *1527-1538* (1977).

Aulhorn, E. & Harms, H. Early Visual Field Defects in Glaucoma. Glaucoma, *151-186* Karger, Basel/New York (1967).

Author's address:
Department of Ophthalmology
Hyogo College of Medicine
1-1 Mukogawa-cho, Nishinomiya-shi
Hyogo-ken 663, Japan

Docum. Ophthal. Proc. Series, Vol. 19

THE NASAL STEP: AN EARLY GLAUCOMATOUS DEFECT?

M. ZINGIRIAN, G. CALABRIA & E. GANDOLFO

(Genoa, Italy)

ABSTRACT

The nasal visual field was examined both with kinetic and static perimetry. The nasal step can be a physiological sign of the anatomic and functional asymmetry of the retina. In this case it is of a small degree and changeable. Sometimes it is an artifact. The nasal step can also be a glaucomatous defect. It is sometimes late as a sign of the distal edge of the arcuate scotoma, but often is an early sign, because it is the result of the different susceptibility between opposite hemifields. It is easy to discover by kinetic perimetry because of its typical shape and invariable location and easy to check by static perimetry. If it is an early sign, it is possible to reverse. In pratical terms, the nasal step is an early characteristic glaucomatous field loss like the isolated scotomas of the Bjerrum area. Unfortunately it can be observed also in normal visual fields and in other pathological conditions. Besides it may be easily detected, well analyzed in the assessment phase of perimetry and used as a sensitive marker in the follow up of glaucomatous damage.

INTRODUCTION

For many years there has been disagreement between those authors who consider the nasal step an initial pathognomonic sign of glaucoma (Drance 1969; Leblanc 1976; Leblanc & Becker 1971; Procksch 1927; Rønne 1909; Rønne 1909), and those, on the other hand, who consider it an unspecific perimetric change which can be found in the most widely different pathologies and also in normal subjects (Dubois-Poulsen 1956; Dubois-Poulsen & Magis 1953).

According to the first group of authors the upper and lower temporal fibres possess, characteristically, a differing susceptibility to an increase of I.O.P. (Drance 1962, 1969; Dubois-Poulsen 1952; Harington 1964; Procksch 1927). For the second group, on the other hand, many other pathogenic 'noxae' can also influence the sensitivity of the two nasal sectors of the visual field in varying degrees. In fact the temporal fibres receiving stimuli from the nasal visual field maintain their individual and separate arrangement at the level of the retina, of the disc and of the whole optic pathway as far as the occipital cortex.

* This study was supported by a grant from the Consiglio Nazionale delle Ricerche, Roma, Italy.

These authors of the second group detected the presence of a Rönne nasal step in chorio-retinal and papillary diseases, in optic pathway disorders and in cases of refraction errors, etc. (Dubois-Poulsen 1956; Dubois-Poulsen & Magis 1953; Kommerell 1969).

The issue is still unresolved and the subject of debate.

We have therefore carried out a detailed investigation into the frequency and variability of the nasal step in glaucomatous and normal subjects, and also in relation to the I.O.P. variations, in order to evaluate the efficacy of the sign in the early diagnosis of glaucoma.

MATERIAL AND METHOD

We examined 40 normal eyes and 40 glaucomatous eyes; of the latter 20 had ocular hypertension without perimetric defects detectable by standard perimetry; 20 had ocular hypertension and marked visual field defects.

For each eye we carried out first a standard kinetic perimetry with 3 isopters on the Goldmann perimeter. Afterwards the investigation of the nasal step was carried out according to the following procedure:

1 *Kinetic analysis*: 3 different stimuli were chosen in order to be liminal at approximately 15°, 30° and 45° eccentricity on the nasal hemimeridian. Each of the stimuli was presented 4 times along 8 horizontal trajectories contained in a band of 5 angular degrees above and below the 0-180°

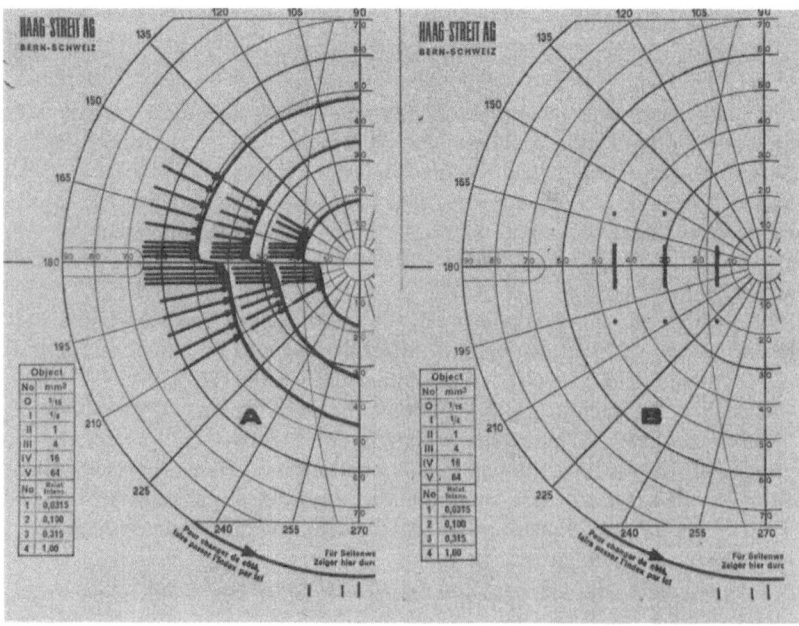

Fig. 1. (See text).

meridian. These stimuli were also used to define other threshold points on 5 oblique meridians located 10°, 15°, 20°, 25° and 30° above and below the horizontal meridian (fig. 1, A).

2 *Static analysis*: a serial static examination along 3 axes perpendicular to the horizontal meridian at 15°, 30°, 45° eccentricity on the nasal side was carried out. 13 positions were studied on each axis: one at the intersection with the horizontal meridian, six above and six below, each 1 angular degree from the other, apart from the outside ones which were 15 angular degrees from the horizontal meridian (fig. 1, B).

RESULTS

A. *Normal subjects (40 eyes)*

In none of these subjects did the standard kinetic examination show a nasal step.

A detailed study of the distribution of the threshold points obtained with our kinetic analysis (see Method) showed three types of behaviour (fig. 2).

1. *step distribution*: the threshold points dispersion is narrow and there is a sharp sensitivity gradient between the two nasal hemifields;

2. *oblique distribution*: the points dispersion is wide and the sensitivity gradient between the two nasal hemifields is not very pronounced;

3. *regular distribution*: the points dispersion is fairly narrow and no sensitivity gradient is in evidence.

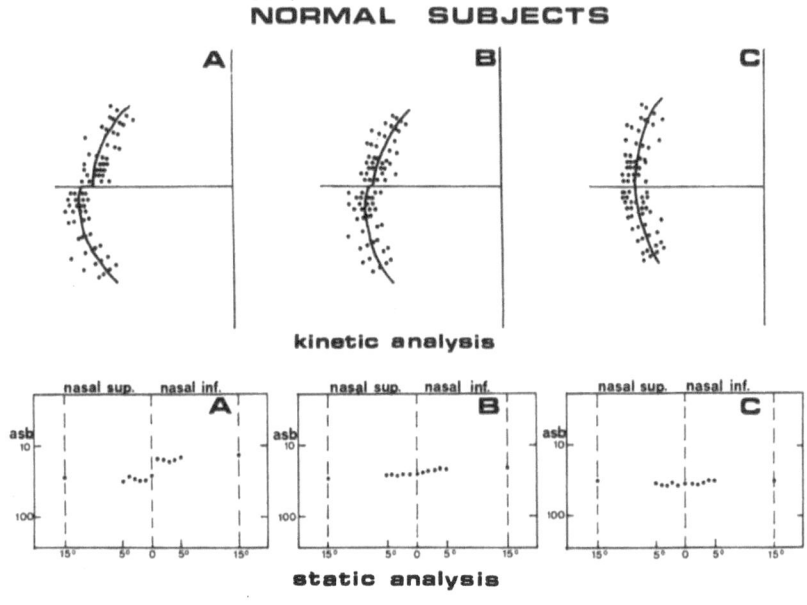

Fig. 2. (See text).

275

The behaviour of type 1) must be considered a *true nasal step*. The true nasal step is usually of limited width, at most 4°; it is more often detected in the external isopters (45°) than in the internal ones (15°, 30°). We observed it in 4 eyes.

The behaviour of type 2) which we observed in 8 eyes, can be considered a *dubious nasal step*. In fact this type of distribution can easily cause false results, either positive or negative, in the detection of a nasal step, and also explains the variable morphology of the defect and the inconsistency in its detection.

The behaviour of type 3) is an absolutely normal finding.

The static analysis of the 4 eyes with a true nasal step confirmed a sudden decrease in sensitivity crossing the nasal hemimeridian.

The static analysis of the 8 eyes with a dubious nasal step confirmed in 3 cases only the above mentioned decrease in sensitivity. Therefore we must consider the nasal step in the other 5 cases an artifact.

B. Glaucomatous subjects (40 eyes)

In the 20 eyes with ocular hypertension but no defects detectable by standard kinetic perimetry, our kinetic analysis (see Method) revealed 16 nasal steps, of which 13 were true nasal steps, because of the typical threshold points distribution, and 3 were dubious nasal steps with the characteristic oblique distribution and wide dispersion of the threshold points.

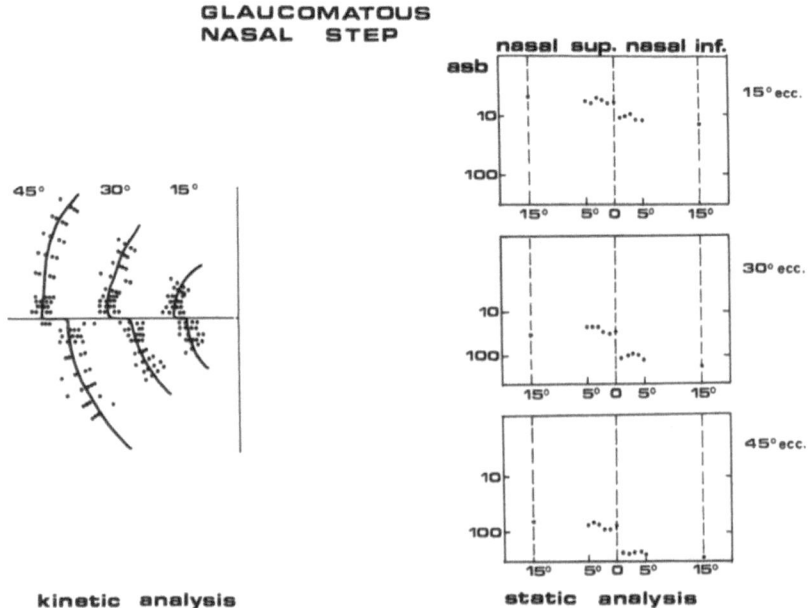

Fig. 3. (See text).

The true nasal step has variable width, but usually more than 4°; it does not show a preference for any one of the 3 examined eccentricities (15°, 30°, 45°) and is often present in all three (fig. 3).

In all the 16 eyes which showed a nasal step on kinetic examination the serial static exploration always revealed a decrease in sensitivity passing from one nasal hemifield to the other.

Where it was possible to normalize the I.O.P. by therapy the nasal step was reduced in width and sometimes disappeared completely.

In the 20 eyes with ocular hypertension and marked visual field defects our kinetic analysis (see Method) revealed the following.

In the case of narrowing of the nasal visual field the typical nasal step morphology was usually found only at the innermost isopter (15°) (3 cases). The nasal step was often the isopteric evidence of the distal edge of an arcuate scotoma (6 cases).

In no case did the normalization of the I.O.P. modify the dimensions or morphology of these nasal steps.

The static examination carried out on the same batch of 20 eyes always confirmed a sharp difference in sensitivity between the two examined hemi-fields.

C. Eyes with raised ocular pressure (12 eyes)

The artificially induced raising of I.O.P. (by ophthalmodynamometric com-pression at about 40 mmHg or by water drinking test with hypertension of about 30 mmHg) provoked in all cases the occurence or the accentuation of a nasal step.

This happened both in normal and glaucomatous eyes.

COMMENT

From the results of our investigation the following may be deduced:

The nasal step can be a physiological sign of the anatomo-functional asymmetry of the retina in relation to the horizontal meridian.

In this case it is of small degree and variable.

Sometimes it is an artifact which can easily be recognized as such by static exploration.

The nasal step is often a glaucomatous defect, in as far as it express a different susceptibility of the two nasal hemifields. In this case it is of greater degree and more easily reversible the earlier it is detected.

Both the physiological and the glaucomatous nasal steps can be accentu-ated by induced ocular hypertension.

In conclusion, the nasal step is an early, frequently detected sign, which is characteristic of glaucoma, but not pathognomonic, as it can be caused by different 'noxae' which damage the retina, the disc or the optic pathway.

However, it is not necessarily a pathological sign, and in fact can also be observed in normal subjects.

When it is a glaucomatous sign it acquires the same significance as an isolated defect of the Bjerrum area: compared to the latter it has the advantage of being more easily detectable due to its invariable location and of being easily analized in the assessment phase.

Finally, the value of the nasal step is that of being a sensitive marker in the follow-up of functional damage due to glaucoma.

REFERENCES

Drance, S.M. Studies on the Susceptibility of the Eye to Raised Intraocular Pressure. *Arch. Ophth. A.M.A.* 68: *478-485* (1962).

Drance, S.M. The early visual field defects in glaucoma. *Invest. Ophth.* 8: *84-91* (1969).

Drance, S.M. The glaucomatous visual field. *Brit. J. ophth.* 56: *186-200* (1972).

Dubois-Poulsen, A. Le champ visuel. Paris, Masson & Cie (1952), p. 687

Dubois-Poulsen, A. Reproduction expérimentale du ressaut de Rønne et du scotome de Bjerrum. *Ann. Oculist.* 189: *37-52* (1956).

Dubois-Poulsen, A., Magis, C. Caractère non pathognomonique du scotome arciforme de Bjerrum et du ressaut nasal de Rönne. *Bull. Mém. Soc. Franç. Opht.* 70: *115-125* (1953)

Harrington, D.O. The visual fields. St. Louis, Mosby (1964) ed. 2nd, p. 198.

Kommerell, G. Binasale Refraktionsskotome. *Klin. Mbl. Augenheilk.* 154: *85-88* (1969).

Leblanc, R.P. Peripheral nasal field defects. *Doc. Ophth. Proceedings* 14: *131-133* (1976).

Leblanc, R.P., Becker, B. Peripheral nasal field defects. *Amer. J. Ophth.* 72: *415-419* (1971).

Procksch, M. Beitrag zum Glaukomgesichtsfeld. *Z.f. Augenheilk.* 61: *344-347* (1927).

Rønne, H. Ueber das Gesichtsfeld beim Glaukom. *Klin. Mbl. Augenheilk.* 47: *12-33* (1909).

Rønne, H. Über die Form der nasalen Gesichtsfelddefekte beim Glaukom. *A.v. Graefes Arch. Ophth.* 71: *52-62* (1909).

Author's address:
University Eye Clinic
Viale Benedetto XV
16132 Genoa
Italy

DISCUSSION OF THE SESSION ON GLAUCOMA

CHAIRMAN S.M. DRANCE

Drance: The discussion which will now take place will be in two parts. We will spend one half of the allotted time on the *early visual field defects* and then the second half of the discussion on *reversibility*. It is however realized these are not independent aspects of the subject and there maybe some overlaps.

You may also address yourselves to the topic as opposed to the paper because what I would like to achieve at the end of the session is a consensus of 1978 not as to what is the earliest visual field defect in glaucoma, but rather what we think the earliest visual fields of glaucoma are at the present time.

It is quite clear that those are entirely different issues and anything that we may in fact agree to as a result of a consensus is obviously working guideline type of idea as to where we stand at this moment in time and it can serve us in terms of future studies and how we perform perimetry and what we demand from the makers of the perimetry equipment in order to be able to do the tasks which we think are necessary to manage the early phases of chronic open angle glaucoma. And so without inhibiting the discussion anyway now I will ask you then to address yourselves to the first topic in the earliest visual field defects in glaucoma.

Friedmann: This question is directed primarly to Dr. Greve, Dr. Dannheim, but also to Prof. Aulhorn, and also to the people who spoke about nasal defects. Now essentially static technic is a profile technique and what is done is similar to histological section.

Dr. Dannheim shows very interesting results by doing a circular motion with his targets. My question to these people is: If one is going to use static technics why not, perhaps after you have done your meridional section to find where your lesion is, so that one gets a better topographical idea, why not then go in a circular motion. Would this perhaps not show defects where people who showed only nasal defects, would this not show defects in the central field?

Dannheim: It is just a question of probability to find a defect to choose the right meridian for the detection and the defects in the Bjerrum area are in a arcuate arrangement so the chance to hit than is maximal if you are choosing the direction of your profile rectangular to the longitudinal pattern of the disturbance which means meridionally in the Bjerrum area. The situation for the nasal step is completely different. There the distribution is more horizontally so the chance to pick some changes or to get the maximal amount of differences between the undisturbed area and disturbed area will be if you cut the field rectangularly to this line which is than circular; doing circular static perimetry in the Bjerrum area does not make any sense.

Fankhauser: Two aspects, when scanning the visual field need to be considered (Greve's detection- and assessment phase): 1. The scotomata need to be detected, 2. the scotomata need to be defined in depth and extent. One single strategy cannot be appropriate for 1. and 2. For detecting glaucomatous scotomata in the Bjerrum area, detectability along meridional profile sections may only be efficient if continuous concentric defects are present (not so however for scattered spot-like defects). Once scotomata of either kind are found, for the definition of the scotomata, a concentric distribution of the scanning points may be more efficient (such as performed by Ourgaud) because the probability of a stimulus hitting the scotoma (ta) is much larger than in a meridional scan.

Greve: I think in this respect we should distinguish between the first phase where we want to detect something and the phase once you have detected something; what you are going to do then?

It is true what Franz says that the best probability of detection is by more or less even distribution of stimuli over the visual field, including the peripheral nasal field and probably in certain instances also including the temporal field, in cases of glaucoma. The question whether one should use meridional or circular static perimetry depends on what one finds in the detection phase. If you want to demonstrate that there is a difference in sensitivity in the nasal area between the upper and lower half it makes sense certainly to do circular static perimetry.

Drance: In fact Dr. Friedmann the answer from Vancouver would be: that is precisely what is being done.

That one combs by means of limited circular static perimetry the nasal area where these visual field defects are likely to occur but not in one part but in a number of places.

Greve: The two are not opposed to each other. It depends on what gives the best result in certain defects.

Friedmann: Perhaps I have been misunderstood. I was talking about the detectability. I think this is not all what concerns us but for the moment let us restrict the remarks to that we have.

The common place for field defects are paracentral defects and you cannot be sure where they are going to be how many meridians you are going to take. Would it not be better taking one or perhaps two meridians and one or two circular.

You see you are giving me an either or one of these and I think you're wrong about it. I think that you should do both.

Drance: I think you misunderstand the screening technic completely. Not yours but obviously what the rest, some of us are doing. As Dr. Fankhauser said the Armaly selective screening like yours concentrates on the inner 25 degrees where the majority of these paracentral defects occur but the technic also includes a particular search for nasal steps in the central portion of the visual field and a modified technic goes, after screening central field, all the way out towards the nasal periphery and the temporal side is examined as well.

Friedmann: Yes, you described the selective perimetry but I am talking about people who do not do selective perimetry. Who do a much more intensive investigation; who would pick up things on the profile that you would not find in your selective perimetry. You see I was asking you where you were setting your sides, you are all limiting sides and I am asking you: shouldn't we in fact extend further, but I accept your answers.

Armaly: The statement I think is that you find what you are looking for. It was said yesterday by Dr. Drance and it is worth repeating.

And in the case of earliest defects of open angle glaucoma it depends on the method you use, the modality of function that you are testing and within the range of sensitivity you detect what is earliest for your technique. We have seen a variety of earliest stages that range from an increase in variance of threshold determination to deep absolute or maximum luminance scotomas.

But throughout all this I think we have been inhibited by the term nerve fibre bundle and I would like to raise an appeal that we forget about this. For a very good reason; morphology is powerful; once you have put in a form you're fit in and you're stuck.

We have heard that tests that have nothing to do with nerve fibers begin to show information that is abnormal much earlier than the modalities of functions that we have used before. The method of Dr. Enoch or brightness sensitivity or colour sense, these are modalities we have not explored before and I think we have neglected because of our blind adhearance to nerve fiber bundles and hopefully in the future we can have some good anatomist with us so that they can explain the progression of the early to the late defect. We impose a certain obligator on the field progression from a small scotoma to a Bjerrum scotoma and we speak of it as if it is going along the nerve fiber bundle. Nothing could be further from the truth. Where is the nerve fiber bundle? Is it at the level of the retina as we have been shown by our Japanese colleagues with very beautiful photographs (which I am afraid, I have not been able to find as frequently in my data of slits) or is the nerve fiber loss at the level of the disc where the only way to explain what we do is to force the nerve fiber bundle to die in depth from periphery towards the center.

Now that is extremely important. I think we have the technology now to examine this in progression and to be able to tell where the lesion is and second whether really a nerve fiber bundle deficit is the earliest change that we encounter in glaucoma.

How does one explain contraction on the basis of a nerve fiber bundle defect? Colour change, brightness discrimination, summation problems and I think as we move from here onward we should begin to debark ourselves and be prepared for a more non specific programming to look for all modalities of the visual field.

Dannheim: It is just easier to detect changes that are following the nerve fiber course but there are other changes that we may find with other more sophisticated techniques. You are completely right. If you are doing a serial sections of the visual field by meridian static testing you will be able to follow the nerve fiber pattern for instance in the wedge shaped defects that Erik Greve has so nicely shown to us. But there are still some patients that do not have small isolated changes from the nerve fiber pattern but a more widely distributed change often producing small nasal steps. These cases are not obviously disturbed at the level of the nerve fiber layer in the retina since we cannot see it as for example Frisén has yesterday shown to us. There might be an explanation for this, that single nerve fibers are dead within normally functioning nerve fibers so the intergral function that we might obtain by threshold measurements or by a more supraliminal testing like for brightness or colours or visual receptive field like properities, might show up a relative defect. This might explain the discrepancy in these cases and some patients do have in one half of the field the type with punched out isolated changes following the nerve fiber pattern and in the other half of the field or in the fellow eye the more widely disturbed type of defects and at the present there is no explanation for this discrepancy of the two types.

Fankhauser: When one does not know anything about the distribution of sensitivity loss in the visual field, only a non-biased scanning strategy, such as a random distribution of the scanning points is able to give a realistic description of the damage. Any other strategy will distort the truth: if the search is carried out over a specific region or along one meridian, the probability of damage detection is very much larger over these areas or lines than anywhere else. Obviously, the recorded damage distribution will then greatly differ from the true damage configuration.

Frisén: I would like to agree with Dr. Armaly about the difficulties of seeing nerve fiber layer defects in many cases of glaucoma. I think that this is because we quite unnaturaly emphasize focal defects in function and focal defects in the nerve fiber layer when we think about this disease. Personnaly I don't have much experiences with glaucoma but I have a lot of experiences with the disease that produces very similar visual field defects, namely drusen of the optic nerve head and it is a common occurence in these patients to find focal nerve fiber layer defects but there is also, in all of them, very severe diffusely distributed loss of nerve fibers, and I think by neglecting the fact that this may also occur in glaucoma we put ourselves in a difficult diagnostic situation. We need a more embracing type of method for estimating function and should not only be looking for focal deficits, steps and levels of different function because in my mind these focal steps are quite randomly distributed. It just so happens that one patient may have them but other patients with a similar lack of nerve fibers but a slightly different distribution lacks the focal defects.

Hayreh: I think optic nerves are involved in a large number of disorders, and that we can get all sorts of defects. The investigation of the optic nerve function with the visual field is one of the modalities. But visual field is not the only modality which can give us the information on disfunction of the optic nerve. Colour vision, luminosity functions, Pulfrich phenomeon are the well known examples. And the other thing we tend to think is, that in glaucoma a particular bundle is going to drop off. It may be more diffuse loss. That is why one can have a cupping of the disc without any vision loss, without any detectable visual field defect.

If we have a sophisticated way of picking up the function of the nerve we may be able to detect a defect. Let us take neuritis. The patient with optic neuritis recovers 6/6, vision butt still, since the disease is in one eye, there is a difference in the quality of vision between two eyes e.g. in stereopsis. They cannot find their way when they are walking down the steps.

I think we tend to get channeled into tunnel vision.

We are talking about visual fields so we have to talk in terms of that only. There are many parameters and I don't think that all we have heard in any way excludes optic nerve as a site of disease; I know this controversy: is it retina, is it optic nerve but I think we can explain most of the disorder on the basis of the optic nerve pathology. Let's have a wider way of attacking the whole thing rather then restricting to visual field as the only modality.

Enoch: I don't want to open the optic-nerve-retina debate but I would like to call attention to these tests we are using. We have looked now at quite a range of diseases, certainly not discussed here today and we have seen no single incident or type of disease, where there is a known abnormality within the retina, where we have seen changes in the sustained or transient like function. At the same time whenever we have a disease of the optic nerve from the point where the myelin starts on inward and not necessarily limited to that, we see the very characteristic and different functional responses.

Specially what we are calling a fatigue or saturation like effect. This is consistent and I can think of no exception.

What is tremendously important is that in glaucoma we see the characteristic change that we see in other *retinal* disease.

Frisén: I think we have a major problem here and that is that we understand so little about the connection between anatomical make-up and function. But many things indicate that of the tests that we are talking about, simple contrast-sensitivity demands very little of the visual system, that the visual system so to speak has redundancy as far as this simple test is concerned. We might have better opportunities of recording function in an adequate way if we could understand what we are asking in anatomical terms and one of the few tests that I know off, where we know the anatomical basis, is peripheral visual acuity. Because peripheral visual acuity is exactly proportional to the density of working neural channels. Perhaps this would be one of the tests that Dr. Hayreh had in mind and perhaps that would be one of the few tests that might reveal the diffuse loss of function, a diffuse loss of channels that certainly characterizes this disease.

Greve: I fully agree with that and it does open a wide area of further research. However I should like to split up a little bit the purposes of this meeting here. I think one is the basic question about the earliest possible defect and the method that can detect the defect. And the other is the *practical* approach: how do we in our daily glaucoma practice go about to detect these defects. I think what we have learned this morning is that there are many methods in a experimental stage which are certainly not yet used on routine level but that there are other methods, the wellknown detection and assessment methods, that are now in a position to be used on a much wider scale. These are two different questions.

Armaly: I think the logic of what Erik is saying is obvious, on the other hand it is equally important I think to maintain the boundary low between the two fields so that one cannot prevent progress from one to the next. The importance of remaining or maintaining the uncertainty lies in the fact of selection. What are you or me as we develop experimental methods, going to use for the glaucoma patient. How we are going to select the glaucoma patient? Are we going to select them on the basis of field criteria? As we develop more and more computerized systems we should be able to eliminate our bias and have the criteria of the field depend on themselves and not on any other findings. Or are we going to select these patients on the basis of nerve fiber layer defects, optic nerve heads, high ocular pressures or some other parameters?

The main virtue of the uncertainty is in the future, prevent us from going on too many different channels and therefore not having comparable data. My glaucoma population or what I would select is different from the group that I heard about this morning, in terms of a case for experimental work.

It is important therefore that we indentify the uncertainty so that if any future research is to be done with sophisticated methods we try to eliminate the difference in selection. Every new definition opens up a new population for entry.

Friedmann: I would just like to draw attention to some papers this morning that showed the importance of the time factor. The only way you can tell what you are dealing with to follow-up the cases for one or two or more years and I think that that to some extent will overcome Dr. Armaly's difficulties of defining the cases.

You may not be able to define them when you first see them and perhaps not even in the first year if you took very early cases. It is maybe only after five years that you can solve this. I would plead for long-term research on the same cases here and not for short-term.

284

Drance: I think if I read down Armaly correctly that was the plea he was making, but his additional concern was that you can follow something for ten years, if you have a specific way of following it that precludes the other things, you will not find the other things. This is really I think the gist of what came out this morning not only by utilizing the criteria that have changed due to ‹changes in our understanding of sensory physiology but also because for instance of what we witnessed even in the perimetric field alone.

That a nasal step and non-nasal steps, focal or otherwise changes occur depending how one was doing ones perimetry. So we have already got 20 years of illustration of how different centers may come up with different incidences for instance for early perimetric findings, conventional perimetric findings, merely by utilizing the technique that precludes the indentification of certain things in the visual field and I think that was the plea that Armaly was making if I am paraphrasing him correctly.

May I draw your attention to an unread paper that dealt with pupil perimetry. The paper shows that that particular modality (whatever the pupil response depends on and that it is quite an open question) seems to show a sensitivity again that precedes our standard perimetric differential threshold techniques.

Armaly: Since we are all here doing perimetry and it is nice to expose the various problems that require our attention, I would like to focus on a statistical analysis that came up in an attempt to assess improvement of given visual field defects. I find this of major importance to quantitatively describe and to put some weighted judgement on area, depth and location as we consider improvements of the visual field in glaucoma.

I have not had the opportunity to read Dr. Frisén's analysis of this area but I would like to point out that one can go astray by limiting his attention to the traditional statistics of studying the range and standard deviation of a pair of points where he has maybe 6 points to consider robably we should look for the best fitting lines rather then whether a point was within a standard deviation of 2 or 3 and so on. And here again I think the entire validity of the sensitive methods depends on randomness and as soon as we develop methods of portraying defects in the random fashion so that error cannot account for changes, then I think we should resort to techniques of curve fitting that are most sophisticated and more powerful then looking at the .1 or .2 discrimination techniques. I wonder if any of those present have any experiences in this?

Frisén: I have had the opportunity of speaking at an earlier meeting about this approach, to recognize the minimum abnormality.

The technique for dealing with the isopters of the central visual field is already solved and you can even do it without the computer. Now kinetic perimetry is easier to deal with from this point of view because the apparent shape of the normal isopters goes back to symetric conditions within the eye.

It is fairly easy to define realistic models that you can handle. You can analyse, you can see how well they fit. This remains to be done unfortunately in static perimetry where you deliberately throw out factors like symmetry conditions that can be used to define a plausable model. I would like to extend Dr. Armaly's view a bit and say what we really need to do have to be able to estimate how good our methods are, is a good model of the visual field, that can be handled objectively and a model that can be handled in the computer and I think this one of the ways we have to use in the future if we want to have a standard for comparison. We can no longer go on looking at individual patients and compare our results obtained in one way or another without assertaining by other authors. We need an objective mathematically workable model.

Drance: At the risk of narrowing the discussion for just a few minutes however (and I am not normally a narrower) I think we should at least see whether the standard perimetrists at the moment would like to coach down on their things and maybe just see whether in this morning's discussion they got some ides of what they feel at this time can be accomplished perimetrically in order to at least narrow down the perimetric discord which has existed.

The perimetric discord basically is that our techniques today, that are used as a result of our notions of 15 years ago, limit themselves for instance in perimetric terms just so searching the inner 20 degrees or 25 degrees. Does that make sense in 1978 on nonsophisticated terms? Is this type of discord that I had in mind?

Greve: I don't think that the discord is this much. People have been talking about paracentral defects whether for maximal luminance or whether relative and about nasal steps, giving the impression that this is something totally different. I think that they are almost the same. If we have the relative depression somewhere in the visual field but not along the nasal horizontal meridian, this will give you a relative more or less isolated defect. If it is for maximal luminance it will give you a punched out scotoma or defect. If the same defect happens to be along the horizontal meridian it will show up as nasal step but it is from the perimetric point of view the same type of defect. The discords are not that great and it is efficient to talk in terms of where the location of a relative or maximal luminance defect is. You, Stephen, showed in your slides where you compared static threshold and kinetic threshold, that a step of let's say 5 degrees corresponds with a relative defect in static perimetry of about 0,3 log. unit, if I remember your figures well.

Drance: You must have gleamed something from my slides that I hadn't noticed.

Enoch: Let me follow a point that Erik touched on and in reference perhaps to yours and several others; when one tries to compare paracentral defects or nasal notches in nasal steps with static changes and all. I would think this is very sensitive to adaptational level. That is we are in that part of the field where, shall we say the cut through the visual field is rather flat and it would seem to me that a small amount of change in sensitivity on one side of the horizontal meridian may well be rather sensitive to modest differences in adaption level. I don't know if that's ever been looked at, but it would seem to me that one could ampilify those differences by a little bit of adjustment of the test level.

Aulhorn: I would like to say that I don't think there is a discord but I think it is more a question of definition. You made differentiations between central nasal step and peripheral nasal step and I think your paracentral nasal step is the same as we (Erik and I) call little scotomas or scotomas in the paracentral area. I think there is no discord and I am very happy that now in this meeting here we have both the nasal steps, and the paracentral scotomas in the other region. I also am happy that we have seen that the accuracy and the quality of the investigations improves from time to time, from the first symposium in Marseille to Tübingen and from Tübingen to Tokyo and I think in Bristol or in Vancouver it will be even better.

Phelps: I like to address a question to Dr. Yamazi who gave a fascinating paper on the relationship between the diurnal variation of retinal sensitivity and intra ocular pressure and my question is whether there is always a straight line relationship between the level of intra ocular pressure and sensitivity as he seemed to show in the graphs. I also extend the question to Erik Greve: whether the variation you find in your early wedge shaped defects correlated with the IOP at the time the field was measured.

Drance: If Dr. Yamazi is here I would like to add an question to the question and that is: could he define for us also what he meant in his context of what the critical pressure meant in terms of his definition because that is published in the Japanese literature I see from his paper but I have not had the opportunity of seeing his definition of what he actually meant when he used the term: critical pressure in this context? Dr. Yamazi, can you oblige? Erik would you meanwhile like to answer your part of the question?

Greve: Charles, the best thing we could find of course would be that the defect disappears if the pressure goes down and that the defect reappears again, if pressure goes up. This is what we wanted to investigate in the study on short-term elevation and subsequent drop of pressure. Unfortunately we didn't find a clear correlation in this material. We also, studied the effect of the level of the IOP on the VF after operations, like you also mentioned in your presentation, and there was not a clear cut relation between IOP and behavior of the field, indicating that other factors are involved.

Armaly: I would like to add another question to Dr. Yamazi. Is there a diurnal variation of retinal sensitivity?

Drance: Now there is a question. Would you like to speak to it?

Fankhauser: Is there any diurnal variation of the contrast threshold? Variations of the contrast threshold over shorter and longer time periods do exist

(L. Ronchi and L. Barca. biological rhythms and rhythms of performance, and annotated bibliography. Fondazione 'Giorgio Ronchi' XL). In order to take these variations in perimetric determinations into account, a practical, simplified procedure had to be found. It is to discriminate between short-term, long-term and total fluctuations (H. Bebie et al.: Static perimetry: accuracy and fluctuations. Acta Ophthal. 54: 339 (1976)). The total fluctuation is on the average 1.5 times larger than the short term fluctuation. This factor should not be neglected when comparing perimetric results which have not been obtained during the same session.

Yamazi: I would like to answer to the first question. The critical pressure means the limiting pressure which produces a visual disturbance in the individual glaucoma case. If the IOP increases above the critical pressure over a long time, then the visual function will decrease.

Drance: Fine. Now the second question was one posed by Dr. Phelps about the diurnal variation in your sensitivities.

Phelps: The question was whether the relationship between the IOP and retinal sensitivity was always linear. You measured IOP 5 or 6 times during the days I recall. Yet the graphs you showed showed only 2 points on a straight line and I got lost on the transition between the measurements on the graphs. Where do the other points fall? Do they always fall in a straight line or?

Yamazi: The diurnal variation of the IOP was measured at AM 6.00, 9.00, 12.00, PM 3.00, 6.00, 9.00 and 12.00. The visual sensitivity with Tübingen perimeter was measured three or four times when large differences of the IOP level were present. The decrease of visual sensitivity in the figure of the estimation method of Pc means the difference between logarithm scale of threshold of brightness of each IOP levels and that of minimum IOP.

Drance: Thank you very much for your translating efforts and I would suggest to Dr. Yamazi and to Dr. Phelps that on the way to Fuji tomorrow they should sit together and actually spend the first half hour of that journey to get that point absolutely cristal clear and then report it in the proceedings.

Enoch: In my dissertation many years ago I was drawn into a consideration of the variable blur and I learned at that time that this is one of the most confounding variables in visual sciences. It is what I might call a dirty variable in the sense that the effort differs tremendously from person to person. In all of our techniques in Gainesville we utilize a simple stigmatoscopy procedure. That is we put the image of the point tested on the retina with a degree of shortness. We don't refract every point on the retina. But if one is talking about reliability of determinations at a given point on the retina (and its rather important to know if some sensitivity is changing) it becomes rather important to control blur and if you do so it is amazing how much you reduce variance in determinations. That does not mean you eliminate the natural variance of any threshold. Nor does it mean that you eliminate the effects of a change in pupilsize although modest degrees of this can be handled by working on the data portion of the response curve. But it is terribly important if you are worrying about the variance to control blur and in general to work at as high a level as you can.

Frisén: I would like to aks Dr. Enoch one thing in connection to this: I assume that his decreased variance would apply between persons and not for one and the same person. Is that true?

Enoch: There is tremendous difference in the effect of blur in any single observer. Some observers show very little effect in the presence of blur. Other showed tremendous variance in the presense of blur. Once you have eliminated or minimized (let me use the word minimize because none of us are going to eliminate it because we are not going to carry this to its logical conclusion) the amount of blur you find that the variance between the individuals goes down remarkably also.

Fankhauser: Optical blur should be avoided because it leads to apparent loss of sensitivity and hence simulates disease of the neuro-visual system. The easiest way to suppress the effects of blur is by using large stimulus target sizes. (Because, when the size of the target's retinal image increases, the ratio of the circle of least confusion/retinal image size decreases; hence the effects of blur upon sensitivity for large retinal images are less.) Using stimuli of larger size may be the only way to suppress blur effects when the latter is caused by increased light diffusion (e.g. in retinal edema) as compared to blur originating from a defocussed system, which may well be eliminated by correcting glasses. L. Sloan (Vis. Res. *1*: 121 (1961)) has shown that the blur attenuating action of a 30′ diam. target is already considerable. Larger targets may be even more effective.

Lichter: I would like to ask you Dr. Drance if your question about the friendly discord was answered as to the use of techniques. Could you be more specific?

Drance: No I think basicly I posed the question in general terms and from our discussion I noticed that there is no discord and that it is ready for summing up.

Lichter: The reason I asked the question was from the point that Dr. Greve made about the practical issue versus the theoretical and research issue. When we are meeting here there is a group of people interested in perimetry and in glaucoma. Our techniques and methods and interest most likely exceed those of the clinicians who are seen by far most of the patients. And I would wonder if this organization would not want to come up with the statement as to what the clinician should look for in the earliest visual field defect. For we have of course other parameters, that we use, including the pressure and the disc and so on. But in doing the visual field we ourselves know (those of us who have seen many referals) that the visual fields done in the average clinicians office are far inferior to what we would feel is the bare minimum. So I would wonder whether this group could not come up with a way to teach the clinician to do the bare minimum. Not necessarily tell him that there is a defect of so many apostilb and so much of a region; that goes far beyond him but perhaps leave those things for certain discussions and then come up with some answers in the practical.

Drance: You mean what we should do in 1978 and foreseeable future. The question that you have raised I was going to raise in my summing up. It is only 10 minutes to go and I hoped to be able to challenge the group with precisely that.

Frisén: I think the best thing you could do to improve the results of today's examination is to complete your diagnostic armanentarium with a handcalculator. It is all a game of statistics. What we should speak about is really not is there a defect or is there not. It is all a question of probabilities and we need to define some probabilities from various types of investigations when we want to make a diagnosis with a reasonable certainty. The nasal step of this and that size might be pathological with the probability of perhaps 80%. Relative central scotoma with a depth of 0.3 log. units has a probability of being pathological of let us say 20%. Combine the probabilities of these related examinations and you can arrive at a very logical and discussable measure of security.

Armaly: I think the trend that Paul Lichter wanted us to address is very important. But nothing could be more harmful then for us to try and describe what is necessary for a clinician. We can describe our findings. We can describe what everyone has reported which is not comparable. We heard today all sorts of reports about sensitivity in the Bjerrum area correlating with the nasal steps, about perimetry, selective perimetry without going into details as to what the stimulus was or how was the difference between the stimulus and threshold of the area being tested. We heard about static perimetry profiles. We heard data from the Friedmann Analyser. So I don't think that the data that we heard is so comparable that it would permit us to describe it given dictum to what the ophthalmologists should do perimetrically for the glaucoma patient. We can describe in general terms. We can see that the large majority of cases have their abnormalities located somewhere within 15 degrees or 20 degrees of fixation. That is not all abnormalities. That if an abnormality would be found there, he will detect somewhere between 56 and 80% of cases, if you limit your attention to that. In fact it could probably be more. But is that what we want to describe? We should highlight the fact that it is only 75% and not the 100% or it is 80% and there are some defects that cannot be found unless you go searching for them around 50, 60 or 70 degrees and this is how I feel we can best serve the detection of glaucoma.

Drance: I think Paul Lichter meant it even in such general guidelines, if I read him correctly, because even that hasn't sunk yet to the practising profession.

Aulhorn: I think there are two things: the detection of a scotoma and the follow-up of a scotoma that need nearly two methods. I know how difficult it is to detect small scotomas but to follow them and to say this change is a real change, is a deterioration or an improvement, is much more difficult than to detect them.

Ernest: As I sit here listening to the papers and the questions it seems to me that the first half of the discussion has been devoted to careful measurements and the second half has been devoted to show how unreliable measurements are. And I like to ask just one question so that I can take home something: Are absolute scotomas in glaucoma reversible or are they not?

Aulhorn: It is a funny thing that absolute defects can be reversible in cases of low tension glaucoma. But in high tension glaucoma I never have seen that an absolute defect disappears.

Drance: When you say reversible Dr. Aulhorn, you mean improvable or really reversible so there is nothing left?

Aulhorn: I think that a relative defect may change.

Drance: But he is talking about absolute.

Aulhorn: But absolute maximal luminance.

Drance: I think the answer seems to be 'no' except Dr. Aulhorn suggested that in low tension glaucoma this may occur which is a fascinating finding.

Furuno: I agree with Dr. Aulhorn. If we used single stimulus static perimetry or kinetic perimetry for studying of progression, the scotoma will wander along the nerve fiber pathway and that is why I utilized multiple stimulus static perimetry. I use the Friedmann Visual Field Analyser for my study because multiple stimulus static perimetry is much more steady than kinetic and single static perimetry. And if an early relative depression is going to develop into an absolute defect, the relative defect will no longer wander along the presumed nerve fiber pathway. Also I can find reversibility in very early stages of glaucomatous change but not in the absolute scotoma or punched-out defect.

Phelps: Very brief. I think that both Dr. Armaly and I this morning showed examples of defects that were absolute to the V/4^e testing on the Goldmann perimeter, that improved. They may not be absolute but with the brightest stimulus they would be found at first.

Drance: It seems that you are using the term reversibility just as improvement as opposed to disappearance.

Phelps: One of them totally disappeared. This is a very rare phenomenon but it does happen.

Docum. Ophthal. Proc. Series, Vol. 19

SUMMARY OF SESSION II: GLAUCOMA

CHAIRMAN: S.M. DRANCE

'Before summing up the deliberations of the Glaucoma Research Group I would like to thank Dr. Matsuo for the excellent local arrangements of this meeting and also for the excellence and willingness of his many young co-workers in providing us with hospitality and excellent services.

I would like to thank the invited opening speakers of the two glaucoma topics for the readiness to rise to the challenge of my invitation by preparing original work or background philosophy to the two topics. They were joined by many who have participated by presenting free papers and non-read papers at these sessions.

The discussions have shown that even the earliest perimetric defects in glaucoma may not be the earliest evidence of damage of the sensory elements which may be affected in this disease. The work presented on receptive field-like functions, the work on color disturbances, the work on pupilography and possibly also the work reported on gratings, all point in this direction. It is also possible that a pressure-dependent constriction of isopters which has been reported by many in the past, could be associated with this type of disturbance.

There appears to be a concensus on the early perimetric defects of open angle glaucoma which embodies some of the older and some of the newer concepts. Observations of patients at risk who developed field defects in previously normal visual fields confirms the presence of early localized paracentral scotomata, relative depressions of the arcuate bundles, resulting in central nasal steps, mid-peripheral as well as peripheral nasal steps with the appropriate scotomas that are causing them. It was shown that many of the nasal steps, even towards the periphery, have very definite localized scotomata associated with them. The presence of peripheral changes by themselves appears to be more common than previous cross-sectional studies of Harms and Aulhorn, Armaly, and others, suggested. These changes were reported by Becker and LeBlanc in the literature. Attention has also been drawn and reconfirmed to the occasional, but nevertheless important for the patient, early involvement of temporal and other unusual sector defects. Two papers have shown that peripheral and central nasal steps may occur in normal visual fields but that they are smaller and not reproducible. The work of Professor Zingirian was not read at the Congress but presented in a paper which suggests that these steps are always less than 4°. This was confirmed in an opening paper. Nasal steps could be as large as 14° by chance alone but are never reproducible.

Depending on the technique used for screening of the visual field, the frequency of the earliest defect varies between observers but only to a degree. During the Symposium slight relative disturbances measured by qualitative disturbances with supraliminar stimuli, increased localized scatter of responses, wedge-shaped defects, pupilographic disturbance and subtle differences between two eyes were also reported. Such disturbances often show considerable fluctuation.

The second topic dealt with reversibility of visual field defects. In modern terms, with current care for technique of perimetric analysis, Armaly has redrawn our attention to this phenomenon. He indicated the many pitfalls which must be avoided when studying reversibility. Other factors, in addition to intraocular pressure, must be considered. It would appear that reversibility is more likely to occur in younger individuals, in those in whom no disappearance of nerve fibres in the retina can be ophthalmoscopically seen, in those in whom the neuroretinal rim of the optic nerve head does not go all the way to the disc margin and in people in whom the intraocular pressure is high and amenable to great reduction, either by medical or surgical means. It was also noted that not all of even the earliest disturbances are reversible, which is of great importance in the management of the disease. The currently more conservative approach to the management of intraocular pressure should not be based on reversibility of visual field defects. It was also realized that reversibility and spontaneous fluctuation occur under similar circumstances and it must therefore always be borne in mind in studies of reversibility that fluctuation must be taken into account.'

Docum. Ophthal. Proc. Series, Vol. 19

THRESHOLD FLUCTUATIONS, INTERPOLATIONS AND SPATIAL RESOLUTION IN PERIMETRY

F. FANKHAUSER & H. BEBIE

(Switzerland) Berne

ABSTRACT

The detrimental effect of threshold fluctuations upon detectability of sensitivity loss is emphasized. The only remedy seems to consist in the application of averaging methods, thereby attenuating threshold noise with computer methods. Two scanning methods directed at a rapid and accurate detection of scotomata are considered. In the first, the scanning points are distributed as a rectangular grid. In the second, the points are aligned along meridians. The average detectability of the first method is rated superior and is therefore preferred. Furthermore, particular consideration is given to the role of interpolation procedures played in perimetry.

INTRODUCTION

It has been claimed that with the development of automated perimeters we have entered a new era of investigations. In a number of respects this may well be true. However, some fundamental problems encountered in the analysis of any perimetric method (conventional or automated) have remained the same. Though some of these problems may be found in the older literature, they had to be reformulated in the past two or three years for the purpose of creating automated examination procedures. It is the aim of this discussion to emphasize some of the problems centered around notions of accuracy, choice of examination grid, graphic representation of the results of visual field examinations, interpolation procedures, significance and interpretations and the like. Our method is necessarily based on statistical considerations.

ACCURACY OF PERIMETRIC EXAMINATIONS

The inaccuracy of perimetric threshold determinations and the consequential implications are notoriously underestimated. Estimation of the individual fluctuation σ at a point of a given visual field may be obtained by comparison of repeated determinations; σ is defined more precisely as the root mean square deviation of the results of independently repeated measurements. — Fluctuations of perimetric thresholds have been analysed by a number of authors: see, e.g., Krakau (1969), Niesel (1970), Ronchi (1972),

Bebie et al. (1976), Koerner et al. (1977) and Spahr et al. (1978).

It is well known that the main source of errors stems, in careful determinations of the static visual field, from the statistical nature of patient responses. The threshold luminance can only be statistically defined, namely as that luminance which is perceived with a 50% probability. In order to raise the probability of a 'seen' response from 16% to 84% the stimulus luminance has to be raised by a factor of approximately two to four. Consequently, the accuracy of thresholds derived from five to seven stimuli, which is routine in static procedures, will necessarily be poor.

Apart from these procedural imperfections, the individual spread σ which characterises the ability of a subject to reproduce the same threshold result is slightly increased by reversible long-term fluctuations of the true threshold. Though, by definition, σ includes all noise sources, we shall use the term 'measurement error' for brevity throughout this paper.

Table 1 gives the mean fluctuations as derived from repeated determinations of the visual field of 45 mostly elderly experienced patients with various pathological disturbances. Independent examinations were separated by an interval of several days. For kinetic perimetry, σ has been obtained by transforming isopter displays to profile sections and comparing these for several independent examinations.

These figures may strike one as surprisingly high. They reflect, nevertheless, reliable values, provided that experienced subjects with pathological disturbances of the visual field are involved. The conclusions to be drawn for the evaluation of visual fields will be worked out in the following section.

DETECTABILITY OF VISUAL FIELD DEFECTS

The detection of defects, which are either small in their spatial dimension, or which exhibit only minor sensitivity reductions, is an extremely difficult task. A critical discussion is intimately connected with the measurement error together with geometrical considerations concerning the examination grid.

Table 1. Measurement error of standard procedures. Derived from repeated determination of 45 pathological visual fields. σ: mean of individual error (and standard error of the mean σ). d: population distribution of individual error. Numerical values are in dB (1 dB = 0.1 log unit). Spahr et al. (1978).

	σ	d
Automated static perimetry (Octopus)	3.0 ± 0.1	3.0 ± 0.8
Conventional static perimetry (Goldmann perimeter)	3.8 ± 0.2	3.8 ± 1.3
Kinetic perimetry (independent examiners)	3.4	3.4 ± 1.8

The relevant quantities are defined in figure 1. D denotes the depth of a scotoma relative to normal threshold. As pointed out in the preceding section, the result D' of a single static determination (consisting of some up- and down-procedure) usually does not reflect the true threshold; instead, the results of such determinations, repeated independently, will be distributed about the true threshold with a rms deviation denoted by σ. Some criterion Δ ('critical deviation from normal threshold') has to be introduced in order to interpret a measured deviation D' either as 'normal' (D' $<$ Δ) or as 'pathological' (D' $>$ Δ). The shortcomings of any criterion set up for the purpose of recognizing true deviations are obvious: depending on its severity, either true defects will be overlooked (ms) or apparent defects (ps) will be accepted as real, whereas they are nothing more than fortuitous manifestations of the measurement error.

A statistical description of the situation in one single point of the examination grid is given in figure 2a. Curve N represents the distribution of the results of repeated determinations, assuming normal threshold; its standard deviation corresponds to the measurement error σ. If, instead, a scotoma is present, the curve has to be shifted by the magnitude D of the defect (curve P). In our numerical analysis, Gaussian distributions will be assumed, which is a satisfactory approximation to our actual records.

In figure 2a, the shaded areas to the right and to the left of the criterion chosen represent the probability w_{ps} of producing a pseudoscotoma and the probability w_{ms} of missing a true defect, respectively. These probabilities are complementary to each other in the sense that less defects are missed, if the criterion is relaxed but more pseudoscotomata are picked up at the same time. Alternatively, a more stringent criterion will depress the number of pseudoscotomata, but, of course, at the cost of missing more true defects.

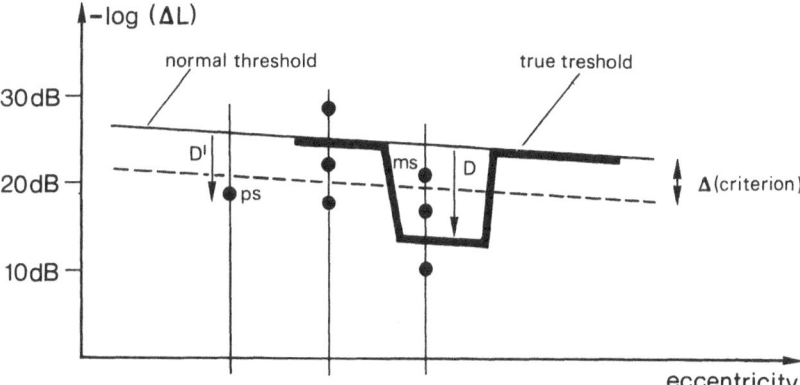

Fig. 1. Profile section: Dashed line: criterion. Dots indicate possible results of perimetric threshold determinations. ms: missed scotoma. ps: pseudoscotoma. D: true depth of defect.

The dependence of w_{ps} and w_{ms} on the choice of the criterion is plotted in figure 2b for a particular signal-to-noise ratio ($D = 2\,\sigma$). Numerical values for arbitrary parameters D, Δ, σ may be obtained from the following formulae:

$$w_{ps} = \frac{1}{\sigma\sqrt{2\pi}} \int_{\Delta}^{\infty} dD' \, e^{-(D')^2/2\sigma^2} \tag{1}$$

$$w_{ms} = \frac{1}{\sigma\sqrt{2\pi}} \int_{-\infty}^{\Delta-D} dD' \, e^{-(D')^2/2\sigma^2} \tag{2}$$

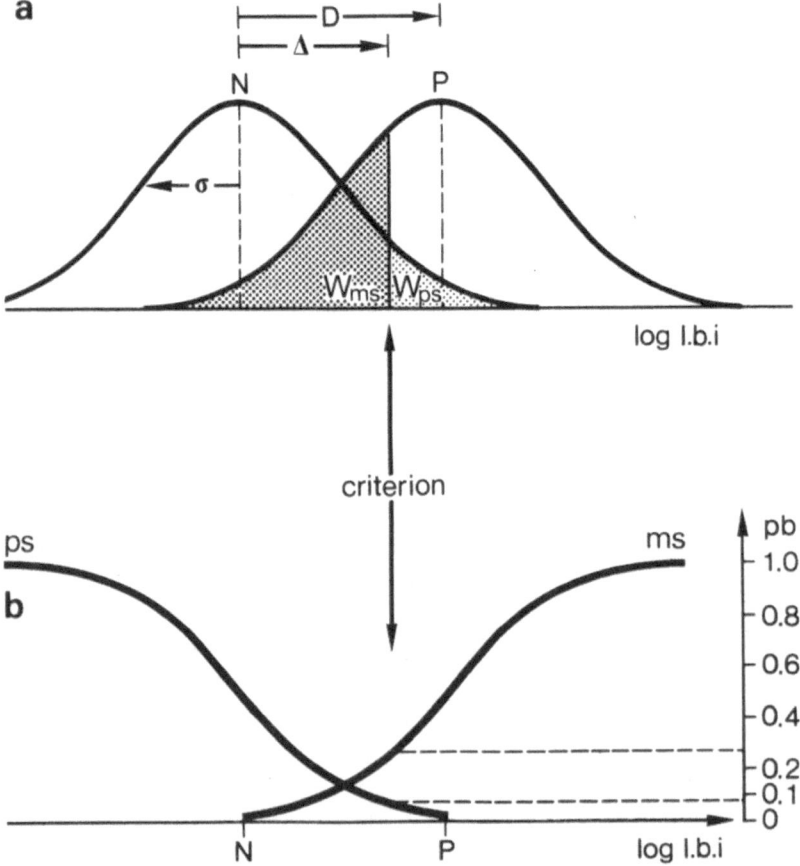

Fig. 2. Statistical decision in one point of a visual field: Probability w_{ps} of producing a pseudodefect and probability w_{ms} of missing a true defect (dept D). 2a: Probability densities of perimetric results (N: normal threshold. P: pathological threshold). 2b: w_{ps} and w_{ms} as functions of the criterion. Assumed signal-to-noise ratio: $D/\sigma = 2$.

The average number n of false scotomata produced in an examination of N = 64 points of a visual field is listed in Table 2 as a function of the ratio Δ/σ. For $\sigma = 3$ dB, e.g., and setting the criterion at $\Delta = 6$ dB, 1.4 false scotomata would be produced per examination, which is an unacceptable high figure. Raising the criterion to $\Delta = 7.5$ dB, the number of false scotomata drops to a level of 0.4 per examination, which may be entirely acceptable for pathological disturbances with high occurrence, but may still be too high for a less frequent pathological entity.

Since, as a rule, the criterion Δ should be set at least at about 2.5 times the measurement error σ, in order to avoid too many pseudodefects (Table 2), the following discussion of the probability w_{ms} of missing a true defect, assumed to exist in one point of the examination grid, may be restricted to this particular case ($\Delta = 2.5\ \sigma$). The missing probabilities given in Table 3 (as a function of the true depth D of the defect) have been derived from eq. (2). As an example, assume a typical measurement error σ of 3 dB and a corresponding criterion Δ of 7.5 dB; even a depression as deep as 10.5 dB will then be missed with a probability of 16%.

There is one solution to this dilemma: namely by averaging over repeated determinations, whereby the mean fluctuation σ is suppressed by the square root of the number of examinations, i.e. from about 3 dB to about 2 dB for a single repetition. A criterion Δ of about 5 dB might then be adequate,

Table 2. Number n of false scotomata produced per examination of N = 64 points. σ: measurements error. Δ: criterion. w_{ps}: fraction of pseudodefect points, from eq. (1). $n = N \cdot w_{ps}$.

σ	Δ	Δ/σ	w_{ps}	n
3 dB	3 dB	1	0.16	10
3	6	2	0.023	1.4
3	7.5	2.5	0.006	0.4
3	9	3	0.0013	0.08
2	4	2	0.023	1.4
2	5	2.5	0.006	0.4
2	6	3	0.0013	0.08

Table 3. Probability w_{ms} of missing a true defect assumed to exist in only one point of the examination grid. σ: measurement error. Δ: criterion. D: true depth of scotoma. – w_{ms} from eq. (2).

σ	Δ	D	D/σ	w_{ms}
3 dB	7.5 dB	7.5 dB	2.5	0.50
3	7.5	10.5	3.5	0.16
3	7.5	13.5	4.5	0.02
2	5	5	2.5	0.50
2	5	7	3.5	0.16
2	5	9	4.5	0.02

providing on the one hand reasonable suppression of pseudoscotomata, and on the other, offering an almost safe detection of scotomata deeper than 7-9 dB (Tables 2 and 3). This is, apart from other aspects, one of the strongest points of computer perimetry, which is ideally suited for noise-attenuation, i.e. reduction of the measurement error by averaging methods, a capability which is beyond human capacity.

The gain in separability of true defects from pseudoscotomata by averaging over threshold results of two determinations emerges clearly from figure 3, in which the relation between the number n of pseudoscotomata per examination and the probability w_{ms} of missing a true defect is given for three different evaluation procedures. In preparing curve 1, single threshold determinations carried out with an accuracy σ of 3 dB have been assumed. If, instead, the decisions are based on the mean of two such determinations, curve 2 is obtained. Obviously, error probabilities are much reduced. In order to derive curve 3 finally, a scotoma was assumed whenever the result of the first determination, as well as that of the second, exceeded the criterion. Comparison of curve 3 and curve 2 clearly demonstrates the overall superiority of decisions based on the mean value.

Note, that our discussion, so far, applies to tiny scotomata located at only one point of the examination grid. For larger defects, less stringent

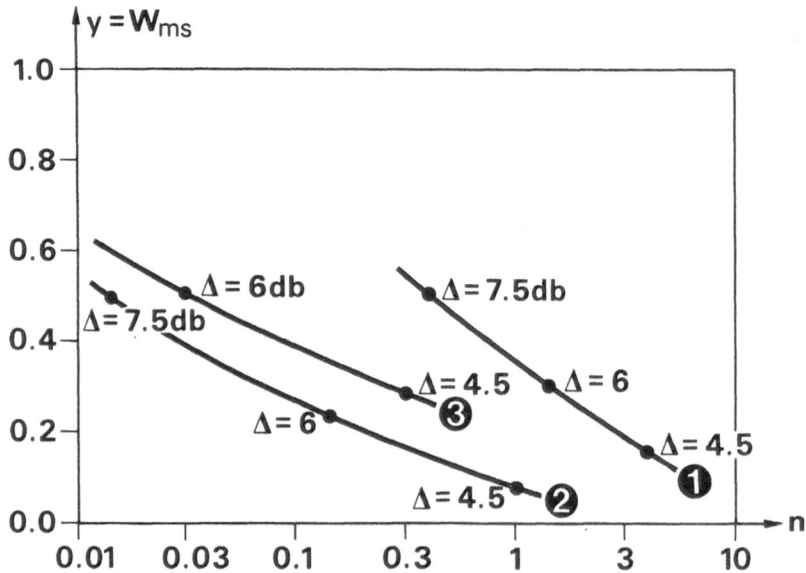

Fig. 3. Performance of decision procedures: Relation between probability w_{ms} of missing a defect and number n of pseudodefects (64 points examined). Assumed depth of defect: D = 7.5. dB. Curve 1: one measurement per point. Curve 2: two measurements; defect assumed, if mean of both results exceeds criterion. Curve 3: two measurements; defect assumed, if both results exceed criterion. – Assumed measurement error: σ = 3 dB.

criteria will suffice for the separation of true defects from pseudoscotomata. However, since now one more parameter is involved (spatial dimension of the defect), no general and simple rule concerning the most appropriate criterion can be offered. Numerical examples listed in Tables 4 and 5 are merely intended as an illustration.

In Table 4 some probabilities related to more extended pseudodefects are given. Obviously, if no pseudodefects can be tolerated (e.g. in case of an apparently almost normal visual field), a criterion as high as $\Delta = 3\,\sigma$ has to be recommended. If, however, one is willing to disregard small defects, covering only one point of the grid, e.g., a more lax criterion, like $\Delta = 2 ..$ $2.5\,\sigma$ may be acceptable.

Finally, probabilities of detecting true defects covering more than one point of the examination grid are listed in Table 5. Surprisingly, even larger defects ($n = 4$, e.g.) may be missed, unless their true depth exceeds the measurement error by a factor of order two. To summarize, even in case of large defects their separation from pseudodefects is more difficult than might be expected on intuitive grounds.

Table 4. Normal visual field: statistics of pseudodefects. N = 64 points examined. Parameter: criterion-to-noise ratio Δ/σ.

Δ/σ	1	2	2.5	3
mean number of pseudodefect points per examination	10.1	1.4	0.4	0.08
probability of producing:				
– any pseudoscotomata	1.00	0.77	0.33	0.08
– 2 or more defect points	1.00	0.43	0.06	< 0.01
– 4 or more defect points	0.99	0.06	< 0.01	
mean number of pseudo-scotomata per examination consisting of:				
– 2 or more connected points	2.2	0.1	0.01	
– 4 or more connected points	0.5	< 0.01		

Table 5. Probability $w_{det}(n)$ of detecting a true defect (assumed to cover n points of the examination grid) in at least one point. Assumed measurement error: $\sigma = 3$ dB. D: true depth of defect. Criterion chosen: $\Delta = 7.5$ dB.

D	n = 1	$w_{det}(n)$ n = 2	n = 3	n = 4
4.5 dB	0.16	0.29	0.41	0.50
7.5 dB	0.50	0.75	0.88	0.94
10.5 dB	0.84	0.97	1.0	1.0
13.5 dB	0.98	1.0	1.0	1.0

DETECTABILITY AND CHOICE OF EXAMINATION GRID

It is a commonplace to note that the probability of detecting small scotomata by static procedures depends essentially upon the number of points examined, in particular the scanning density. Furthermore, any improvement in detectability is possible only by the use of a denser grid, of course at the expense of examination time. Nevertheless, it is sometimes felt that for specific purposes some particular arrangement of examination points is more suitable than others.

Table 6. Detection probability as a function of the radius R of the defect (for the examination grids defined in figures 4a and 4b).

| R | Detection probability (in %) | |
	fig. 4a	fig. 4b
0.17°	0.25%	0.25%
0.7°	4%	4%
1.0°	9%	8%
2.0°	35%	17%
3.0°	79%	25%
4.2°	100%	36%

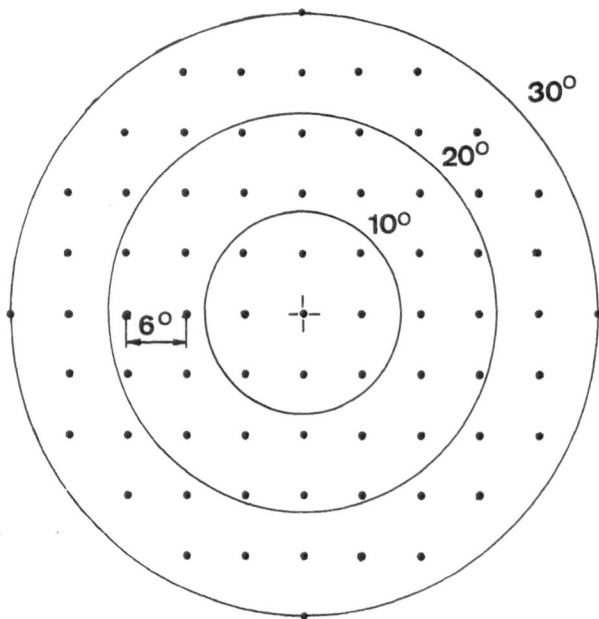

Fig. 4a.

Fig. 4. Scanning grids. Radius of examined area: 30°. *Fig. 4a:* Square grid. Octopus, programme 31. 72 points examined. Resolution: 6°. *Fig. 4b:* Scanning along meridians. 81 points examined. Radial resolution: 1.5°.

Let us consider the two arrangements shown in figure 4. The square grid (figure 4a) is taken from one of the standard programmes incorporated in the automaton Octopus: in this programme the central visual field (out to an eccentricity of 30°) is tested at 72 points, corresponding to a resolution of 6°. In contrast, another arrangement, the one shown in figure 4b, tests the same central area along two meridians; assuming a radial resolution of 1.5°, the number of points examined is about 80. The probability of detection of a circular scotoma of radius R, placed at random anywhere in the central area (out to an eccentricity of 30°), i.e. the probability of detecting it with one scanning point at least, follows for both grids from purely geometric considerations.

From the numerical values, listed in Table 6, some conclusions may be drawn:

— For tiny scotomata, with a radius smaller than 1°, the detection probability is extremely low and is independent of the choice of the grid, the search for such scotomata being almost hopeless anyway. Furthermore, as far as the detection phase is concerned, there is no point in applying test targets smaller than about 0.5°.

— For larger defects, a regular, rectangular grid, such as the square grid provided by the Octopus, is more appropriate. In fact, the difference in the probability of detection for the two compared arrangements is quite impressive.

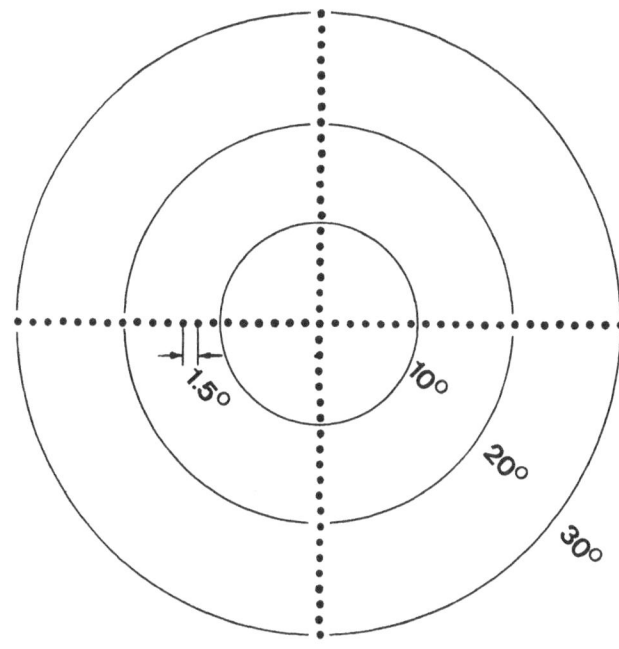

Fig. 4b.

— If, in a case, where there is reason to believe that a defect will be situated along a specific meridian, a search carried out with high resolution along this meridian may be considered. However, in such a case, one must be well aware of the extremely poor interazimuthal resolution.

Actually, many investigators have adopted the following procedure: routinely, a preliminary examination of some kind is performed which provides the justification for choosing one or several meridians for subsequent scanning. It would, however, be erroneous to believe that a preexamination of low resolution may be compensated by a subsequent high resolution meridional search programme. Obviously, during the second phase, only the detected scotomata define the meridians to be scanned. Although it is true that scotomata, if found during the first phase, may be better defined and assessed by a subsequent high resolution meridional scan, it must be emphasized that scotomata overlooked during the initial phase are lost for ever and will not be detected by a single or only a few meridional scans, based on the

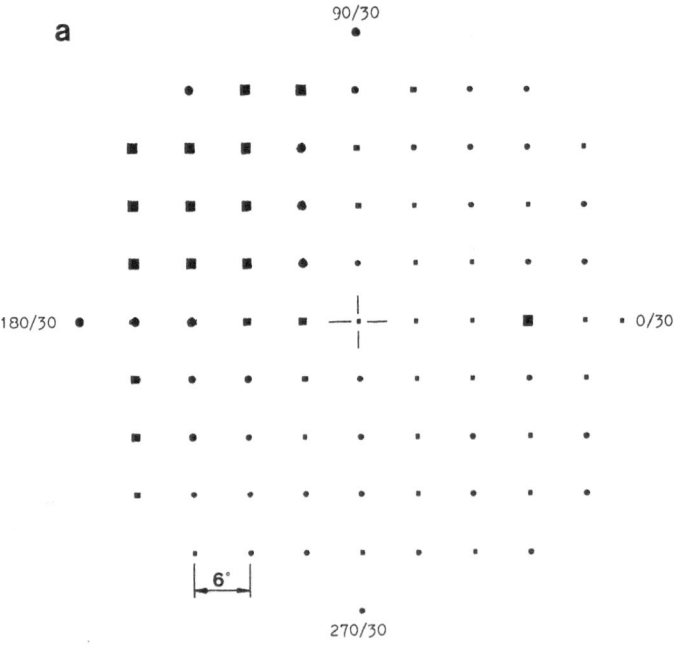

Fig. 5a.

Fig. 5. Results of static field examination. Radius of examined area: 30°. 5a: results of actual measurements (square grid, resolution 6°). 5b: based on actual results as displayed in 5a, but supplemented by symbols obtained from bivariate linear four point interpolation (original Octopus half-tone display, programme 31).

304

results of an initial low-resolution examination. An exception are those scotomata which are detected by chance by the meridional scan. This, however, may be considered an infrequent event unless a multitude of meridians is explored.

As a consequence of the divergence of the polar coordinate points – in contrast to the method involving a rectangular scanning grid – meridional perimetry has the additional disadvantage that the interazimuthal resolution of sensitivity loss drops with increasing eccentricity; this introduces an uncontrolled element of distortion which may reach extreme degrees in the far periphery and is overlooked most of the time.

GRAPHIC DISPLAY AND INTERPOLATION PROCEDURES

In kinetic perimetry, points actually determined are connected by solid lines in the hope that these would represent some probable course of the isopters.

Symb.									
dB	51 – 36	35 – 31	30 – 26	25 – 21	20 – 16	15 – 11	10 – 6	5 – 1	0
asb	0,008 – 0,25	0,31 – 0,8	1 – 2,5	3,1 – 8	10 – 25	31 – 80	100 – 250	315 – 800	1000

1 asb = 0,318 cd/m²

OCTOPUS® interzeag

Fig. 5b.

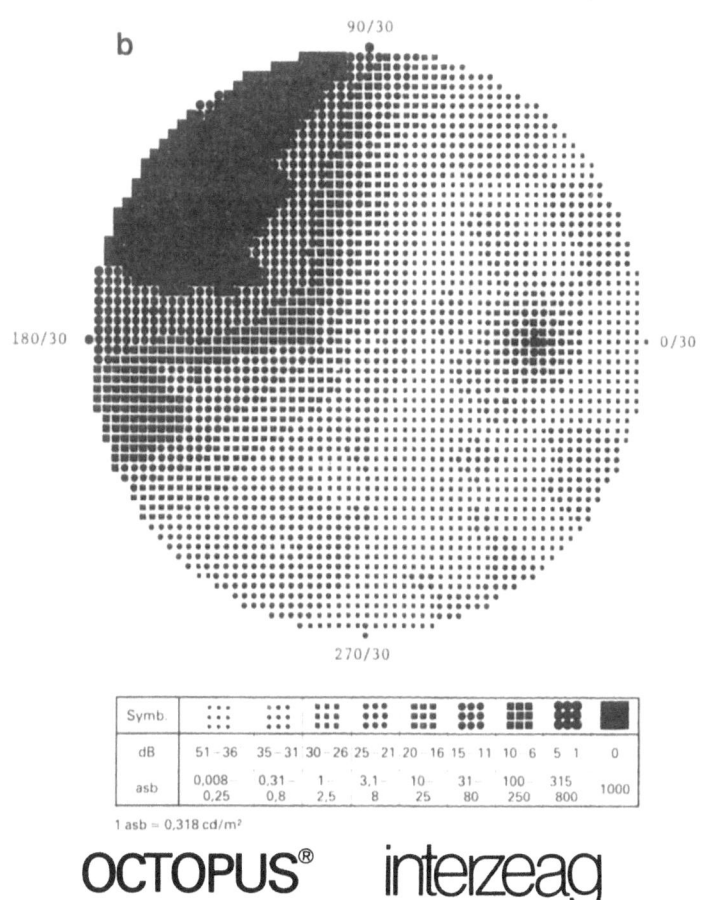

Because of a lack of definite knowledge, restricted examination time has to be substituted by a reasonable guess; this procedure may be called interpolation.

In the graphic display of automated visual field determinations, the role of the interpolation procedure, carried out over a two-dimensional grid of examination points, is illustrated in figure 5. The homogeneous half-tone display (figure 5b) is an original Octopus printout. The points actually determined are shown in the auxiliary display (figure 5a), with a grid constant of 6° in this particular example. Measured sentitivities are transformed into graphic symbols, each symbol corresponding to a specific sensitivity range in steps of 5 dB (0.5 log unit), as explained in more detail in the legend; again, the actual results are reported in figure 5a. In the original Octopus printout (figure 5b), based on identical measurements, the gaps have been filled by symbols corresponding to interpolated sensitivities; more precisely, interpolated sensitivities are derived from measured sensitivities (in the four neighbouring points) using coordinate differences as weight factors. The actually determined points remain unchanged and, if desired, are still recognizable by means of transparent overlays not shown here.

In a perimetric sensitivity display, of whatever nature it may be, interpolated auxiliary lines or points appear not infrequently in a twilight, which all too often misleads the interpreter. On the one hand, he may realize that interpolated auxiliary lines or patterns are of great help in the understanding of the sensitivity distribution across the entire visual field or just a section of it. This seems to reflect gestalt-psychological mechanisms and points to the fact that information should preferably be funneled into the human pattern-analyzing apparatus in a form which takes advantage of mental routines used during daily life. Connecting lines, such as used in profile sections, isopters or additional points filling up empty space, rather than using isolated determination points, are of considerable help in the interpretative perimetric task; they have always been used in manual static or kinetic perimetry. On the other side, interpolations may be questionable if they represent the truth rather poorly. This danger is particularly acute when improperly marked determinations and interpolations are confounded.

As the importance of representations by isolated values has been recognized, Octopus-routines have been developed displaying the sensitivity as discrete values in the form of figure tables not containing interpolated values.

The fact, however, remains, that visual field analysis by the perimetrist, that is, inspecting single values on the one hand and considering the visual field as a whole on the other, involves different cortical search mechanisms complementing each other.

INTERPOLATION PROCEDURES AND SPATIAL CORRELATIONS

In this section statistical analysis of the mean accuracy of interpolated sensitivities will be given, or, rather, an attempt is being made to determine the difference between true and interpolated thresholds. With regard to

306

practical applications, for pathological visual fields, numerical values, based on empirical material will be presented.

In order to gain a quantitative insight, let us consider four points P_1 ... P_4 of a visual field, forming a square with a side length of $L = 6°$, with centre P. Let the results of single threshold determinations at the corner points and at the centre be denoted by S_1 ... S_4 and S, respectively, and the true threshold at the centre by S_o

Three possibilities may be taken into consideration for the determination of the threshold at the centre:

a) Direct measurement (result S), carried out once (consisting of 4-6 answers).

b) By averaging of repeated determinations the true threshold S_0 may be approached to any desired accuracy.

c) In another attempt, we may estimate the threshold at the centre of the square by an interpolation procedure, namely by computing the average of the results of single threshold determinations at the corner points:

$$S_{int} = \frac{1}{4} \cdot (S_1 + S_2 + S_3 + S_4) .$$

(3)

In order to estimate the quality of the interpolation procedure, we have to compare the mean deviation of S_{int} from S_o with the mean deviation of S from S_o. S deviates from S_o due to the measurement error, its rms value being denoted by σ:

$$\sigma^2 = \overline{(S-S_0)^2} .$$

(4)

S_{int} deviates from the true threshold S_0 for two reasons:
(i) the true threshold S_0 at the centre is not identical with the mean of the true thresholds at the corner points. For normal visual fields, these non-linearities are caused by the natural ripple of the contrast sensitivity as a function of retinal location, and for pathological visual fields, local defects are superimposed on these nonlinearities; (ii) furthermore, the values S_1 ... S_4, inserted into (3), deviate from the true thresholds at the corner points, the rms deviation also being given by the mean measurement error σ. Let σ_{int} stand for the deviation of S_{int} from the true threshold S_o:

$$\sigma_{int}^2 = \overline{(S_{int} - S_0)^2}$$

(5)

We have collected numerical values for σ and σ_{int} by analysing more than 2000 combinations of five points (corner points and centre of a square) spread out to an eccentricity of $30°$ and distributed over 45 eyes, the great majority of which had heavily damaged visual fields due to glaucoma or optic nerve disease. Actually, the visual fields were determined twice by the automated perimeter Octopus, applying programme 31, which has a grid constant of $6°$, thus obtaining sensitivities at the corner points of the squares to be analysed. The same visual fields were redetermined twice by programme 32, which is shifted along the ordinate and the abscissa relative to programme 31 by half a grid constant, thus yielding the sensitivities at the centres of the squares.

From the total of the data material, the following numerical values have been obtained (rms average):

(i)   error of single determination: $\sigma = 3.0$ dB

(ii) deviation of interpolated sensitivity from the true sensitivity: $\sigma_{int} = 3.2$ dB (Note that exact knowledge of S_0 is not necessary in order to estimate σ and σ_{int}; from basic statistics, the determination of S and S_{int}, repeated once, will suffice).

Therefore, when interpolation within a grid having a grid constant equal to or smaller than $6°$, interpolated sensitvities are only slightly worse than direct measurements, at least on the average. From this point of view, a grid constant of $6°$ seems adequate. If actual measurements by means of a denser grid are replaced by interpolations, small scotomata between points actually determined may of course be missed. Keeping this in mind, actual measurements are always preferable provided sufficient time is available if small scotomata are expected. Our discussion aims to indicate the average error to be expected when applying interpolation procedures, if, for lack of examination time, or for economic reasons a denser grid is not available. Keeping this necessity in mind, a series of high-resolution Octopus programmes are being prepared at the present time.

CONCLUSIONS

Due to threshold fluctuations, which occur in the neurovisual system, scotomata are often either submerged in the threshold noise and thus undetectable or else fortuitous threshold shifts may be taken for true pathological sensitivity disturbances. These effects are notoriously underestimated and can only be controlled by statistical evaluation of the threshold fluctuations and by evaluating the magnitude of the sensitivity loss.

The diagnosis of an observed scotoma is always a statistical decision and not an absolute matter, as implied by a number of graphical displays found in the world literature on perimetry.

Averaging methods and statistical decisions, in the domain of computer methods, enable us to detect scotomata which otherwise would go undetected.

The strategies to be followed for a rapid and reliable detection of unknown scotomata distributed over a part or the whole of the visual field depend firstly on the size and the distribution of such sensitivity depressions.

If the distribution of damage is not known, a rectangular scanning grid offers the greatest probability of detection. Other search strategies may be subdivided into a cursory examination providing a first preliminary information followed by a second more detailed scan, which approximates in essence a rectangular coordinate search pattern. This is so, because the first examination phase also provides information about the interazimuthal visual field areas which are usually ignored by meridional profile perimetry.

As a rule, time restrictions limit the density of our scanning grid, i.e. the number of our determination points. Unscanned field areas are advantageously filled up with interpolated values representing the best possible guess of the sensitivity over such areas. A superficial estimate of such interpolated values may dismiss the latter as useless and misleading. However, the analysis of a representative interpolation problem, assessing actual deviations of interpolated from true values shows, that, on the average, interpolation displays true values to a surprisingly high degree. In addition, methods of interpolation are appreciated because isolated, discrete figures or symbols of sensitivity make a comprehension of the distribution of sensitivity difficult.

ACKNOWLEDGEMENT

We are indepted to Dr. R. Markus for his help and advice in preparing the manuscript. The figures were made by Mr. R. Sutter.

REFERENCES

Bebie, H., F. Fankhauser & J. Spahr. Static Perimetry: Accuracy and Fluctuations. *Acta Ophthal.* (Kbh.) 54: *339-348* (1976).

Koerner, F., F. Fankhauser, H. Bebie & J. Spahr. Threshold noise and variability of field defects in determinations by manual and automatic perimetry. Doc. Ophthal. Proc. Series 14: *53-59* (1977).

Krakau, T. On time series analysis of visual acuity. A statistical model. *Acta Ophthal. (Kbh.)* 47: *660-666* (1969).

Niesel, P. Streuungen perimetrischer Untersuchungsergebnisse. *Ophthalmologica* 161: *180-186* (1970).

Ronchi, L. An annotated bibliography on variability and periodicities of visual responsiveness. Atti Fond. G. Ronchi, vol. 17 (1972).

Spahr, J., F. Fankhauser, F. Jenni & H. Bebie. Praktische Erfahrungen mit dem automatischen Perimeter Octopus. *Klin. Mbl. Augenheilk.* 172: *470-477* (1978).

Author's addresses:
University Eye Clinic
Institut für theoretische Physik
University of Berne
CH-3000 Berne
Switzerland

Docum. Ophthal. Proc. Series, Vol. 19

SEMI-AUTOMATIC CAMPIMETER WITH GRAPHIC DISPLAY

SUSUMU HAMAZAKI, TSUNEO YOKOTA, HIROSHI MIENO,
SHINICHI KOIKE, MICHIMASA TAGA, JUNJI HAMAZAKI,
GEN KIKUCHI & HARUTAKE MATSUO

(Tokyo, Japan)

ABSTRACT

Results of perimetry have a tendency to be influenced by tester's technique and subjectivity. We have attempted to provide a new instrument which works automatically under constant condition which multiple pattern stimuli.

At the first step, we made a semi-automatic system. This system is composed of a common television receiving set, micro computer system and audio cassette tape-recorder. Tester's task is only to push the key (indicated numbers, directions, 'go', 'D' etc.) of the micro computer. Subject's task is only to reply numbers and directions of recognized light point(s) according to the instructions and questions displayed on television. The rest of the work (including changes of stimulus intensity) will be carried out by the micro computer. Finally, the result is displayed on television.

INTRODUCTION

In order to produce a simple and economical automatic perimeter system, a recently progressed micro computer system (MC) and a commonly used television receiving set (TV), were utilized. At the first step, production of semi-automatic campimeter with graphic (character) display was tried.

METHOD

The semi-automatic campimeter is composed of MC, TV and audio cassette tape-recorder as seen in Fig. 1. The programme to be memorized in MC for this campimetry has been recorded in the audio cassette tape. Consequently, time and labour to enter programme in the memory of MC at each test were saved.

Before the test begins, the subject is explained how to be tested with several samples. Then, the subject is kept under adapting condition during 5 minutes.

At first, following instruction appears on TV for 12 seconds: '"READY" appears on TV. One light point will appear on the center of TV twice. When you will be looking at that point, several light points will be seen. Then, please tell me the number of recognized point(s).'

The operation-system of the new campimeter consists of 4 Divisions, each of which has several Section's.

Section:

1. Characters 'READY' and central fixation point are shown on TV for 5 sec..

2. The central fixation point lighted for 0.5 sec. is shown twice with an interval of 0.5 sec. (flicker).

3. After the fixation point has disappeared for 0.5 sec., multiple stimuli which have different patterns from one another are shown for 0.5 sec.. (fig. 2)

4. The subject tells the number of recognized point(s).

5. Tester pushes the key of MC corresponding to the subject's reply.

6. MC judges whether the reply is correct or not. If the reply is correct, this section is finished. If not correct, however, re-test is performed as described in 1 through 5.

7. MC judges finally. In case of mistakes, the characters 'Please tell me in which direction(s) you saw, such as above, below, right, left, upper left, down right, etc..' are shown.

8. The subject tells the direction of the recognized point(s).

9. Tester pushes the key of MC corresponding to the subject's reply, according to the rules decided at each pattern.

10. MC memorizes the pattern of this section and the subject's mistaken stimulus point(s). Then, this section is finished.

The first division consists of 15 sections. Each section has a pattern of A

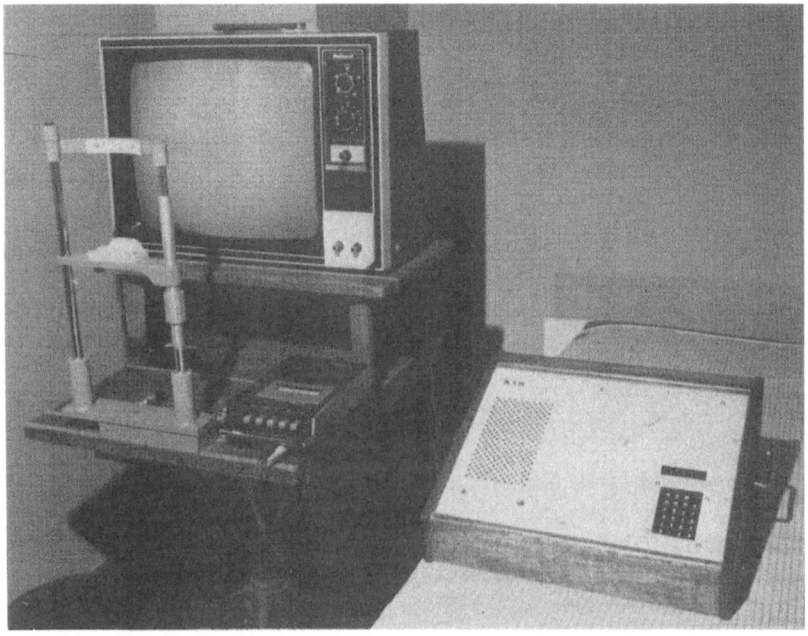

Fig. 1. System of the semi-automatic campimeter.

through P, which are all different. (Fig. 2) These patterns are similar to 15 patterns reported by Shinzatos. Of all four divisions, the first division's stimulus intensity was the lowest.

The second division consists of sections which have the patterns mistaken in the first division. This time, stimulus intensity is one step higher than before.

The third division consists of sections which have patterns mistaken in the second. Stimulus intensity is one step higher than the second.

The final division consists of sections which have patterns mistaken in the third. Stimulus intensity is the highest.

These four divisions are not always tested. When all stimuli points are recognized, except Mariotte blind spot, this test is finished according to tester's judgement.

At the end of each section, the result obtained so far, can be shown by pushing the key 'D'. The point mistaken up to this time is displayed with 'X'. The point recognized for the first time in the second division is displayed with '1'. The point recognized for the first time in the third division is displayed with '2'. The point recognized for the first time in the final division is displayed with '3'.

15 PATTERNS

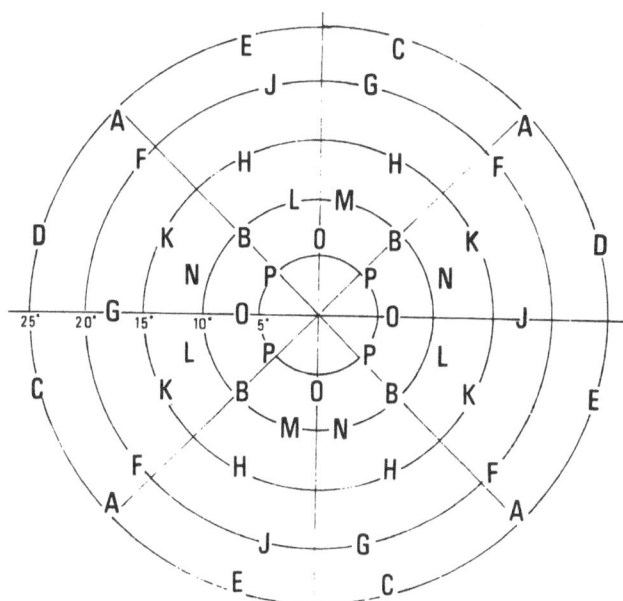

Fig. 2. 15 patterns of multiple stimuli.

In order not to disturb the subject's adapting condition, it is neccessary to separate the subject from the tester. Tester knows the situation of the programme without looking at Braun tube. Because judgement in section, pattern's mark, etc. appear on the display-board of MC.

RESULTS

In normal subjects, after the end of the first division which was tested with lowest stimulus intensity, all points, except Mariotte blind spot, were recognized.

In a case diagnosed as open angle glaucoma, a 56-year-old, female, a depression was found by kinetic perimetry with Goldmann Perimeter as seen in Fig. 3, and several scotomata were found by static perimetry with Friedmann Visual Field Analyser as seen in Fig. 4. From the result of the semi-automatic campimeter, scotomata expressed in characters '1', '2', '3' and 'X' were recognized (Fig. 5). It shows that this campimeter can be useful in practice.

DISCUSSION

The results of not only kinetic perimetry but also static perimetry by single pattern stimulus method were liable to be influenced by tester's technique and subjectivity. It had been even said that perimetry was an art. Then,

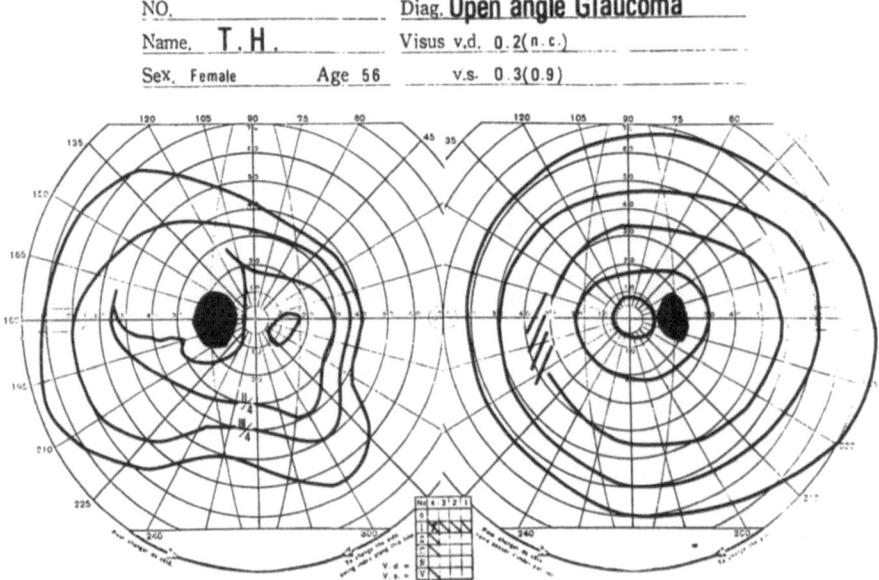

Fig. 3. Result with Goldmann Perimeter in the case of open angle glaucoma.

314

multiple pattern stimuli method was introduced for the purpose of simple perimetry. But this multiple pattern stimuli method has a few weak points influenced by tester's technique and subjectivity. Therefore, many investigators tried to make an automatic perimeter. Aulhorn made the Tübingen Perimeter automated. Fankhauser made the Octopus which was elaborate but expensive. Heijl made an automatic static screening perimeter. These perimeters used the single stimulus method. Greve (1977) reported a remote control semi-automatic perimeter using an oscilloscope. Greve's method incorporated multiple pattern stimuli.

It was considered that multiple stimuli method was more suitable to make a simple instrument and acquire stabilized results, than single stimulus method. Moreover, for the purpose of dissolving difficulty of keeping central visual fixation, a flicker was made at the central fixation point.

The experiment was placed under some limitation of MC which was used at that point of time. For example, only characters can be displayed by this MC. Therefore, one period corresponding to 35 min. of visual angle had to be used as one stimulus point. Stimulus intensity was controlled by change of electric resistance. Because of using ordinary TV, stimulus time was 0.5 sec. duration in order to distinguish stimulus from noise.

If background luminance is modulated at mesopic condition (0.03 asb.), the subject is apt to miss the stimulus by glow remaining after the display of

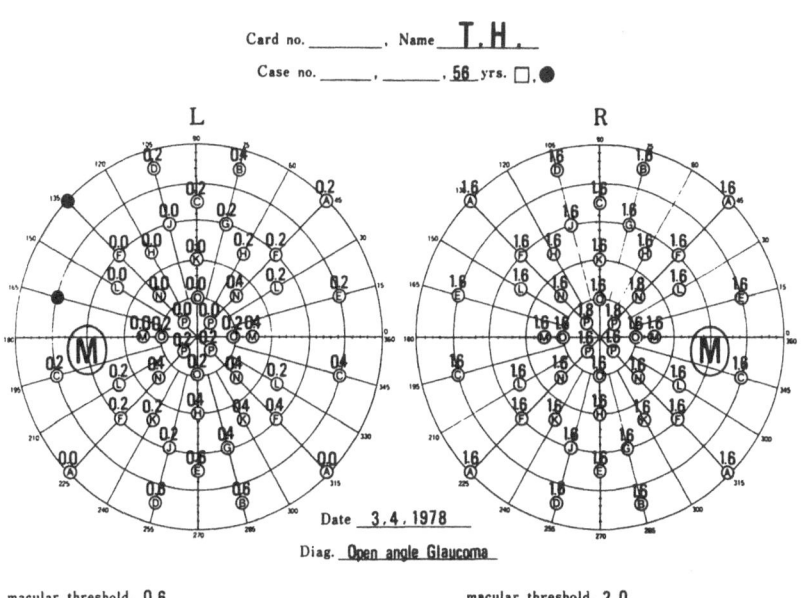

Fig. 4. Result with Friedmann Visual Field Analyser in the case of open angle glaucoma.

315

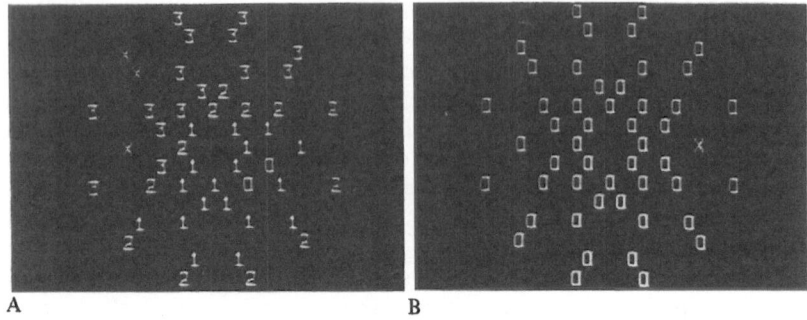

A   B

Fig. 5. Result with the semi-automatic campimeter in the case of open angle glaucoma.

the indicating characters. Moreover, the subject's adapting condition is disturbed by brightness of displayed characters for the instructions and questions. Therefore, background luminance had to be decided at 0.1 asb. same as the condition of Friedmann Visual Field Analyser. This adapting condition is at the maximum of mesopic condition, but the size of stimuli points could not be changed as in Friedmann Visual Field Analyser. Hence, even in normal subjects, difficult points to be recognized were seen at periphery and near by displayed characters. In the future, instructions and questions to the subject, shall be given verbally instead of being displayed on Braun tube. Then, background luminance will be under the mesopic condition in order to acquire same stimulus intensity in periphery and points near displayed characters.

But this time, it was possible to give instructions and questions with constant timing and method. This experiment made it possible to make the automatic perimeter.

CONCLUSION & SUMMARY

Production of simple and economical automatic campimeter was tried. At first, using micro computer which has been recently progressed and commonly used television receiving set, multiple pattern stimuli was displayed on Braun tube of TV as we considered the method was suitable for automation. Instructions and questions were also displayed. Even though, there are many problems to be solved, campimeter can be measured semi-automatically.

REFERENCES

Aulhorn, E. & Durst, W. Comparative investigation of automatic and manual perimetry in different visual field defects. *Docum. Ophthal. Proc. Series* 14: *17-22* (1977).
Fankhauser, F., Spahr, J. & Bebie, H. Three years of experience with the OCTOPUS automatic perimeter. *Docum. Ophthal. Proc. Series* 14: *7-15* (1977).
Greve, E.L., Groothuyse, M.T.H.J.N. & Bakker, P. Simulated automatic perimetry. *Docum. Ophthal. Proc. Series* 14: *23-29* (1977).

316

Heijl, A. & Krakau, C.E.T. An automatic static perimeter, design and pilot study. *Acta Ophthal.* 53: *293-310* (1975).

Shinzato, E., Suzuki, R. & Furuno, F. The central visual field changes in glaucoma using Goldmann Perimeter and Friedmann Visual Field Analyser. *Docum. Ophthal. Proc. Series* 14: *93-101* (1977).

Authors' address:
Dept. of Ophthalmology
Tokyo Medical College Hospital
6-7-1 Nishishinjuku, Shinjuku-ku
Tokyo 160
Japan

Docum. Ophthal. Proc. Series, Vol. 19

AUTOMATIC COMPUTERIZED PERIMETRY
IN NEURO-OPHTHALMOLOGY

H. BYNKE, A. HEIJL & C. HOLMIN

(Lund, Sweden)

ABSTRACT

115 eyes of 63 patients with neurological diseases were examined with an automatic computerized perimeter. Manual kinetic perimetry with Goldmann's instrument was used for comparison. In 92 fields the automatic method disclosed all defects that had been found by manual perimetry. Furthermore, in 8 fields it revealed small defects that had been missed at the initial manual examination. The remaining 15 fields were normal using both methods. In 22 pathological fields of 12 patients both examinations were repeated during the course of the disease and showed parallel improvement, deterioration or unchanged defects. It was concluded that the automatic method is superior to manual kinetic perimetry in detecting visual field defects of neurological origin, and that it may replace the manual method in following up small and medium-sized defects. For large defects it is not suitable.

INTRODUCTION

An automatic computerized perimeter has been constructed at the Department of Experimental Ophthalmology in Lund (Heijl & Krakau 1975, Krakau 1978). A pilot study has shown this method to be superior to manual kinetic perimetry in detecting visual field defects of neurological origin (Bynke & Heijl 1978). The instrument has now been used in a greater number of cases. The purpose of this work was to evaluate its ability to reveal and follow up neurological field defects.

MATERIAL

The material consists of 115 visual fields of 63 patients with intracranial tumours, cerebrovascular and other cerebral lesions, and optic nerve disease, who had been referred to the Department of Neuro-Ophthalmology in Lund. 37 patients were male and 26 female, and their ages ranged between 9 and 74 years. The material comprises a selection of small and medium-sized bitemporal and homonymous hemianopias and quadrantanopias, central and paracentral scotomata, arcuate defects and normal fields.

METHODS

The automatic computerized perimeter (AP) used has 64 static test points located in the paracentral visual field inside 25 degrees of eccentricity (Fig. 1). These stimuli can be lit at 16 intensity levels, the ratio between two consecutive levels being 1:2 (Heijl & Krakau 1975, Krakau 1978). A test programme requiring an examination time of approximately 8 -9 minutes per eye was applied (Test logic I, Heijl 1977). The examination is entirely automatic, i.e. the perimeter needs no attendance while the examination is carried out.

The control method was the kinetic manual perimetry with Goldmann's instrument (MP), which is routine in this hospital. In most cases this examination was performed prior to the automatic perimetry by specially trained technicians. Additional methods in some cases were tangent screen examinations and confrontation tests. 93 visual fields of 51 patients were examined with AP and MP on one single occasion. 22 fields of 12 patients were examined during the course of the disease on two, three or four occasions. Eleven of these 12 patients had suprasellar tumours.

The visual fields recorded by means of Goldmann's instrument were interpreted as is generally done in clinical work. Thus isopter irregularities and scotomata were given more attention than a general depression of sensitivity. A more stringent type of interpretation was used for the automatic fields. Generally, a decrease of sensitivity surmounting two intensity steps in multiple adjacent points was considered pathological.

RESULTS

In 92 visual fields the same defects were revealed both by MP and AP. In 15 fields no defects were found by either method.

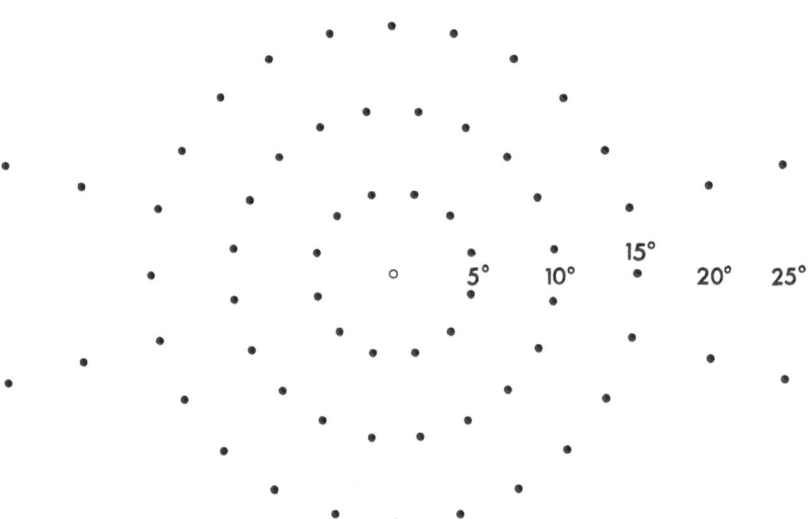

Fig. 1. Test point pattern of the perimeter. Each point represents one test point.

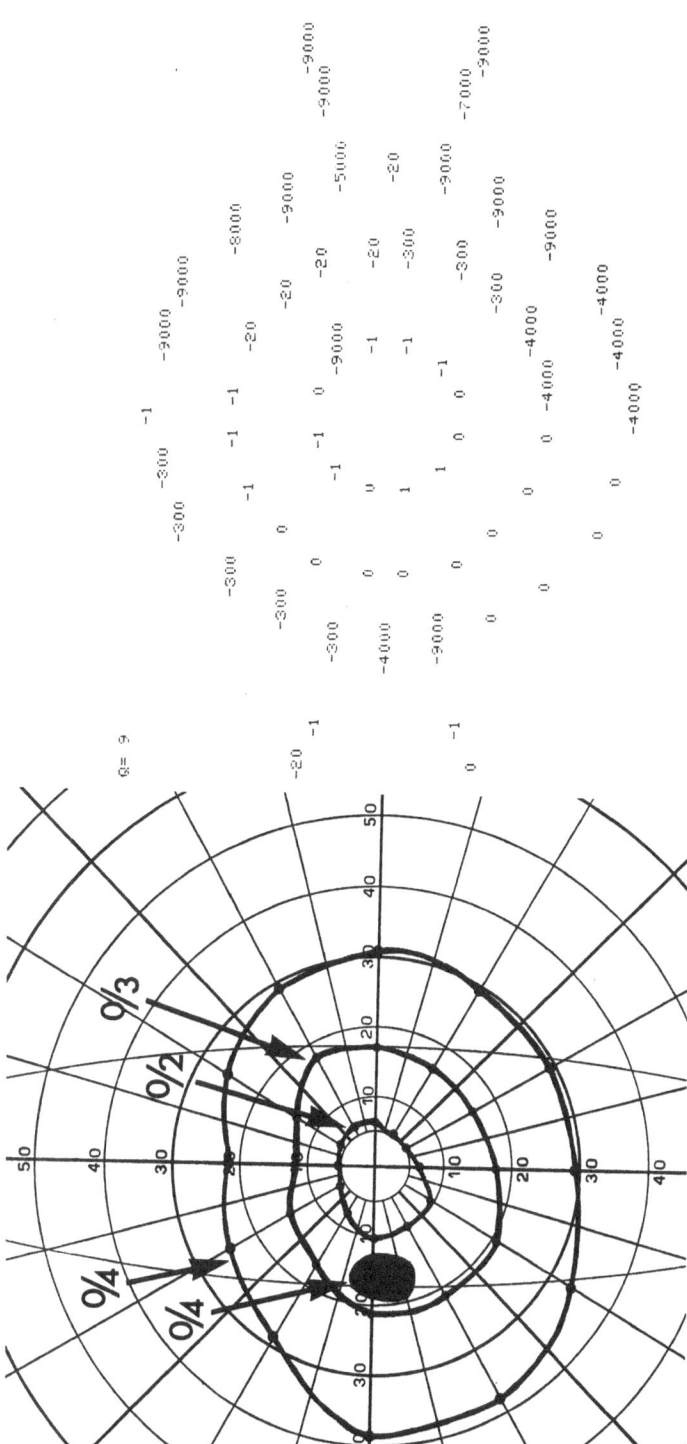

Fig. 2. Left visual field in a patient with homonymous hemianopia. The defect was missed at the first manual examination but revealed at automatic perimetry.

In the automatic field charts each figure represents the threshold value in a test point as compared with Q. Q is the most frequent threshold value (mode).

In the plotting of the chart the computer uses the formula $P_N = T_N - Q$, where T is the threshold value and P is the plotted volume in a point N. Thus, a zero in the plot represents a threshold value that equals Q. A negative figure means lower sensitivity. If the strongest stimuli have not been seen ($T_N = 0$) P_N will be $- Q$.

Zeroes are added to the negative values so as to let the defects stand out more strikingly.

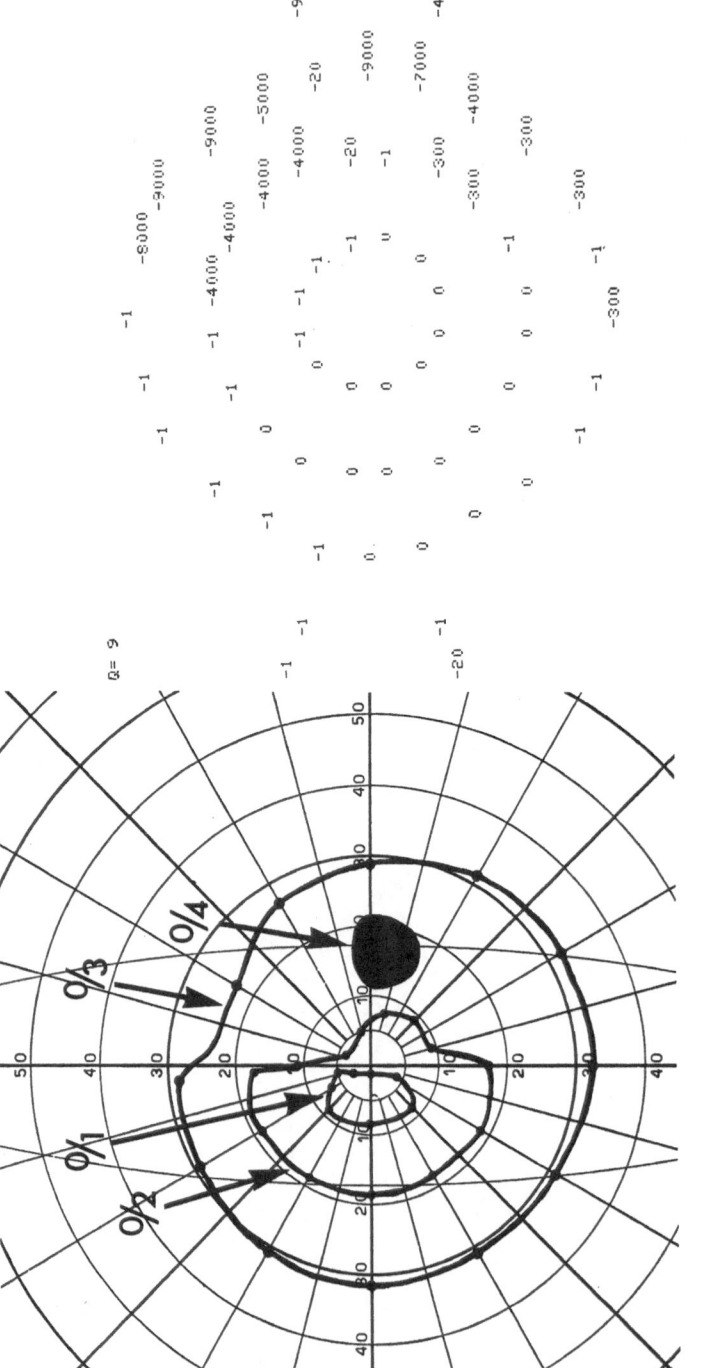

Fig. 3a.

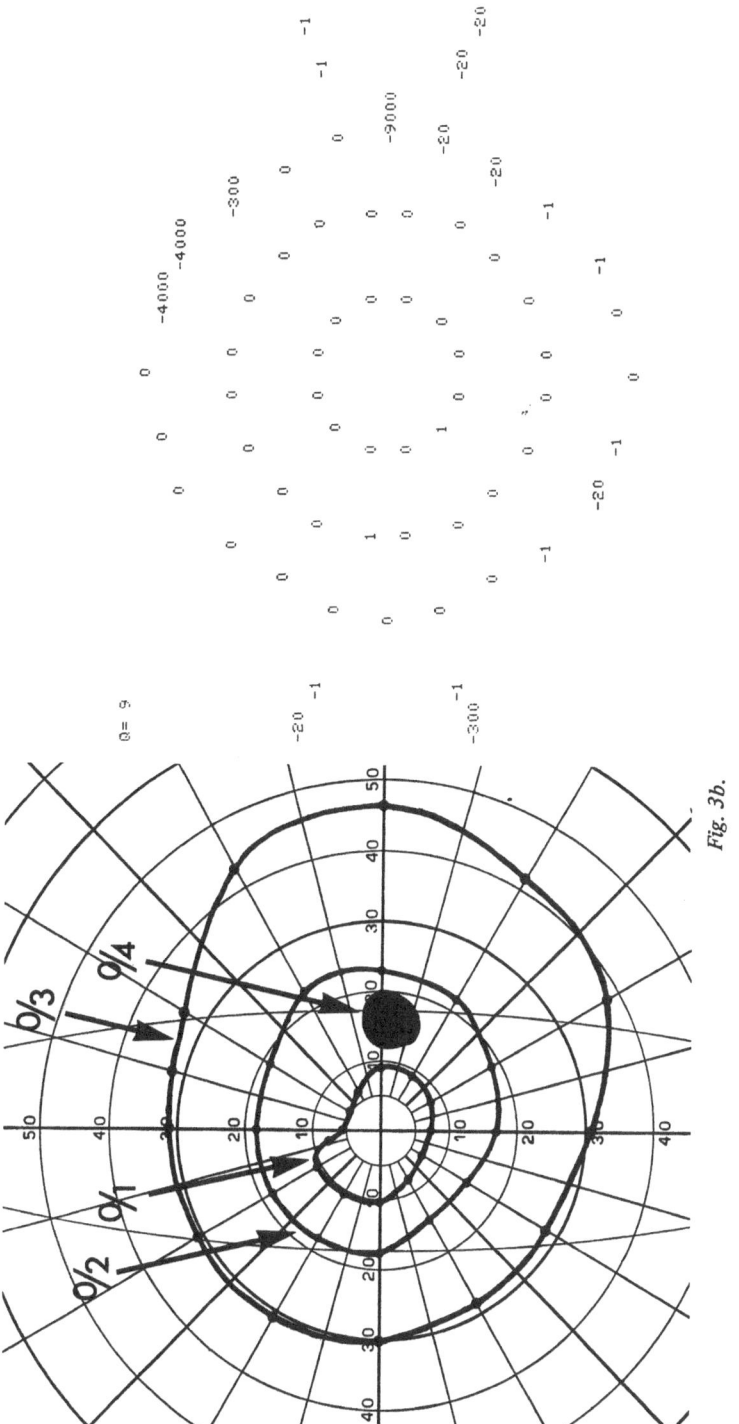

Fig. 3. Right visual field in a patient with bitemporal hemianopia due to a pituitary adenoma. The visual field was examined before (3 a) and after (3 b) the operation. The defects were revealed and the fields showed consistent improvement both at manual and at automatic perimetry.

Fig. 3b.

In the remaining 8 fields of 5 cases, small defects were missed by MP but disclosed by AP. One of these patients had a paracentral scotoma corresponding to an old choroiretinitis and another one a small bitemporal hemimnopia due to an empty sella after treatment of a pituitary adenoma (Bynke & Heijl 1978). Other defects missed by MP but detected by AP were a small temporal hemianopia in one field of a patient with a pituitary adenoma and homonymous hemianopia in a case of cerebrovascular lesion (Fig. 2). The defects of these four patients were verified at subsequent manual examinations performed by the authors.

The fifth case was a 9 year-old boy with small paracentral defects in both fields because of retinal dystrophy with optic atrophy. These defects were not verified by MP but the appearance of the fundi made their existence highly probable.

In the 12 patients in whom the examinations were repeated during the course of the disease, both AP and MP showed improvement in 7 fields (Figs. 3 a and b), deterioration in 6 fields and unchanged defects in 9 fields.

DISCUSSION

AP did not miss any of the field defects disclosed by MP but revealed 8 small defects that had been missed at the initial MP. Consequently, the previous conclusion that AP is superior to MP in detecting neurological field defects (Bynke & Heijl 1978) was supported by this extended study.

At repeated examinations during the course of the disease the two methods showed consistent results. It is evident that AP may replace MP in following up small and medium-sized defects. However, it is not suitable for checking large defects, since it cannot cover the peripheral field and since its maximum stimulus intensity is lower than that of Goldmann's instrument.

As regards the position of the field defects, the concordance of the methods was good. However, several defects seemed larger and/or deeper in the automatic than in the manual charts, and the reverse was true in some fields. This may be explained by the dissimilarity of the methods. The stimuli are of different size and intensity and the background illuminations are not equal. MP is a kinetic method which presents the stimuli in positions that may be more or less expected by the examinee, while AP is static and presents the stimuli at random positions. Furthermore, in MP the length of the test session is influenced by the patient's cooperation and the perimetrist's accuracy but in AP it is kept fairly constant. Thus, AP has the advantage over MP of eliminating errors introduced by the perimetrist.

REFERENCES

Bynke, H. & Heijl, A. Automatic computerized perimetry in the detection of neurological visual field defects. A pilot study. *Graefes Arch. Ophthal.* in press (1978).

Heijl, A. Computer test logics for automatic perimetry. *Acta Ophthal.* (Kbh.) 55: *837-853* (1977).

Heijl, A. & Krakau, C.E.T. An automatic perimeter for glaucoma visual field screening and control. Construction and clinical cases. *Graefes Arch. Ophthal.* 197: *13-23* (1975).

Krakau, C.E.T. Aspects on the design of an automatic perimeter. *Acta Ophthal.* (Kbh.), in press (1978).

Authors' address:
University Eye Clinic
S-221 85 Lund, Sweden

AUTOMATED PERIMETRY:
MINICOMPUTERS OR MICROPROCESSORS?

M. ZINGIRIAN, V. TAGLIASCO & E. GANDOLFO

(Genoa, Italy)

ABSTRACT

Until a few years ago, microprocessors had several disadvantages in comparison with minicomputers: they were not fast process unit; they could implement only small sets of instructions; they could not reach a high number of memory cells; they implemented algorithms of modest complexity; they could control a limited number of peripherals, but had the advantages of very reduced overall dimensions and of reasonable costs.

In recent years the differences between the two process units have notably decreased, due to the increased number of microprocessor-based systems, whose features more and more resemble those of minicomputers. The problems originating from the continuous evolution of process systems could be overcome by the adoption of a digital standard interface, with whom typologically different computers and perimeters could be connected. The perimeter would acquire, in this case, the role of a simple peripheral unit.

PRESENT STATE OF AUTOMATED PERIMETRY

The development of automatic perimetry is at the present moment at a standstill.

In the last years many typologically different prototypes (Aulhorn et al., Crick et al., Greve et al., Heijl and Krakau, Pashley), whose performance usually doesn't go beyond the detection phase, have appeared in the clinical and research fields (Aulhorn 1975, 1977; Fankhauser, Bebie & Spahr 1977; Greve, Groothuyse & Bakker 1976; Heijl 1976, 1977; Heijl & Krakau 1975; Pashley & Bipas 1978).

Few more accurate devices, like Fankhauser and Spahr's Octopus (Bebie, Fankhauser & Spahr 1976; Fankhauser, Bebie & Spahr 1977; Korner, Fankhauser, Spahr & Bebie 1977; Spahr & Fankhauser 1974; Weber & Spahr 1976) and Zingirian et al.'s automated campimeter (Grignolo, Zingirian & Frugone 1977; Zingirian & Tagliasco 1977), permit also the development of the clinical assessment phase, due to their exploration accuracy but as they become available on the market, their diffusion is limited by high costs and by too rapid technological evolution.

This work was supported by a grant from the Consiglio Nazionale delle Ricerche, Roma, Italy.

Finally, as far as the process unit is concerned, the choice of the use of minicomputers or microprocessors is still a matter of controversy.

MINICOMPUTERS AND MICROPROCESSORS

Until a few years ago, microprocessors i) were not very fast process units; ii) they were based on words made up of a low number of bits and so could implement only a small set of instructions; iii) they could not reach a high number of memory cells; iv) they implemented calculations and algorithms of modest complexity; v) they could control a limited number of peripherals, but had the advantages of very reduced overall dimensions and of reasonable costs. These characteristics substantially differentiated microprocessors from minicomputers, which are faster computing and process units, endowed with a larger set of instructions and wide possibilities of reaching memory, and capable of implementing complex algorithms and running various peripherals. The drawbacks of minicomputers were overall dimensions and high acquisition and running costs.

In recent years, the differences between the two units, microprocessors and minicomputers, have notably decreased, due to the increased number of microprocessor-based systems (Klig 1978), whose features (fig. 1) more and more resemble those of minicomputers (their performances are in fact very similar, except for velocity). There are presently available 16-bit microprocessors with a machine language identical to that of minicomputers.

Nowadays one can say that there is no substantial difference between the performance of a sophisticated perimeter based on microprocessors (or rather, on microcomputers) and that based on minicomputers. The latter are mainly used in ophtalmic centers where not only perimetric tests but also other semeiologic procedures can be carried out automatically, such as electroretinography, evoked potentials, ultrasonography, fluorangiography, and so on (fig. 2).

The continuous evolution of computing and process units makes extremely unstable the substratum on which research and prototype design in the area of automated perimetry are based.

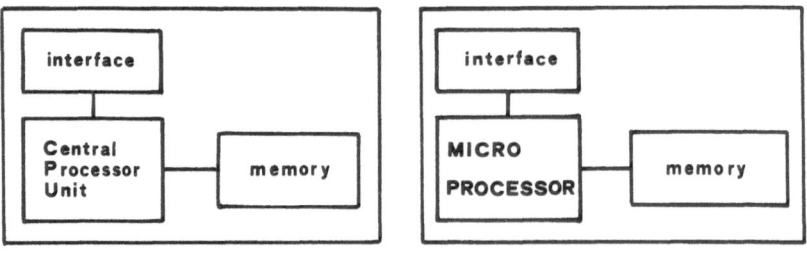

MINICOMPUTER   **MICROCOMPUTER**

Fig. 1. Comparison between minicomputer and micro-processor structures.

328

Historically standardization has constituted a necessary stage in automation development.

In automated perimetry standardization is an essential condition for attaining, at low costs, reliable, repeatable results, which may be compared and transferred from clinic to clinic.

As a contribution towards the achievement of an international standardization, an initial approach might be to isolate from the present systems, especially for kinetic perimetry, three different structures (fig. 3):

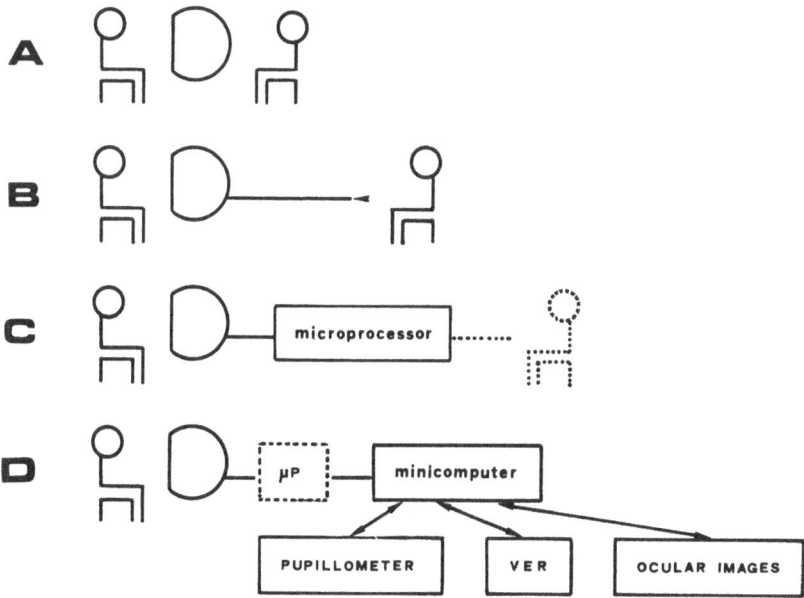

Fig. 2. Evolution of perimetry:
A-Manual; B-Remotely controlled; C-Micro-processor controlled; D-Micro-processor controlled, inserted in a more complex minicomputer-based structure.

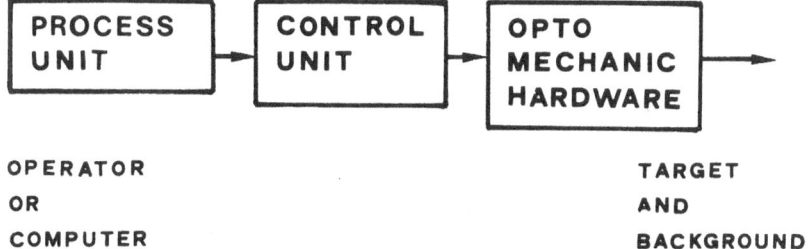

Fig. 3. Hardware and software structures of an automated perimetric system.

1. the opto-mechanical frame (by which it is possible to present to a subject a target with certain assigned geometric and photometric characteristics, on a luminous background);
2. the control unit (which allows us to change the geometric and photometric parameters as well as the position of the luminous target);
3. the process unit (by which particular strategies of target presentation are implemented and the subject's responses are recorded and graphically represented).

By considering 1) and 2) as hardware structures and 3) as a software structure, we can define hardware and software protocols, by which it is possible to characterize both the various types of perimeter available and those which will be developed in the future, on the basis of construction typologies (mechanical, optical, photometric, etc.) and computing units employed.

In order to formulate these protocols, we must first define a standard perimetric unit through its performance and the functions that put it in contact with the two users: the subject examined and the operator.

Thus, we might change from the concept of perimeter as a device to that of 'perimeter status' defined, in static conditions, by the photometric and geometric characteristics of the targets and by the photometric features of the background. Such perimeter status can and must also be considered from a dynamic point of view, when we analyse the strategies of target presentation along particular trajectories (kinetic perimetry) or by orderly sequences of positions (static perimetry).

Thus, automated perimetry could aim at controlling such 'perimeter status' during the examination. Therefore the characteristics and their acceptable tolerances of optomechanical hardware and the electrical inputs and outputs of the control unit should be standardized; above all digital interface standard between control and driving units should be defined. In the last few years, digital interface standards have come to prominence, such as IEEE 488 (Loughry & Allen 1978) and IEEE 583, along with mini- and microcomputer diffusion. Should this philosophy be accepted, the perimeter would play the role of the real peripheral, which could be included in existing computing units not limited to any particular system.

Finally, in case a standardization proposal of this type should be accepted, we might study the opportunity to achieve standardization of target presentation procedures, of strategies and of results representation techniques (in both static and kinetic perimetry), which would then be reduced to classical software problems.

In Italy a special Programme in Biomedical Technologies is now developing and there is a trend towards applying these concepts of digital standard interface to medical instrumentation. As far as concerns ophthalmology, our philosophy is to promote the adoption of these standards, not only for visual field examination, in order to avoid the overwhelming role of continuously changing computer-based devices.

REFERENCES

Aulhorn, E. Ueber die Automatisierung der perimetrischen Untersuchung. Die Wahl der Untersuchungsstrategie aus augenärztlicher Sicht. *Biomed. Tech. (Stuttg.)* 20 (1975).

Aulhorn, E., Durst, W. Comparative investigation of automatic and manual perimetry in different visual field defects. Proc. 2nd Int. Visual Field Symp. Tubingen, 1976 *Doc. Ophthalmol.* 14: *17-22* (1977).

Aulhorn, E., Gauger, E., Karmeyer, T. Die Steuerung des Tübinger Perimeters mit einem frei programmierbaren Kleinrechner. *Biomed. Tech. (Stuttg.)* 20 (1975).

Bebie, H., Fankhauser, F., Spahr, J. Static perimetry: Accuracy and fluctuations. *Acta Ophthalmol. (Kbh.)* 54: *339-348* (1976).

Crick, J.C.P., Ripley, L.J., Crick, R.P. The principles involved in the design of a visual field computer and automatic transcriber. Proc. 1st. Int. Symp. Visual Field. Marseille, 1974 *Ann. Thér. Clin. Ophthalmol.* 25: *355-363* (1974).

Fankhauser, F., Bebie, H., Spahr, J. 3 years of experience with the OCTOPUS automatic perimeter. Proc. 2nd Int. Visual Field Symp. Tübingen, 1976 *Doc. Ophthalmol.* 14: *7-15* (1977).

Greve, E.L., Groothuyse, M.T. & Bakker, P. Simulated automatic perimetry. Proc. 2nd Int. Visual Field Symp. Tübingen, 1976 *Doc. Ophthalmol.* 40: *242-254* (1976).

Grignolo, A., Zingirian, M. & Frugone, P. et al. The visual field examination and its automatization. Symp. on Bioengineering in Ophthalmology. Haifa, 1975 *Doc. Ophthalmol.* 43: *45-50* (1977).

Heijl, A. Automatic perimetry in glaucoma visual field screening. A clinical study. *A.v. Graefes Arch. Ophthalmol.* 200: *21-37* (1976).

Heijl, A. Studies on computerized perimetry. *Acta Ophthalmol. (Kbh.) Suppl.* 132: *1-42* (1977).

Heijl, A. & Krakau, C.E.T. An automatic perimeter, design and pilot study. *Acta Ophthalmol. (Kbh.)* 53: *293-310* (1975).

Klig, V. Biomedical applications of microprocessors. Proc. IEEE 66: *151-161* (1978).

Korner, F., Fankhauser, F., Spahr, J. & Bebie, H. The interpretation of threshold noise and variability of bi-temporal field defects followed with manual and automated perimetric techniques. Proc. 2nd Int. Visual Field Symp. Tübingen, 1976 *Doc. Ophthalmol.* 14: *53-59* (1977).

Loughry, D.C., Allen, M.S. IEEE Standard 488 and microprocessors synergism. Proc. IEEE 66: *162-172* (1978).

Pashley, J.C. BIPAS-Binocular Instantly Programmable Automatic Screener. Proc. 2nd Int. Visual Field Symp. Tübingen, 1976 *Doc. Ophthalmol.* 14: *47-45* (1977).

Spahr, J., Fankhauser, F. On automation of perimetry. Problems and solutions. Proc. 1st. Int. Symp. Visual field. Marseille, 1974 *Ann. Thér. Clin. Ophtalmol.* 25: *337-347* (1974).

Weber, B., Spahr, J. Zur Automatisierung der Perimetrie. Darstellungsmethoden perimetrischer Untersuchungsergebnisse. *Acta Ophthalmol. (kbh.)* 54: *349-462* (1976).

Zingirian, M., Tagliasco, V. Probleme der automatischen Perimetrie. *Klin. Mbl. Augenheilk.* 170: *542-546* (1977).

Authors' address:
University Eye Clinic
Viale Benedette XV
16132 Genoa
Italy

DISCUSSION OF THE SESSION ON AUTOMATION

CHAIRMAN: H. MATSUO

Matsuo: I should like to begin with the comments on the report of Dr. Frankhauser.

Mrs. Frisén: Dr. Frankhauser, I enjoyed your talk very much. It stresses very clearly that the random errors of responses in perimetry can not be neglected. Even with a good procedure as yours the probabilities of falsely detecting a non-existing scotoma or missing a scotoma is considerable. If we combine the information from your paper and consider that each response is to be compared with a, with various random errors we will see that the situation is very bad indeed. To me it suggests that one should add any additional information in the objective analysis. The information could either be general such as 'normal isopters' are elliptical in shape or it could be specific for each patient.

Fankhauser: I fully agree with you.

Frisén: I would like to come back to the discord that sometimes comes up to with regard the values of static perimetry and kinetic perimetry. Franz, you have given us numbers comparing the standard deviation of two different methods measuring quite different things. Do you think that these values, these standard deviations really can be used to inform in the relative value of two different procedures?

Fankhauser: I didn't quite catch your question?

Frisén: Well actually I am referring to page 2 of your manuscript where you list calculated standard deviations for conventional static perimetry, automated static perimetry and kinetic perimetry and you conclude that they may indicate on unrealisticaly low error of kinetic perimetry, providing a too optimistic picture of the method. But my point is, you can't really compare standard deviations of two different visual functions. You could calculate standard deviations of visual acuity and for the error scores in the 100 Hue test for instance but the comparison would not be very meaningfull. I think, it is the same here.

Fankhauser: We do not pretend having proved that generally threshold fluctuations, obtained in kinetic perimetry are larger than in manual static perimetry. We have only pointed to the fact that this may be so.

Matsuo: Any other comment on Dr. Fankhauser's paper? No. Then comments on Dr. Hamazaki's paper.

Dannheim: Well can I make one remark? This is: single stimulus presentation is an easier task for the patients since he has to respond only to one stimulus and not to look whether it is 2, 3 or 4 whereas in the Friedmann you run into problems as soon as there are defects, where he has to make up his choice, whether he has seen 1 or 2 or in which direction so the Friedmann VFA is easy in normal fields and single stimulus presentation is easier when there are defects.

Enoch: Dr. Hamazaki I noticed in your presentation that you turned off your fixation light $\frac{1}{2}$ sec. before the presentation of the multiple stimuli; since the latency for saccadic eyemovements is of the order of $\frac{1}{4}$ sec., you are allowing time for two eyemovements before the stimulus is presented. I wonder if this is not contributing to some of your errors.

Greve: I would like to ask Dr. Hamazaki how he standardizes his instrument. As you know we are using an H.P. oscilloscope for our automatic perimeter. We found that the main problem with such screens is the standardization both of background and stimulus.

Hamazaki: To Dr. Enoch: the central fixation point lights up for 0.5 S; after the disappearance of the second presentation of the fixation point, stimuli appear on the TV screen. There is an after glow of the fixation point which makes it easy to keep central fixation.

To Dr. Greve: the background luminance is the same as in the Friedmann VFA. The stimulus intensity I controlled with my own eye. We cannot measure it accurately at present.

Frisén: It was very interesting to observe the difference in results between manual kinetic perimetry and automatic perimetry. Dr. Bynke said that in no less than 7 cases there were negative findings in kinetic perimetry in positive findings in automatic perimetry; he also showed one example where unfortunately picture contrast was too poor to analyse the numbers, but it seemed to me that this was a case of complete hemianopia in the automatic machine and a pretty normal field in kinetic perimetry. This suggests to me that these methods measure quite different things and certainly several aspects can be indentified in which there are differences. One is kinetic, the other one is static; one is achromatic and the other one is chromatic; adaptation level differences and so on. I think before we can conclude that one method, so dissimilar to an other, is superior we need much more material and we need to control these differences. Will you comment to that?

Otori: I should like to know what is the exposure time of your automatic perimeter. I should like to add that in flicker field we can detect the same sort of findings.

Bynke: May I answer the last question first. It is half a second. To Lars Frisén I can say that of course it is very difficult to compare two methods.

334

You are completely right. The case that you refer to, had a very small hemianopia. It was not found by the technician and this may be partly due to the fact that this technician was not very good in visual field examination; much depends on who is the perimetrist. An other technician we have, is very good and he practically never missed a field defect that was found by the automatic method. So there are so many varying things to discuss in this respect. An other thing is that the stimulus intensity is lower in our automatic method than in Goldmann's methods so therefore the defects stands out more strinkingly with the automatic methods than with the Goldmann method. But I should also say that I have been very much in doubt about the automatic methods some years ago, but now I have worked with several machines for several years and I am completely convinced that the automatic method will the only one that we are discussing in about 10 years. All other methods will be disregarded. Another thing that makes the automatic methods very good is the random presentation of the stimuli. We can not make statistics in any way in field defects if we don't present the stimuli at random.

Matsuo: Any comment on Dr. Aulhorn's paper?

Werner: I would like to ask Dr. Aulhorn if she feels that rotational problems are due to the torsion of the globe or if this reflexes different positions of the patient's head from examination to examination and if it is head position would an improved method for fixing the head in the machine be of any benefit?

Aulhorn: I am sure that it is not due to the position of the head in the holder. Also if the head is exactly in the same position the eye rotates a little bit.

Fankhauser: Threshold determinations in the region of the blind spot obtained by computer perimetry confirm the findings of Aulhorn and collaborators. We have also found marked inter-individual differences. However, we have not observed systematic trends, simulating increase of the blind spot. We believe that increasing scanning density in the region of the blind spot is important and should be observed when designing strategies (i.e. scanning programs).

Enoch: Is it possible to control ocular rotations by special design of the fixation target, e.g., by using a vertical line with a spot in the middle. There is great sensitivity to vertical orientation. (e.g., see recent studies of hyperacuity by Westheimer, or other recent analysis of John Lott Brown).

Drance: I would like to ask Dr. Aulhorn whether she has actually measured the amount of rotation. We have all been finding this. It is extremely important in designing screening procedures to know how far the horizontal meridian is likely to rotate, the range of its fluctuations, so that one can then design the target positions to make appropriate compensation.

Friedmann: Dr. Aulhorn said that one would need an infinite number of fixed stimuli to measure changes due to eye-movement. I do not think you need an infinite number; I don't know what the number is and I don't think anybody does, but I should imagine it would be a very definitely finite number.

Ernest: I would think that tilting of the head would not have any effect on the rotation of the eye. I would think it would be compensated but I would be curious just how much headtilt is tolerated before the eyes rotate.

Aulhorn: I think the different types of fixation points have no great influence. We measured with 4 points and with 1 point in different sizes, and there was no difference in rotation. And the question of Drance. Yes I did investigate not very exactly the rotation on a large number of patients. I have made the measurements on my technicians and then I found a rotation so big that the blind spot shifted 5 degrees upwards. Perhaps the rotation can be bigger. In the first publication of Rössler he found nearly 6° or 7°; I found only 5°. And to Friedmann. Yes I think not infinitive but the more the better. As far as the mechanism of the rotation is concerned: I know that if you turn a little bit the head the eye makes a compensation or can make a compensation rotation. We can measure this. But I know that in our perimeter the head cannot change so much that the head rotation has an influence. Only if you fix the head very badly.

Matsuo: Any comment on Zingirian's report?

Fankhauser: The standardization within the world of robots (automated perimetry) is just as badly needed as the standardization within the world of humans (manual perimetry). The Research Group on Standardization is beginning to shift its emphasis upon standardization of procedural aspects and strategies in manual perimetry. By consequence, computer routines and strategies should be standardized at a reasonable level, since otherwise exchangeability of perimetric data, originating from computer perimetry, will be seriously compromised.

Besides, according to our experience, we are convinced, that todays microcomputers are very well suited for the specific needs of a complex automated perimetric system.

Harms: I want to make a general remark. I don't agree with Dr. Bynke in his view of the future. I think we have to differentiate between the tasks of automatic perimetry and manual perimetry. And one reason is the patients and an other reason is our clinical view. At first we are interested to detect whether these is any defect in the field and for this purpose I think automatic perimetry is very usefull and that it is an important progress. But secondly we are interested to follow up the deterioration of the patient and this is an individual problem. It is impossible to make an exact programme which is capable to deal with each individual situation. And therefore I think we must have a combination: we must detect with automatic perimetry and then we must follow up and control with manual perimetry. I think this in the interest of the patient.

Bynke: Yes. Dr. Harms I have had the same opinion as you have now two years ago. But of course you are right at present we have not any automatic method that can follow up all types of defects but I think it will be possible in the future to make such methods. And there is something that is good with the automatic methods even in following up and that is the constant relations: for example the lengths of examination-time is constant. A very good perimetrist takes about 15 minutes to make a field/ a new perimetrist takes about 45 minutes for the same task and the new one will have much larger defects because the patient will be fatigued by the length of the examination. So the automatic method gives us constant relations in many respects and this will help us even in the follow up of defects in the future, not now.

Harms: Yes, I know these difficulties and I agree with you but there is an other difficulty and that is the patient. The patient is not constant and therefore we must have sometimes an adaption to the patient. We should not compare automatic perimetry with a young perimetrist, but with well experienced perimetrists. I know it is very hard and difficult work and much experience is necessary. But then I think the experienced perimetrist will do better in different types of patients.

Bynke: I agree fully that all patients can not be examined with automatic methods. You may use your hands to show their defects.

Critical notes on 'Threshold fluctuations, interpolations and spatial res-olution in perimetry, F. Frankhauser and H. Bebie'

by E.L. Greve

In their excellent paper on the fluctuation of perimetric thresholds, the distribution of stimulus positions, and their consequences for defect – de-tectability the authors explain the train of thoughts that brought them to the present construction of their automatic perimeter: the Ocotopus. They also defend and explain their interpolation method for graphic display of the results.

Papers like this that bring perimetry from the unreliable clinical impres-sion to the accurate area of statistical evaluation are extremely important. It is time that we realize exactly what we are measuring in perimetry, specially now that our more or less intuitive way of examination has to be translated in a computer-programme.

The division of their paper is as follows:
– Accuracy of perimetric measurements.
– Detectability of VFD.
– Detectability and choice of ex. grid.
– Graphic display and interpolation procedures.
– Interpolation procedures and spatial correlations.

I should like to comment on some of their ideas briefly: The authors do not separate clearly between normal variation of measurements ('threshold noise') and pathological variation. It is well known that the normal variation is much smaller than the variation in defects. In the first case the intra-individual variation σ (root mean square deviation) is less than 0.1 log. unit in a trained subject, the 5% to 95% probability range is about 0.3 log. unit. Pathological variation may be as high as 2 log. units (range) but this is not the rule (see Greve 1973, Greve 1978 in this Proceedings). It is unlikely that pathological variation has a Gaussian distribution, so that we prefer to use the term range of measurements.

Fig. 2a of Fankhauser and Bebie shows similar Gaussian curves for normal and pathological variation. This does not seem to be justified.

Detectability of defects on isolated positions as the authors rightly point out, can be expressed in Wms and Wps, being the probability of missing a defect and producing a pseudo-defect or false-negative and false-positive results respectively.

With a grid such as used in the Octopus or Friedmann VFA incorporating fixed positions it is better to have a criterion $\triangle$ (critical deviation from normal threshold) that provides a small probability of false-negative responses. This criterion is based on the *normal* variation and not on the *pathological* variation. If a single measurement falls outside the criterion its significance can be checked by repeated measurements.

The problem of the detection-phase is not so much the production of false-positive results; it is the false-negative that bothers us.

It is logical that the best chance for detection is offered by a grid of stimuli whether evenly or unevenly distributed.

However I do not think it is justified to base every further decision on these scattered measurements only. A position that has shown an increased threshold should be carefully explored, and not only this position but the area surrounding it. This is the value of the assessment-phase after the detection-phase. The authors feel that interpolation of values in there grid (with 6° separation) is justified, whether the results are normal or abnormal. It is my opinion that in a normal area the number of examined positions should be increased (between the originally examined positions) in order to avoid false-negatives.

This is a very quick and easy procedure. There is no reason for interpolation in these cases.

In an abnormal area a careful assessment-phase is necessary including measurements with great spatial accuracy (fine grid).

The assessment-phase is the basis for the follow-up examination. It is our experience (with the Friedmann VFA, using a grid comparable to the Octopus-grid) that for the follow-up the wide spread scattered measurements are not sufficient.

Interpolation does not provide any new values. Actual measurements between abnormal positions cannot be avoided, specially not in a sophisticated instrument like the Octopus.

The procedure of examination as I prefer it, should then be:

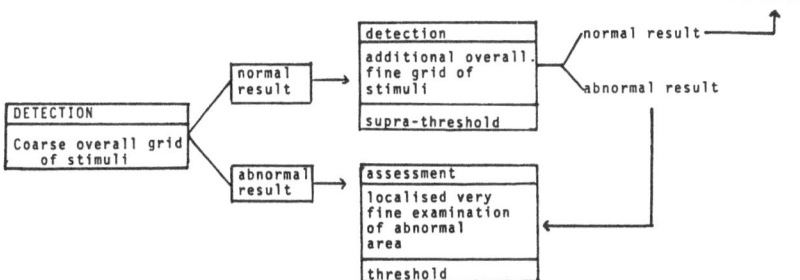

Notes in reply to Dr. Greve's 'Critical notes on-Threshold fluctuations, interpolations and spatial resolution in perimetry by F. Frankhauser & H. Bebie.

F. Frankhauser & H. Bebie

We are well aware of the fact that normal variations and pathological variations in general do not take on the same numerical values. As a matter of fact, data on this subject have been published by our group (F. Koerner et al., Doc. Ophthal. Proc. Series 14: 53-59 (1977)). It is true that this difference, if known exactly, has to be taken into account in certain situations, at, however, the cost of an additional and unfruitful complication of the mathematical model. However, since the probabilities w_{ps} and w_{ms} have been discussed separately, and since numerical values have been given for different criterion-to-noise ratios, the general conclusions drawn, being of a qualitative nature, are not affected at all.

Besides, Dr. Greve considers Gaussian distribution of intra-individual variations in pathological areas as unlikely. We do not agree. Furthermore, it is not clear to us, on what kind of statistical material his claim is based.

Dr. Greve points to the fact that the production of pseudoscotomata is not the main concern in the detection phase. We fully agree. Since a more stringent criterion will be appropriate in the assessment phase, we have treated the criterion as a parameter (see Tables 2, 3, 4). Everybody is free to choose the criterion according to his specific situation and to produce as many pseudoscotomata as he likes.

Dr. Greves comments on the examination grid support our views. We have stated in our paper that 'our discussion aims to indicate the average error to be expected when applying interpolation procedures, if, for lack of examination time, or for economic reasons a denser grid is not available', and that 'actual measurements are always preferable'. We fully admit that an increase of the number of examined positions is favorable. This is a matter of time and cost. – Note that the automatic perimeter OCTOPUS provides an examination program (61) which analyses any desired area with a high resolution, thus living up to the philosophy of the assessment phase.

339

SUMMARY OF SESSION III: AUTOMATION

CHAIRMAN: H. MATSUO

Prof. Fankhauser said in his summary of Automation session at the 2nd IPS symposium as follows:
'Computers will slowly or rapidly invade almost all spheres of human activity and perimetry will not be the last conquest.'
In fact, for these two years we have been living right in the midst of the computer era. This is the same with the field of medicine. Today, Prof. Fankhauser told that statistical method is essential in making exact decisions of visual field defects and that nothing answers this purpose so satisfactorily as computer system. In general, in conventional perimetry we have, off course, used the statistics to analyse masses of measured visual fields. However, in the individual clinical case, many limitations are found in calculating the results of manual perimetry.

Moreover, Prof. Fankhauser proposed the rectangular scanning grid method for a rapid and reliable detection of scotomata and the interpolation procedures as its supplementary method. Speaking of the grid in visual field examination I am always reminded of Prof. Amsler's grid. His grid has caught a lot of fish called 'information' in the sea of central visual field. This grid is, so to speak, something like a casting net and Prof. Fankhauser's grid will make a better and larger catch suitable for the age of computer.

It is appreciated by every one that automatic perimeter has many advantages in perimetry. However, there is still one difficulty, that is, the problem of cost.

I hopefully expect that the remarkable speed with which electronic engineering has been progressing will solve this problem in the near future. The same thing can be said with the data processing system proposed by Prof. Zingirian.

Dr. Hamazaki's system, though it may be still a prototype, is an economical method of automation which is expected to be further developed. Dr. Holmin (whose paper was read by Prof. Bynke) reconfirmed us that Heijl's auto-perimeter has advantages over conventional perimetry by comparing results of measurements of both perimetry.

Prof. Aulhorn pointed out the fact that spontaneous eye-rotation has influence upon the decision of small scotomata and discussed how to avoid this influence.

I deeply appreciate her indication of the fact, which has never come up to my thoughts before.

With this, I would like to conclude my summary for this session.

Docum. Ophthal. Proc. Series, Vol. 19

FUNDUS CONTROLLED PERIMETRY

The relation between the position of a lesion
in the fundus and in the visual field

KAZUTAKA KANI & YOJI OGITA

(Nishinomiya, Japan)

ABSTRACT

New instrument for fundus controlled perimetry was presented. This instrument is composed of an infrared television ophthalmoscope, cathode ray tube for test object, background and fixation target. The light passes through the central part of the pupil. Perimetry was carried out by the instrument in normal subjects and in some clinical cases.

INTRODUCTION

Fundus controlled perimetry is useful in patients who have small retinal or choroidal lesion or who have poor central fixation. Trantas (1955), Meyer (1959) and Awaya et al. (1972) have used a Visuscope or an Euthyscope for this purpose. Inatomi (1977) has modified a fundus camera and measured visual field in hemianopic patients, coincidentally taking fundus photographs. In the Second International Visual field Symposium two methods for quantitative fundus controlled perimetry have been reported. Isayama et al. (1977) used a fundus camera in which a test object projector (size, intensity and duration changeable) was set. The author (Kani, Eno, Abe & Ono 1977) has presented a fundus controlled perimeter which was composed of an infrared television fundus camera and a perimeter.

In this paper, a new fundus controlled perimeter is shown and some examples of visual fields are presented.

INSTRUMENT

The block diagram of the new instrument is shown in Fig. 1. A cathode ray tube was used for making the test object. The fundus, the vidicone tube and the cathode ray tube were set at conjugate positions. The examiner points a desired retinal position with a light pen, observing the fundus on the television monitor. The object is presented on the cathode ray tube with the aid of a microcomputer. The object can also be moved by the light pen for kinetic perimetry.

Visual fields were measured under the following conditions: background 10 asb, white; test object 7 min in diameter, white, 200 msec in duration; fixation target 10 min in diameter, red.

A. Fundamental approach on the normal fundus

Normal visual fields are shown in Fig. 2-5. A deep angioscotoma of a large vein is shown in Fig. 3. At the center of the vein, visual sensitivity is about 1 log unit lower (1/10) than the surrounding area. Along both sides of the vessel, there are very narrow zones where the sensitivity is slightly depressed. As the vessel becomes narrow, the scotoma becomes shallow (Fig. 4). It was possible to follow a small vessel (about 10 min in diameter) by the instrument. Blind spots of Mariotte were measured in normal subjects (Fig. 5). Not only within the disc but also in the conus, an object of 0 log unit (1000 asb) was invisible. As the test object approaches the margin of the disc or the conus, the sensitivity falls down gradually in a very narrow range and suddenly it becomes blind as soon as the object enters the disc or the conus.

B. Clinical application in a certain cases

Case 1. A 46-year-old male lost consciousness on Dec. 31, 1977. He came to our clinic because of blurred vision. The visual acuity was right 0.9 (1.2x + 0.5D), left 0.7 (1.2x + 0.5D = +cyl 0.5D Ax 180°). Bilateral choked disc was noted. A right fronto-temporal subdural hematoma was found by means

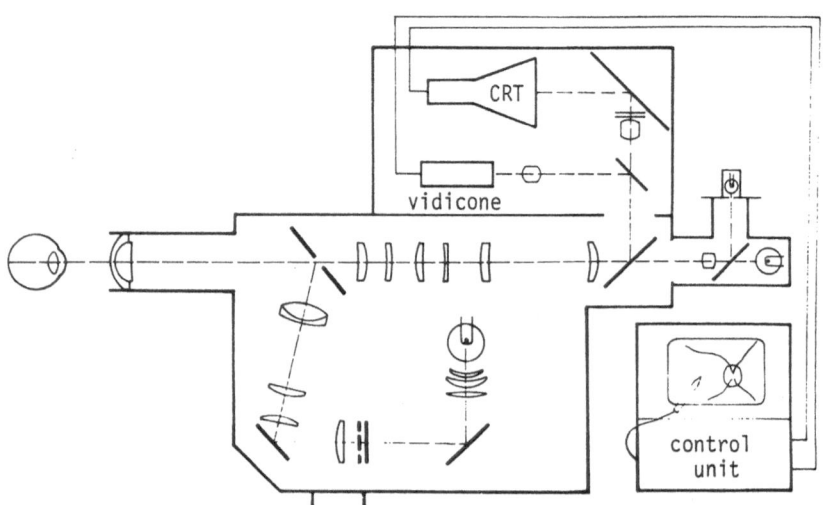

Fig. 1. Block diagram of the new fundus controlled perimeter.

of C.T. scan. By fundus controlled perimetry, test object of 1000 asb could not be seen within the dotted lines (Fig. 6).

Case 2. This 33-year-old man had been treated as chronic renal failure since 1971. The visual acuity was right 1.2 and left 1.5. Nephritic retinopathy was noted. At the retina with hemorrhage the visual sensitivity was depressed and at the cotten wool patch severely depressed (Fig. 7).

Case 3. A 39-year-old female noticed a paracentral scotoma on the right eye on June 27, 1977. One of the retinal arteries showed occlusion and

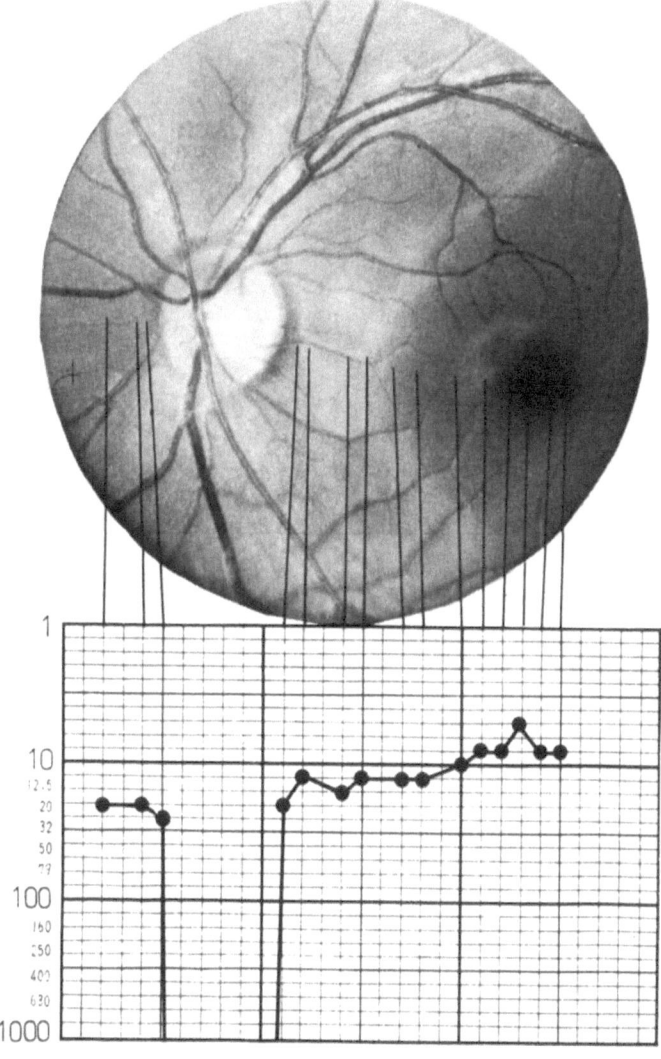

Fig. 2. Static measurement was done at the end of each line in normal subject.

retinal edema was seen. The visual acuity was 1.0. She could not see 1000 asb within the dotted line (Fig. 8).

Case 4. A 66-year-old male had noticed a left central scotoma since Jan. 1977. The visual acuity was 0.03 (n.c.). Exudation, edema and small hemorrhage were seen within the macula. Central scotoma with gentle slope was measured (Fig. 9).

Case 5. This 46-year-old male noted ocular discomfort of the left eye in Jan. 1978. He consulted an ophthalmologist who found a tumor. The visual acuity of the left eye was 0.7 (1.2x − 1.0D = −cyl 0.25D Ax 90°). A very steep edged scotoma was measured at the location of the tumor. (Fig. 10).

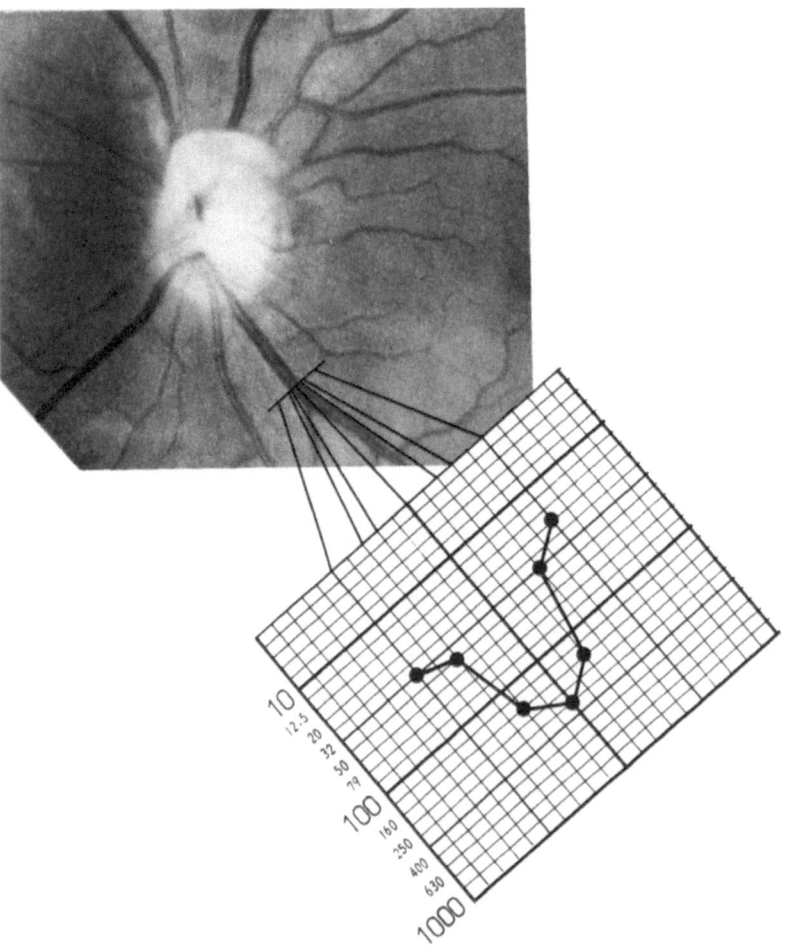

Fig. 3. Angioscotoma in normal subject. Static measurement was done on a line across the vein.

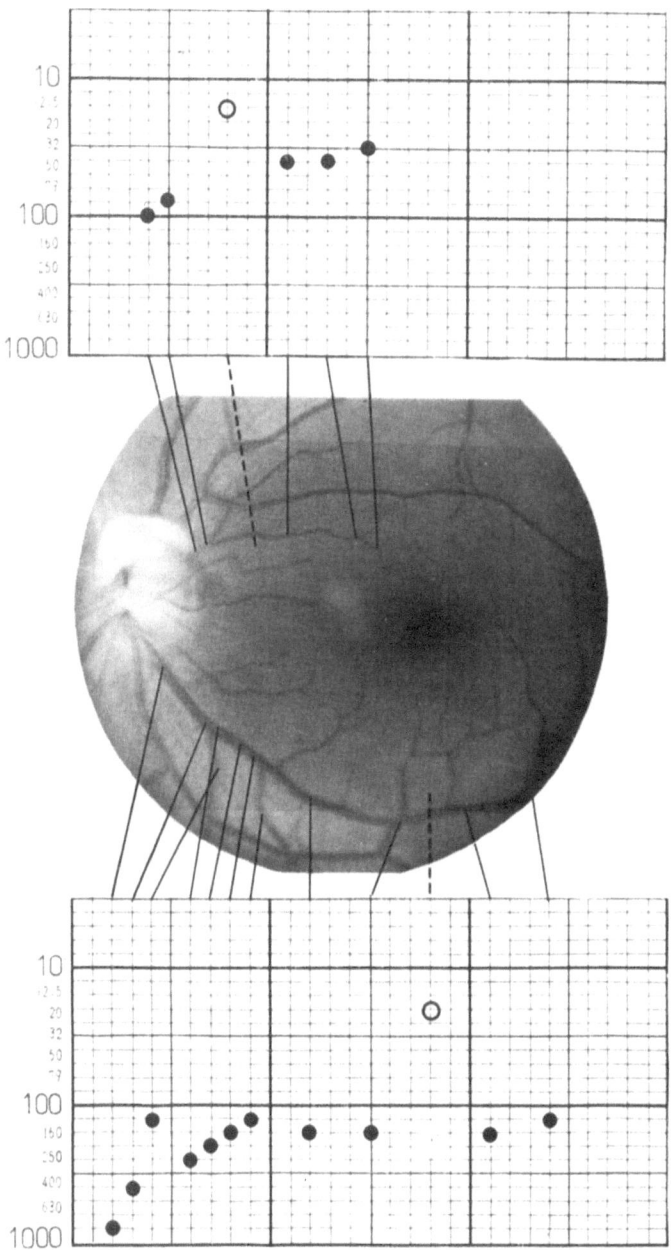

Fig. 4. Angioscotoma in normal subject.
• sensitivity on the vessel, ○ sensitivity on the vessel-free retina.

DISCUSSION

In the new fundus controlled perimeter, an infrared television is also used for fundus observation. The optic disc, vessels, choroid and lesions with pigmentation or hemorrhage are clearly shown, but the macula, edema or whitish lesions are difficult to distinguish because of the characteristics of the infrared ray. A cathode ray tube was used for the test object. Place, size and duration of the test object were controlled by a light pen and a micro-computer. The television system works according to NTSC. The stimulating light emerges every 16.7 msec.

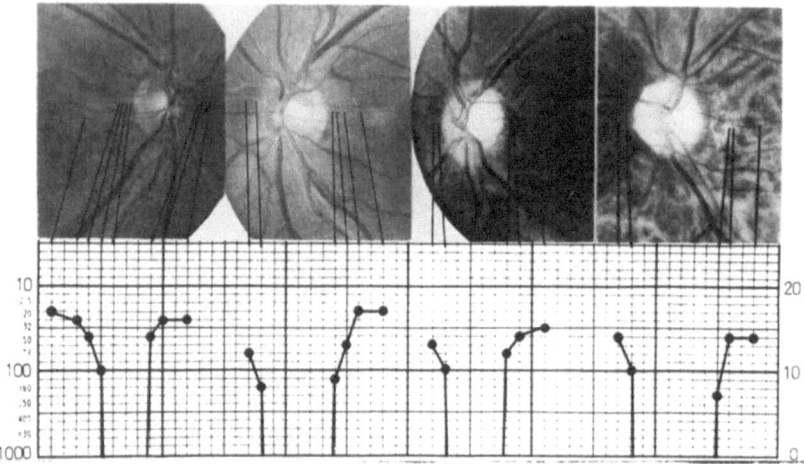

Fig. 5. Blind spot of Mariotte in normal subjects.

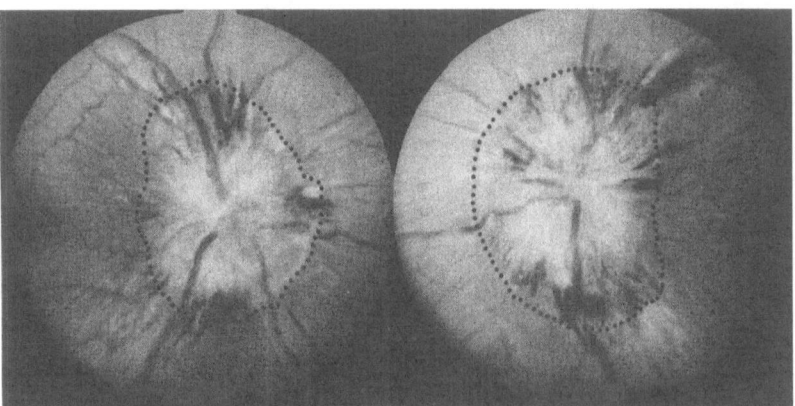

Fig. 6. Choked disc. (Case 1)
Test object of 1000 asb is invisible within the dotted line.

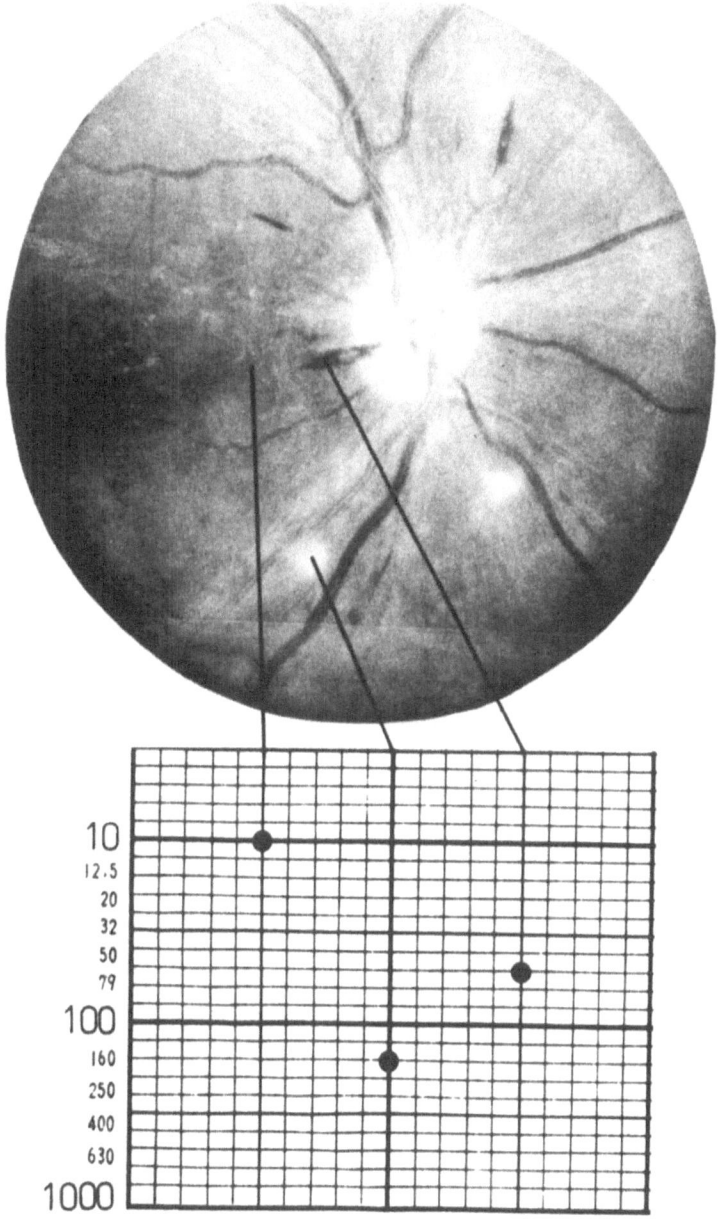

Fig. 7. Nephritic retinopathy. (Case 2)

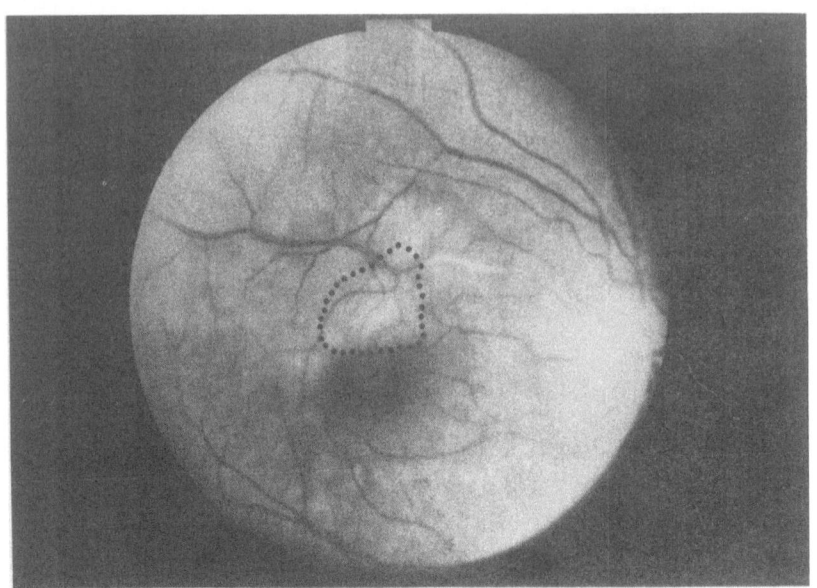

Fig. 8. Occlusion of arterial branch. (Case 3)

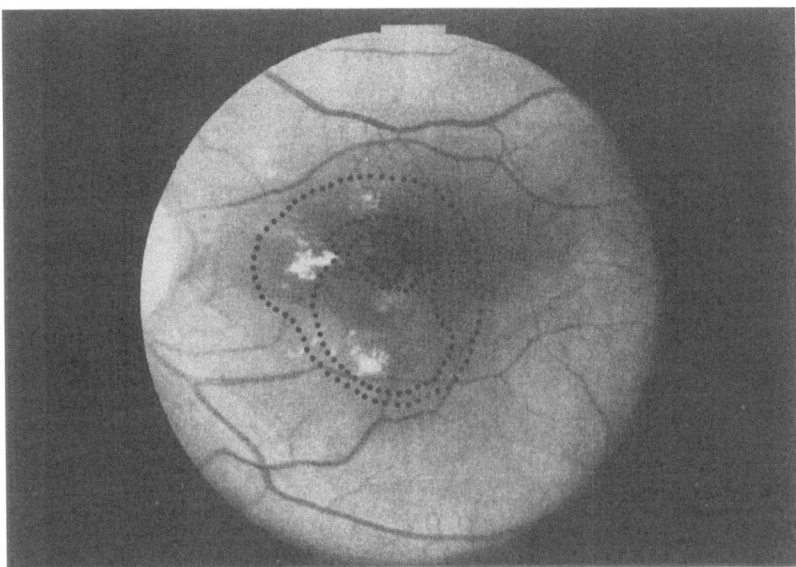

Fig. 9. Central retinochorioiditis, toxoplasmosis suspected. Dotted lines are isopters of scotoma, from outside to inside, 63, 100, 125, 160 asb respectively.

As mentioned above, the measurement was done with a background of 10 asb. In this condition, perimetry could be performed with an ordinary pupil. Even if the pupil is dilated, the retinal image of the test object is clear because the light passes only the central part of the pupil (Maxwellian view). Moreover, retinal illumination is not influenced by pupillary movements.

Fundus controlled perimetry is useful not only for localized lesions on the fundus but also for optic nerve disease. It is difficult to measure central scotoma accurately by traditional method. By fundus controlled perimetry, isopters are easily drawn on the fundus picture. The sensitivity of a certain point of the retina is measured irrespectively of a minor eye movement namely microsaccade, drift or tremor.

This instrument is also appriciated for observation of ocular movement or central fixation.

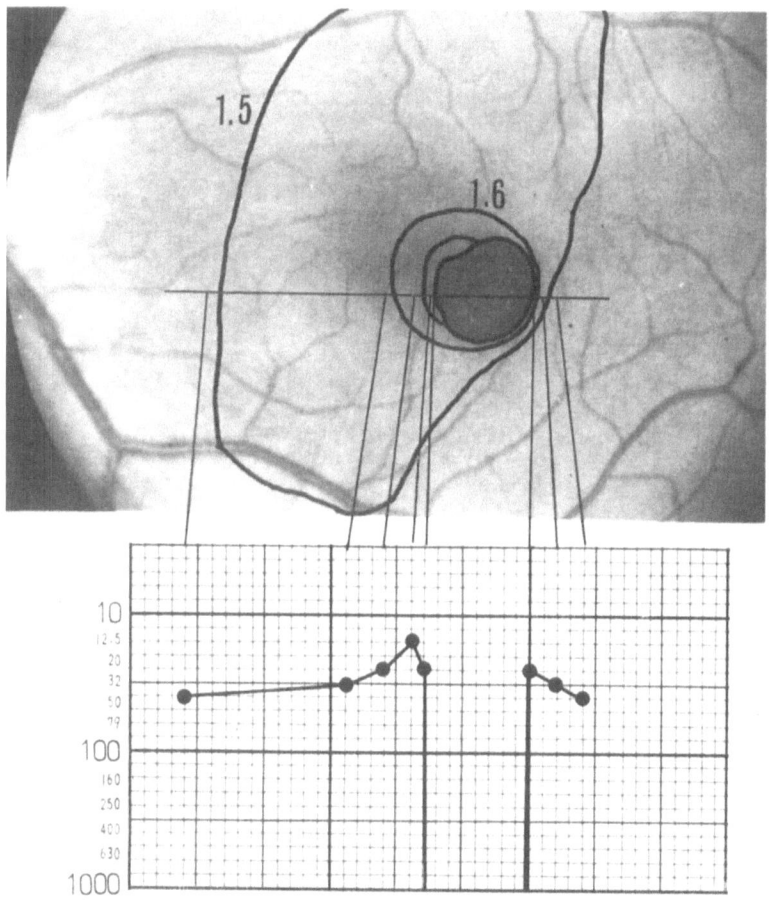

Fig. 10. Melanocytoma? Malignant melanoma?
Isopters are, from outside to inside, 32, 25, 20 asb respectively.

ACKNOWLEDGEMENTS

The authors would like to thank Konan Camera Research Institute and Ono Camera Laboratory for making the instruments.

REFERENCES

Awaya, S., Ohashi, T. & Asano, T. Spot scotometry – a new method to examine scotomas under direct ophthalmoscopy by using Visuscope (Euthyscope). *Jpn. J. Ophthalmol.* 16: *144-157* (1972).

Inatomi, A. Fundus perimetry and overlap of the nasal and temporal visual field. *Jpn. Review Clin. Ophthalmol.* 71: *528-532* (1977).

Isayama, Y. & Tagami, Y. Quantitative maculometry using a new instrument in cases of optic neuropathies. *Docum. Ophthalmol. Proc. Series* 14: *237-242* (1977).

Kani, K., Eno, N., Abe, K. & Ono, T. Perimetry under television ophthalmoscopy. *Docum. Ophthalmol. Proc. Series* 14: *231-236* (1977).

Meyers, M.P. The use of the visuscope for mapping a 'field' of retinal function. *Amer. J. Ophthalmol.* 47: *677-681* (1959).

Trantas, N.G. Applications et résultats d'un moyen simple d'examen de la photosensibilité de la rétine. *Bull. Soc. Opht. Fr.* 55: *499-513* (1955).

Author's address:
Department of Ophthalmology
Hyogo College of Medicine
Mukogawacho 1-1, Nishinomiya
Hyogo-ken 663, Japan

EXPERIMENTAL FUNDUS PHOTO PERIMETER
AND ITS APPLICATION

YASUO OHTA, TADASHI MIYAMOTO & KAYOKO HARASAWA

(Tokyo, Japan)

ABSTRACT

With a purpose of photographing both the fundus and the visual field with one single exposure under direct observation, we developed a photo-perimeter. Fundus camera with infra-red TV was so modified that you might photograph fundus after plotting visual field with a target in response to a subject through a monitor TV screen, and that the plot-marks might be superimposed on a same film, Polaroid or 35 mm size, simultaneously for recording. The measurable area is approximately 25 degree of the central area, and any of the factors such as background illumination, fixation target, luminance of the target (visual angle; 19') can be easily controlled.

With this instument, we have examined central scotomata, coeco-central scotomata, hemianopsia and other visual field defects due to various fundus diseases, both kinetically and statically, to make a comparison study with other perimeters.

This instrument may be applicable widely to various studies such as for fixation test for the amblyopia.

INTRODUCTION

It is probably needless to say that there has been marked progress in recent years in the techniques for quantitative measuring the visual field both in the kinetic and static methods. This study is, therefore, one of the essential means today for diagnosing the fundus and the visual pathway lesions.

To see how a measured visual field is directly plotted on the retina is in itself interesting study, and is so important that it is being widely carried out in various ways by many researchers. We have made an experimental fundus photo perimeter with which a subject's isopter can be exactly registered on film. This is achieved by monitoring the fundus and the target through a TV screen.

MEASURING INSTRUMENT & METHOD

Fig. 1 shows that optical diagram of the instrument. An infra-red fundus camera, by the Canon Inc., was modified in such a way that the target projected on the retina could be recorded on film. Both the target-knob and the isopter recorder are set on a plate so as to be manipulated in a parallel way. The isopter, a series of dots, can be exposed on film as it is on the

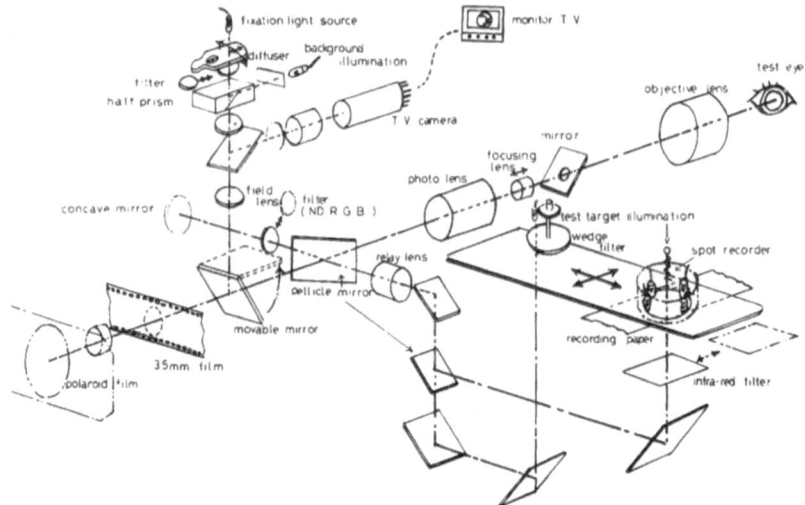

Fig. 1. Optical diagram of the experiment F.P.P.

retina after flipping up an infra-red filter. The light-source for the target is tungsten, and is controllable with a built-in wedge-filter.

Fig. 2 shows the experimental fundus photo perimeter in use. Monitoring the fundus and a target through TV, the examiner can move the target in any direction with a knob. At the same time, the luminance of the target can be controlled as is neccesitated by turning the knob either clockwise or counterclockwise. After having perforated a series of dots, isopter, on a recording card to the subject's threshold responses, the examiner can superimpose the isopter on film with the fundus photograph simultaneously.

The measurable angle for the visual field is approximately 25 degrees wide. The luminance is made controllable each case, i.e. 380 - 28,000 asb. for the target, 450 - 1,000 asb. for the fixation, and 6.3 - 1,000 asb. for the background. The visual angle for the target is 19 minutes wide.

For all the experiments, the luminance for the background was kept to 6.3 asb., while the luminance of the target was controlled each case to the optimum to detect scotoma by disease. All the subject were treated with mydriatica prior to the experiments. The bias-lines drawn on the photographs are for easy discrimination.

Fig. 3 shows the visual field of heredodegeneration of macula, plotted with Goldmann perimeter, while Fig. 4 shows the same visual field plotted with the experimental fundus photo perimeter. The target luminance was 28,000 asb..

Fig. 5 shows the visual field of typical retinal pigmentary dystrophy, plotted with Goldmann perimeter, while Fig. 6 shows the same visual field plotted with the experimental fundus photo perimeter. The target luminance was 28,000 asb.

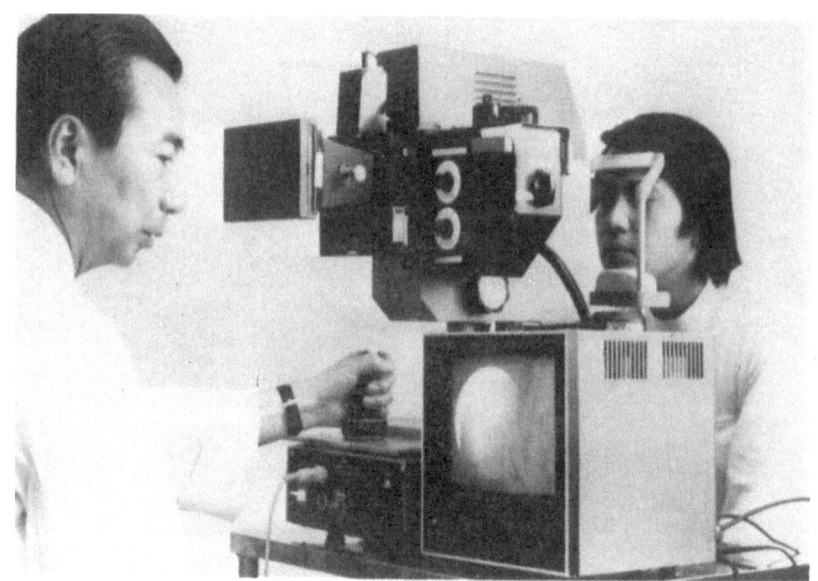

Fig. 2. Experimental F.P.P. in use.

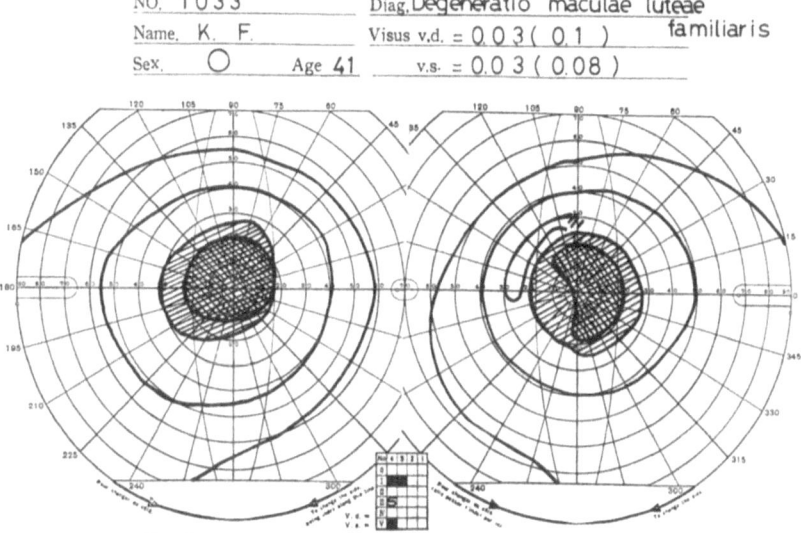

NO. 1033   Diag. Degeneratio maculae luteae

Name. K. F.   Visus v.d. = 0.0 3 (0.1)   familiaris

Sex. O   Age 41   v.s. = 0.0 3 (0.08)

Fig. 3. Heredodegeneration of macula, with Goldmann P.

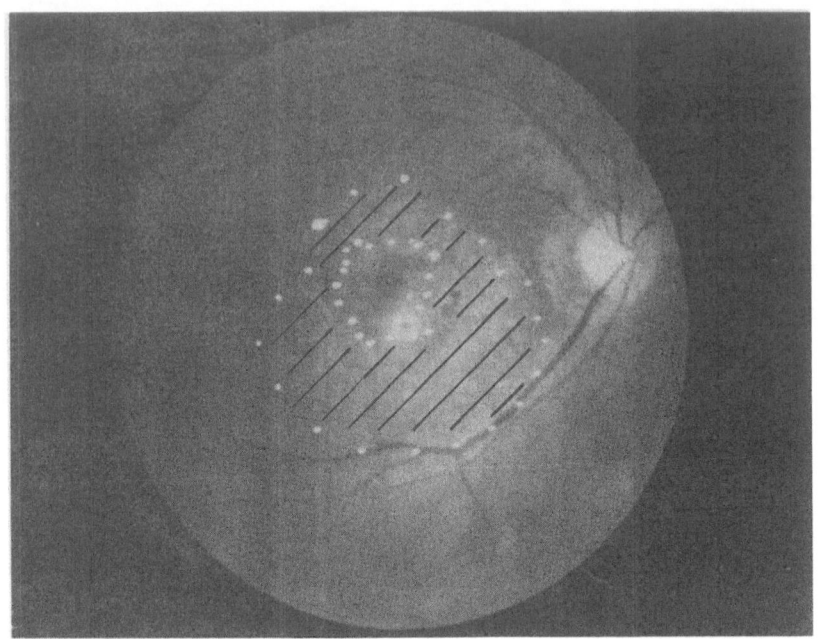

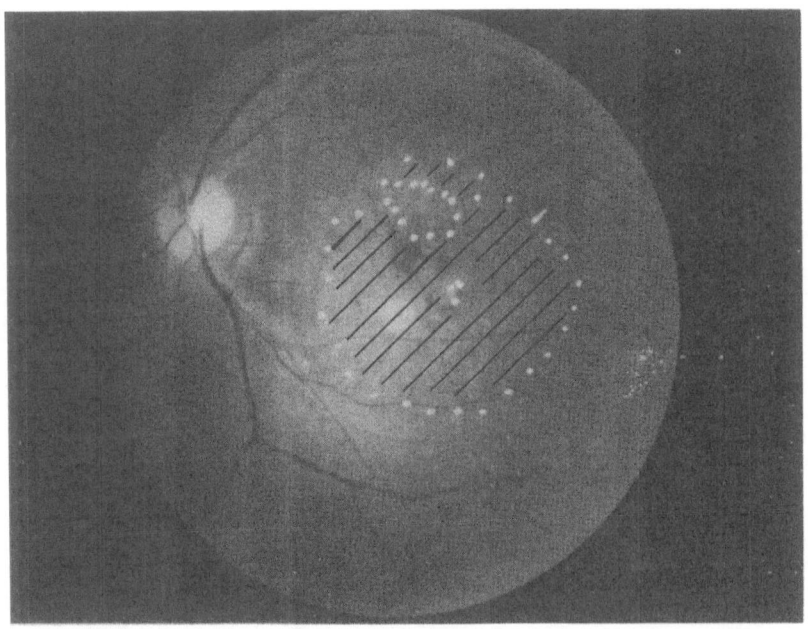

Fig. 4. Heredodegeneration of macula, with the experimental F.P.P.

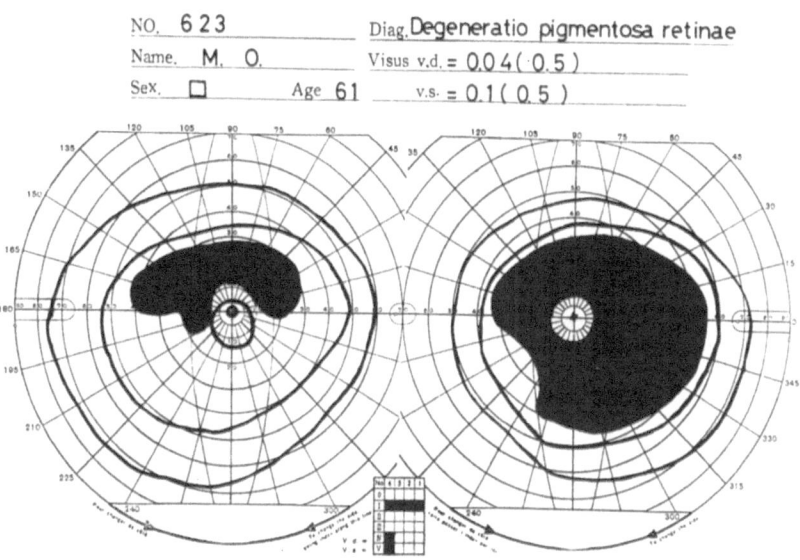

NO. 6 2 3   Diag. Degeneratio pigmentosa retinae
Name. M. O.   Visus v.d. = 0.0 4 (0.5)
Sex. ☐   Age 61   v.s. = 0.1 (0.5)

Fig. 5. Typical retinal pigmentary dystrophy, with Goldmann P..

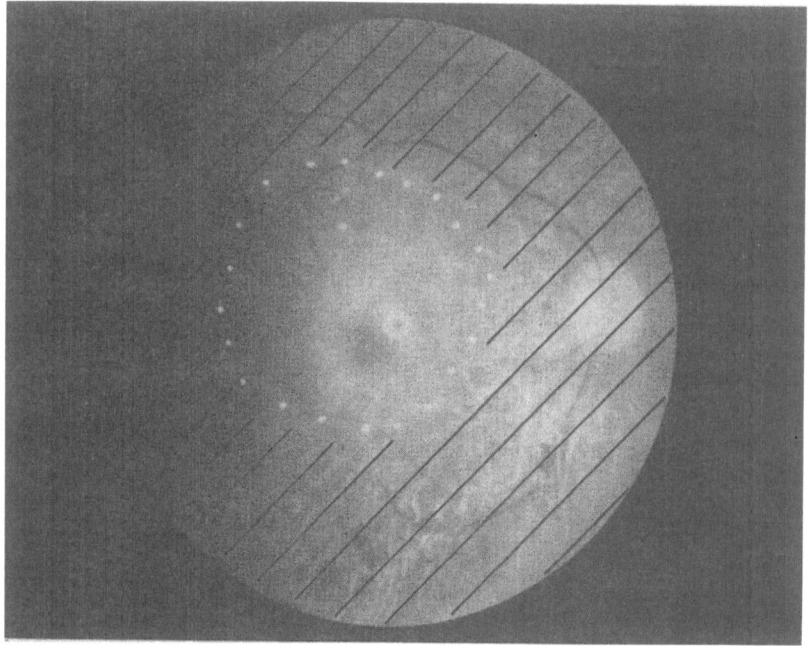

Fig. 6. Typical retinal pigmentary dystrophy, with the experimental F.P.P. for right eye.

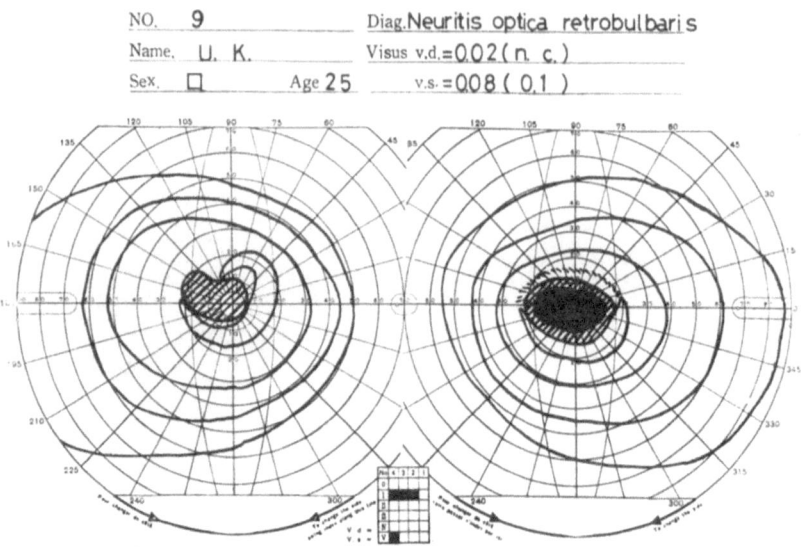

NO. 9   Diag. Neuritis optica retrobulbaris

Name. U. K.   Visus v.d.=0.02(n. c.)

Sex. ☐   Age 25   v.s.=0.08 (0.1)

Fig. 7. Retrobulbar neuritis, with Goldmann P..

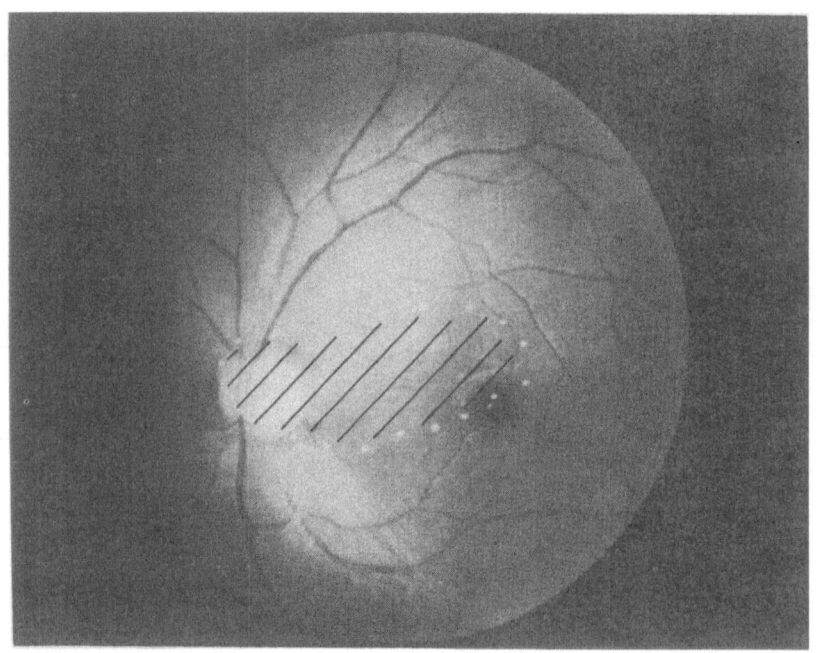

Fig. 8. Retrobulbar neuritis with the experimental F.P.P. for L eye.

356

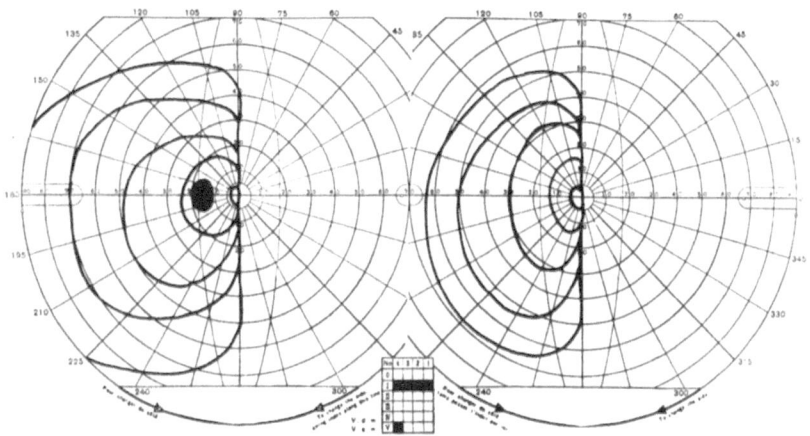

Fig. 9. Homonymous right hemianopsia, with Goldmann P..

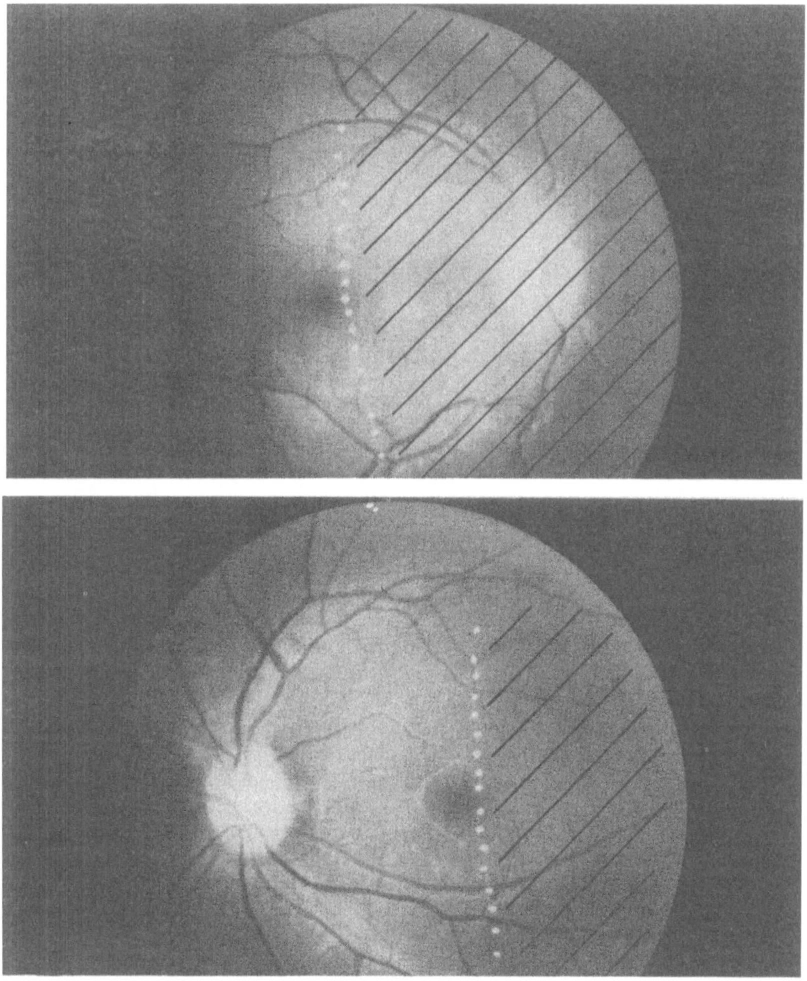

Fig. 10. Homonymous right hemianopsia, with the experimental F.P.P. for R and L eye.

Fig. 7 shows caecocentral scotoma plotted with Goldmann perimeter in a case of Retrobulbar neuritis, while Fig. 8 shows the scotoma plotted with the experimental fundus photo perimeter.

Fig. 9 & 10 are of a case of Homonymous right hemianopsia. Diagnosed as Glioma of the left frontal region of the head, the subject had been operated 4 months before. The target luminance was 28,000 asb.. The lined areas on all the above photographs were put in for easy identification.

RESULTS

In perimetry, there are many experimental cases of direct observation of the fundus. Reports such as those by Trantas, Inatomi and Awaya. To gain more accuracy in the quantitative study of the visual field either kinetically or statically, Kani, Isayama-Tagami made furthermore effort. As a result of their studies, a great deal of progress has been made with direct fundus observation.

By monitoring the fundus as well as a target through a TV screen for manipulating both the target and the luminance, we have succeeded in the quantitative measuring of the visual field, and also in superimposing the visual field accurately on the fundus photograph simultaneously by means of photo-techniques.

In order to improve this method of the quantitative indication, and to clear the relations between those results with experimental fundus photo perimeter and those with all the other perimeters, we will continue our studies.

SUMMARY

1. An infra-red fundus camera by the Canon Inc., was modified, with which we have succeeded in superimposing the isopter on the fundus photograph directly by monitoring the target as well as the fundus through a TV screen.
2. The results from our experiments conducted on various fundus and visual pathway lesions with the experimental fundus photo perimeter were related.

REFERENCES

Awaya, S. Spot scotometry – A new method to examine scotomas under direct ophthalmoscopy by using visuscope (euthyscope). *Jap. J. Ophthal.* 16: *144-157* (1972).
Inatomi, S. Fundus perimetry and overlap of the nasal and temporal visual field. *Jap. Clin. Ophthal.* 71: *528-531* (1977).
Isayama, Y. & Tagami, Y. Quantitative maculometry using a new instrument in cases of optic neuropathies. *Docum. Ophthal. Proc. Series* 14: *237-242* (1977).
Kani, K., Eno, N., Abe, K. & Ono, T. Perimetry under Television ophthalmoscopy. *Docum. Ophthal. Proc. Series* 14: *231-236* (1977).
Trantas, N.G. Applications et résultats d'un moyen simple déxaman de la photosensibilité de la rétine. *Bull. Soc. Ophthal. Fr* 55: *499-513* (1955).

Author's address:
Department of Ophthalmology, Tokyo Medical College
6-7-1 Nishi-shinjuku, Shinjuku-ku, Tokyo 160. Japan

A SIMPLE FUNDUS PERIMETRY WITH FUNDUS CAMERA

AKIHIRO INATOMI

(Shiga, Japan)

ABSTRACT

1. A technique was devised to measure the visual field with an insertion of a test object into a fundus camera, and designated as 'fundus perimetry'.

2. No sparing of the macular lutea could be demonstrated with this technique in cases of hemianopsia. The boundary line of the visual field, however, was slightly deviated toward the non-seeing side. Based on the above findings, it was suggested that the temporal and nasal fields might overlap each other.

INTRODUCTION

Generally, the best way for the exploration of topographical relation between the visual field and the ocular fundus would be to measure the visual field under direct ophthalmoscopy. In 1952, Transtas (1955) carried out the perimetry by use of an ophthalmoscopy, and a similar technique was used by Meyers (1959). In Japan, we first applied this principle to patients with hemianopsia using the visuscope in 1964 (Inatomi 1967). We newly devised a technique with a fundus camera for precise recording. Later on this technique has been developed by Awaya et al. (1972), Isayama & Tagami (1977), and Kani et al. (1977) until today.

The present report describes the simplest method of perimetry using a fundus camera, and gives some information obtained from the patient with hemianopsia.

MATERIALS AND METHOD

A rectangular slit is opened at the lower side of the objective lens-barrel of a fundus camera. A fixation target and a test object for perimetry are inserted through this slit (Fig. 1). The test object is adjusted at the conjugate point, so that it can be seen by the subject as a black dot in a light background. In the mean time, the examiner observes the topographical relation between the ocular fundus and test object together. When the subject is ordered to gaze fixedly at the top of the test object, the foveola will coincide with the top. While making the subject gaze at the fixation target without moving the eyeballs, the examiner measures the visual field with the movable test object. Photographs are taken of the reactions of the subject.

The fixation target is of $2°$ in size, and the movable test object is of $1°$.

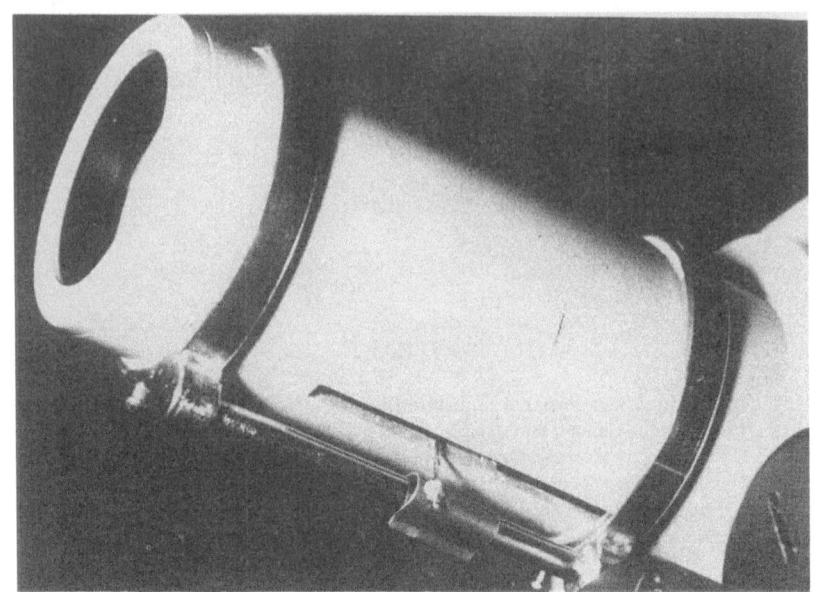

Fig. 1. (See text).

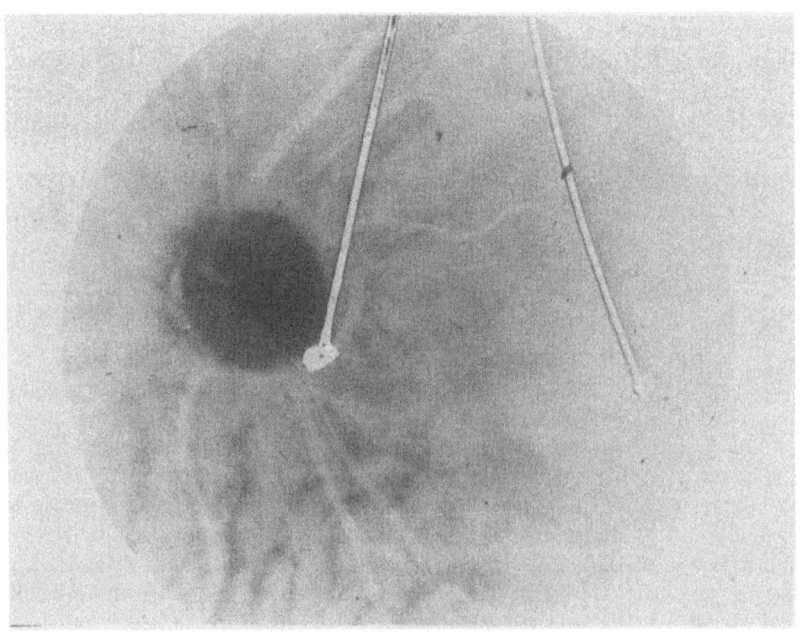

Fig. 2. (See text).

360

Photographs are taken under the illumination of 45,000 rlx, but it would better be taken under 10,000 rlx through a blue filter, because the former illumination is so dazzling. Even under the lower illumination, it could be photographed with monochrome films without a Strobo flash. Fig. 2 shows an actual picture in which the blind spot was detected by this technique.

CASE REPORT

The case concerned a male, 64-year-old patient with right hemianopsia. The result of the fundus perimetry of the patient is shown in Fig. 3, which illustrates the schematical drawing of the ocular fundus superimposed with isopter. There was no remarkable sparing of the macula lutea. Similar results

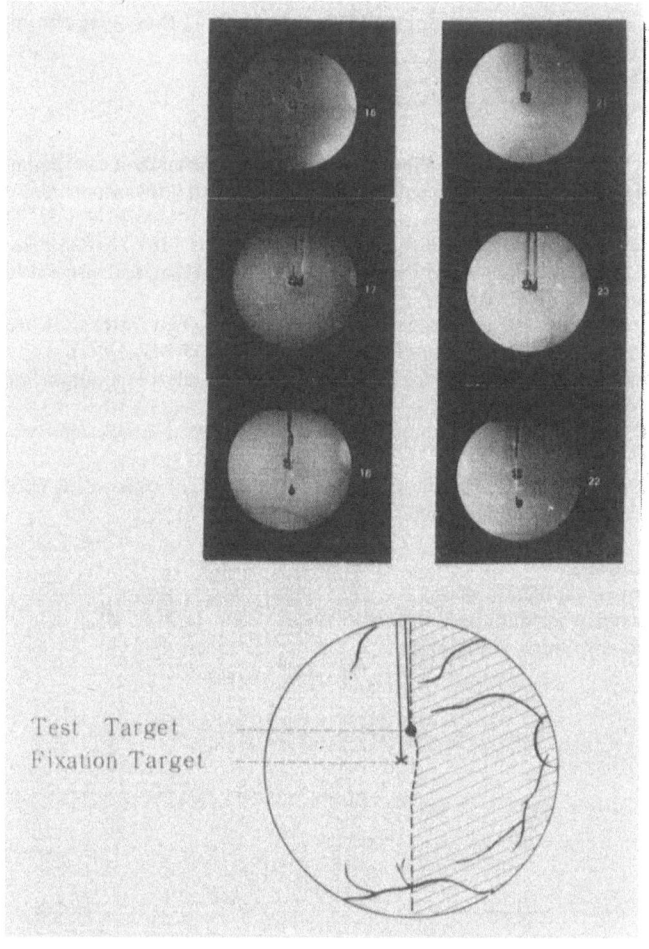

Test Target

Fixation Target

Fig. 3. (See text).

were obtained from several cases of hemianopsia. The boundary line between seeing and non-seeing portions of the visual field was vertical. Further, the line did not pass the foveola, but was deviated by a few degrees toward the nonseeing side from the foveola.

CONCLUSIONS

Awaya et al. (1972) described a sparing of the macula lutea by 1° to 2° in all cases of hemianopsia by drawing isopters on fundus photographs using a direct ophthalmoscope. In the present study, however, no macula sparing was demonstrated, which was due to the different conditions of measurement. Rather, a more interesting finding was that the boundary line of the visual field was deviated from the foveola toward the non-seeing side in all cases of hemianopsia. Based on these findings, it is suggested that the temporal and nasal fields physiologically overlap each other near the macular area.

REFERENCES

Awaya, S., Ohashi, T. & Asano, t. Spot scotometry: A new method to examine scotomas under direct ophthalmoscopy by using visuscope (euthyscope). *Jpn. J. Ophthalmol.* 16: *144-157* (1972).

Inatomi, A. Fundus perimetry. *Jpn. J. Clin. Ophthalmol.* 21: *1109-1110* (1967).

Inatomi, A. Fundus perimetry and overlap of the nasal and temporal visual fields. *Jpn. Review of Clin. Ophthalmol.* 71: *528-532* (1977).

Isayama, Y. & Tagami, Y. Quantitative maculometry using a new instrument in cases of optic neuropathies. *Docum. Ophthal. Proc. Series* 14: *237-242* (1977).

Kani, K., Eno, N., Abe, K. & Ono, T. Perimetry under television ophthalmoscopy. *Docum. Ophthal. Proc. Series* 14: *231-236* (1977).

Meyers, M.P. The use of the visuscope: For mapping a 'field' of retinal function. *Am. J. Ophthalmol.* 47: *677-681* (1959).

Trantas- N.G. Applications et résultats d'un moyen simple d'examen de la photosensibilité de la rétine. *Bull. Soc. Opht. Fr.* 55: *499-513* (1955).

Authors' address:
Department of Ophthalmology
Shiga University of Medical Science
Seta, Ohtsu-shi, Shiga-ken, Japan

Docum. Ophthal. Proc. Series, Vol. 19

THE INFLUENCE OF SPONTANEOUS EYE-ROTATION ON THE PERIMETRIC DETERMINATION OF SMALL SCOTOMAS

E. AULHORN, H. HARMS & H. KARMEYER

(Tübingen, F.R.G.)

ABSTRACT

In perimetric control-examinations at fixed points in a given field of examination, misleading or erroneous changes in the size and shape of the scotomata may be observed. This occurs because the position of the eye is established through fixation according to height and width only, and not according to the spontaneous rotation of the eye. However, even a slight rotation of the eye can cause an examination-point, which lies inside the scotoma in the first examination, to lie outside the scotoma in the second examination. This occurs even though the scotoma in fact remains unchanged. The perimetric methods with which one can avoid this, are discussed.

In the development of automatically-controlled perimetry, it seems reasonable to let the test-points appear at fixed positions on the test-surface, which have been predetermined in the programme. Here the principle of static perimetry is followed, which is certainly more suitable for exact determinations of light difference sensitivity, than the principle of kinetic perimetry. Automatic control of the test-point at the same time allows the test-point to appear — after time-intervals of varying lengths, too — at exactly the same position in the visual field again, but with a change in luminance. During the interval the test-point can be presented at any other random visual field position. In this way static perimetry is possible whereby, after the first test-point presentation, the patient does not know where the next one will be. In this way he is not induced merely to 'gaze' at the test-point. As a result fixation is more stable with such a random test-point presentation than it is when, with the aim of determining threshold, a test-point is offered repeatedly at the same position in the visual field, as is generally the case with static manual perimetry.

The 'faithfulness' to position by the test-point, made possible by computer-control with good mechanism of test-point adjustment, is one of the big advantages of automatic perimetry, which can scarcely be attained with the same accuracy by manual perimetry. One should, however, be aware of the fact that this 'faithfulness' to position also includes disadvantages, which arise because the eye itself does not remain completely 'faithful' to position. That is to say the position of the eye is fixed as regards the horizontal and vertical lines — but not regarding rotation around the line of sight as the axis. This can be easily proved by systematic studies on the location of the blind spot in repeated perimetry. Rössler was the first to point out the significance of eye-rotation in perimetry. Later examiners in follow-up tests have also confirmed this superior or inferior displacement of the blind spot — sometimes amounting to several degrees — and we have also been able to detect such rotations of the eye.

If an eye-rotation such as this occurs during perimetry, it will cause a displacement of existing scotoma limits, which will manifest itself in check-up examinations in the form of increased scatter in the borderline limits. It becomes lost in the individual scatter, resulting from deviation of concentration during the process of perimetry, and can hardly be separated from this.

However, if a perimetric examination is repeated after days, weeks, or years, it can happen that, compared with the first examination, eye-rotation now can simulate a change in the size of scotoma, if the test-point is once again offered at the positions on the test-surface determined earlier, as is of course always the case with static perimetry.

I should like to demonstrate this with two examples (Fig. 1a and b). In Fig. 1a you can see that in one meridian the profile curve shows a deep absolute scotoma in the first examination, but only a relative scotoma in the second examination. The fact that this only seems to represent an improvement can be clearly seen from the topographical perimetry: the scotoma is the same size in both examinations, only the location has changed, so that the profile curve has been placed through the middle of the scotoma in the first examination and, twenty months later, through the edge of it. The

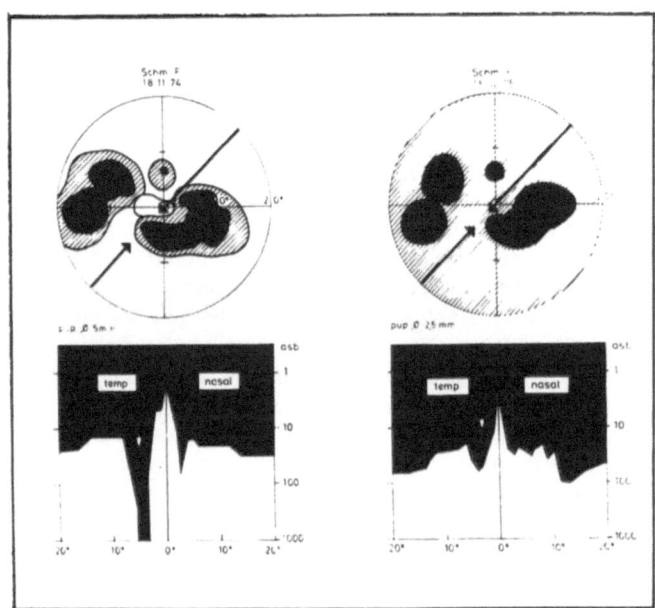

Fig. 1a.

Fig. 1. Two examples of typical displacement of the blind spot and the scotomata in a circular direction due to spontaneous eye-rotation.

364

blind spot has become displaced in the same direction as the scotoma, so that a rotation of the eyeball is confirmed as a result. Fig. 1b shows the same phenomenon of apparent changes in scotoma-size doing profile-perimetry in 3 consecutive examinations.

If in manual perimetry, therefore, static and topographical methods of examination are combined, then the question whether or not a change in scotoma in profile perimetry has occured through eye-rotation alone, or

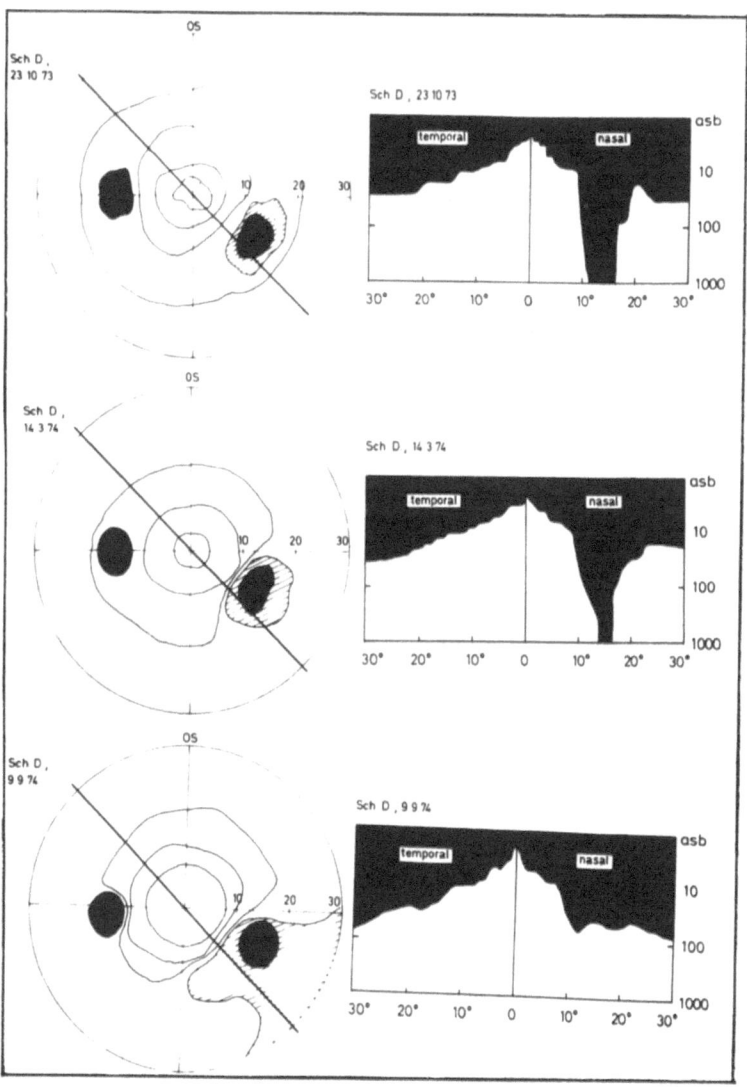

Fig. 1b.

through an actual change in sensitivity, can always be answered on the basis of the topographical visual fields gained kinetically. On the other hand if perimetry is carried out using predetermined examination points, that is statically in the form of screening-perimetry, which is usually the case with automatic perimetry, a control of rotation is not possible, and a scotoma, determined by screening-perimetry alone, must after eye-rotation then appear changed in size.

An avoidance of this fault would only be possible with screening-perimetry, if the test-points could be offered at an infinite number of positions, that is, if one were to make the lines of the examination-screen so close together, that the change in location of the blind spot or of the scotomas would be recognizable. This cannot, however, be reconciled with an examination time of still tolerable length. With such an examination the patient would be so overtaxed, that concentration would quickly decrease and, consequently, the result would be poor.

In our opinion the examination fault, caused by eye-rotation, is not to be avoided in examinations with fixed points; this is easily possible, however, in a manual examination, which as we know must not be done with fixed visual field points, but which can be carried out statically or kinetically.

The description of this possible fault in automatic perimetry is not at all intended as a general attack on automatic perimetry; on the contrary, we are of the opinion that, if applied sensibly, it will be an important improvement in ophthalmological diagnosis. The portrayal of this fault is only aimed at showing the limits of automatic perimetry, and at pointing out that perimetry, using fixed examination points for the exact determination of scotoma size, can lead to false assessments, especially when follow-up examinations are concerned. We believe, therefore, that follow-up examinations, designed to give information as to be possible change in defect limits, must be supplemented by manual perimetry, which serves the purpose of determining the true size of the scotoma — independent of eye-rotation. For this it suffices to determine the limits of the scotoma by moving the test-point slowly out of the scotoma.

The problem in examination caused by eye-rotation is one of the main reasons, why we feel that it is impossible to do with perimetry using exclusively fixed examination points, as in screening-perimetry, but that manual perimetry is necessary in addition. The ideal combination would be as follows: first of all automatic perimetry to recognize, whether or not we are dealing with a pathological or healthy visual field; then a follow-up examination by hand for all diseased cases, where an exact determination of the scotoma size is concerned. Such a double possibility of examination — automatic and manual — is already reasonable from the point of view that not all patients can be examined with an automatic perimeter anyway. Nevertheless, we still think that the introduction of automatic perimetry represents a valuable and, for the doctor, a time-saving supplement of our ophthalmological diagnosis.

366

REFERENCE

Rössler, F. Die Höhenstellung des blinden Fleckes in normalen Augen. *Arch. f. Augenheilk.* 86: *55-86* (1920).

Authors' address:
Universitäts-Augenklinik
Tübingen
GFR

Docum. Ophthal. Proc. Series, Vol. 19

ANALYSIS OF ANGIOSCOTOMA TESTING WITH FRIEDMANN VISUAL FIELD ANALYSER AND TÜBINGER PERIMETER

DR. RYUJIRO SUZUKI & DR. MASAAKI TOMONAGA

(Tokyo, Japan)

ABSTRACT

The authors noticed while measuring the VF with Friedmann Visual Field Analyser (F.V.F.A.) in normal subjects the frequent occurence that a single stimulus point's sensitivity was decreased as compared to remaining stimulus points. In order to clarify this, the visual fields of 592 eyes measured with the FVFA were analyzed and the positions with reduced sensitivity noted (fig. 1 and table 1).

Furthermore the authors have studied fundus photographs (within 30 degrees from fovea) and superimposed a chart of F.V.F.A. over the photograph, to see which point corresponded to a retinal vessel. They also compared the results of F.V.F.A. and Tübinger perimeter.

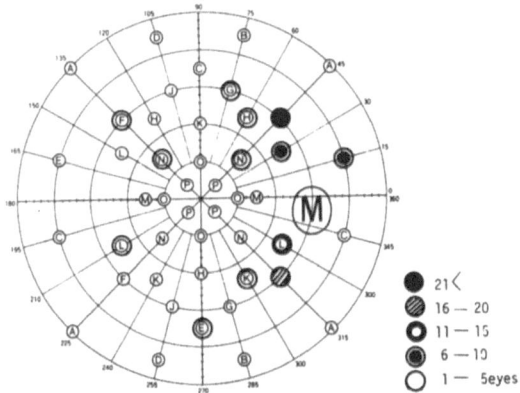

Fig. 1. The incidence of decreased sensitivity points (592 eyes).

Table 1. Diminution Value of the Sensitivity

Decreased Value	Number of Eyes
0.8	6
0.6	14
0.4	44
0.2	32

Authors' address:
Department of Ophthalmology
Tokyo Medical College Hospital
6-7-1 Nishishinjiku, Shinjiku-ku,
Tokyo, 160, Japan

Docum. Ophthal. Proc. Series, Vol. 19

COMPARATIVE EXAMINATIONS OF VISUAL FUNCTION AND FLUORESCEIN ANGIOGRAPHY IN EARLY STAGES OF SENILE DISCIFORM MACULAR DEGENERATION

E.L. GREVE*

(Amsterdam, The Netherlands)

ABSTRACT

Since 1975 a group of patients with early stages of senile disciform macula degeneration (S.D.M.D.) have been investigated at regular intervals. Several stages of development, each with a different clinical significance, have been identified. The results of mesopic-photopic static perimetry and fluorescein fundus angiography will be compared. Mesopic-photopic static perimetry is a highly sensitive method for following changes in the degenerative process.

INTRODUCTION

Since 1975 we follow a group of patients with early stages of senile disciform macular degeneration (SDMD). These early stages comprise drusen, confluent drusen and detachments of the retinal pigment epithelium (RPE) with or without neovascularization or sub neuro-epithelial fluid.

The purpose of this study is to compare visual function with morphology. Secondly we aim at describing several functional stages of the disease and thirdly we want to evaluate the effect of laser therapy. We have used differential mesopic-photopic static perimetry to assess visual function besides visual acuity (Greve, Bos, de Jong & Bakker 1976; Greve, Bos & Bakker 1977). We have worked out a mesopic-photopic ratio (M - P ratio) that indicates the difference in photopic and mesopic intensity of visual field defects in SDMD. This contribution reports on the comparison of visual field defects and results of FFA and on the preliminary results of the follow-up study. The results will be published later in extenso elsewhere including results of laser therapy.

METHODS

All patients with the early stages of SDMD without concomitant fundus pathology who were refered to our clinic underwent general ophthalmological examination, colour fundus photography (F.P.), fundus fluoresceine

---

* Representing the Junius Kuhnt Research group of the Eye Clinic of the University of Amsterdam (D. Bakker, P. Bos, P. de Jong & Versteeg, N.T.).

angiography (FFA) and differential mesopic-photopic static perimetry (DSP). DSP consists of the measurement of static photopic (background 3.12 cd.m^{-2}) and mesopic (background 0.00312 cd.m^{-2}) thresholds along several meridians in the paracentral and central visual field with the Tübinger perimeter. Patients in later stages of the disease who could not fixate were excluded. The position and intensity of visual field defects were compared with the F.P. and FFA. The fluorescein photographs were magnified in such a way that the distance fovea to disc margin corresponded to the distance between the center of the visual field and the normal blind spot on the chart of the Tübinger perimeter. Static perimetric measurements were done while the photograph was on the instrument. (Fig. 1.). The accuracy of the method used is quite sufficient for this purpose. There is hardly any distortion in meridional measurements within the 10° parallel where most measurements take place.

CASE REPORTS

The results will be illustrated with four examples.

Case 1.: Woman of 53 years. (Fig. 1a - d). The FP and FFA of the RE show several drusen, some of them confluent. No leakage. The visual field shows hardly any defects indicating that drusen as such do not necessarily affect differential sensitivity substantially. Only in the 270° meridian a paracentral defect is seen corresponding with confluent drusen. From these photographs one can see that it is difficult to tell from the morphology what the visual function will be. The paracentral drusen in the upper half do not show a different appearance from those in the lower half and yet the lower ones have produced a visual field defect. The defect in the 270° was not predicted from the FP and FFA.

Case 2: A woman of 80 years (Fig. 2a - c). The RE had a visual acuity of 0.75. The FP and FFA showed drusen, a RPE detachment and central edema.

The visual field shows a central defect (M > P) and a paracentral defect (M > P) corresponding with the central edema and the RPE detachment.

The visual field defect is larger than the area covered by the RPE-detachment (225° - 45°). The 135° meridian shows the tip of the RPE-detachment.

Case 3: A man of 67 years was first seen in 1975 (Fig. 3a - c). He had a visual acuity of 0.25. The fundus showed a RPE lesion with edema. FFA showed an area of hyperfluorescense without leakage in the later stages. The four successive static curves in the 120° - 300° meridian show a spontaneous improvement of central sensitivity coinciding with an improvement of visual acuity from 0.25 to 0.8. However they also show the simultaneous development of a paracentral mesopic defect (120° m), while the photopic defect remains approximately the same.

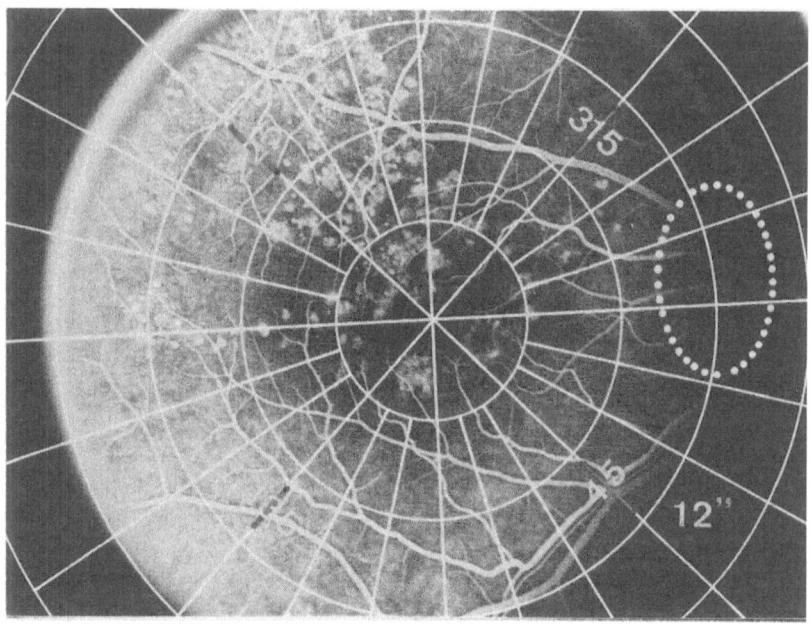

Fig. 1a. Results of FFA of case 1 (12''). The grid indicates the presumed position of the fovea and the blind spot and corresponding meridians. Right eye.

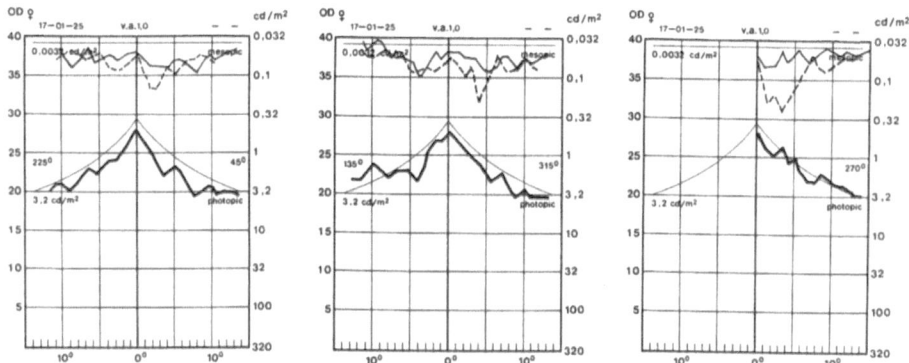

Fig. 1b - d. Results of DSP in 5 meridians (see text). The continuous black (heavy) line indicates the photopic curve of the patient. The continuous black (thin) line indicates the mesopic curve of the patient. The broken line indicates the difference between the intensities of the photopic and mesopic defect. The two very thin continuous lines, one in the shape of a U andd the other one horizontal, are the normal photopic and mesopic curves respectively.

373

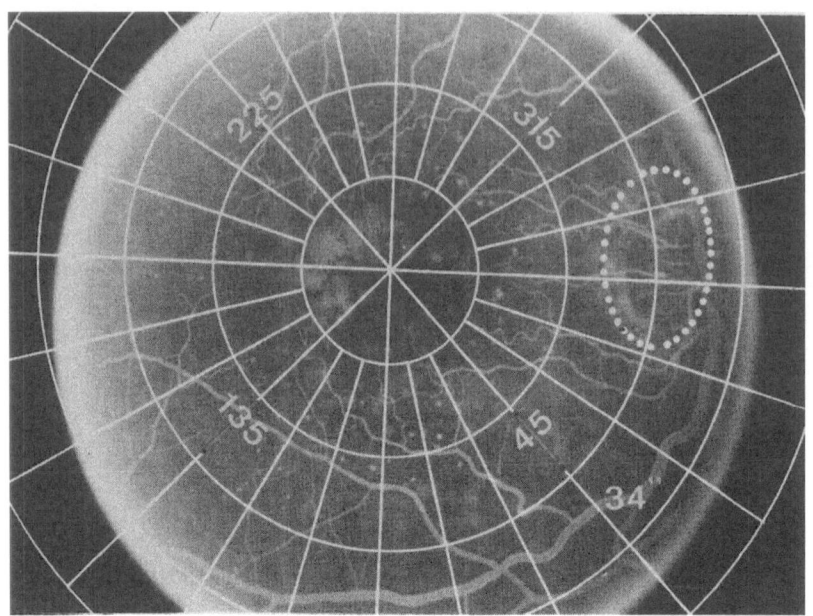

Fig. 2a. Results of FFA of case 2 (34″) see text.

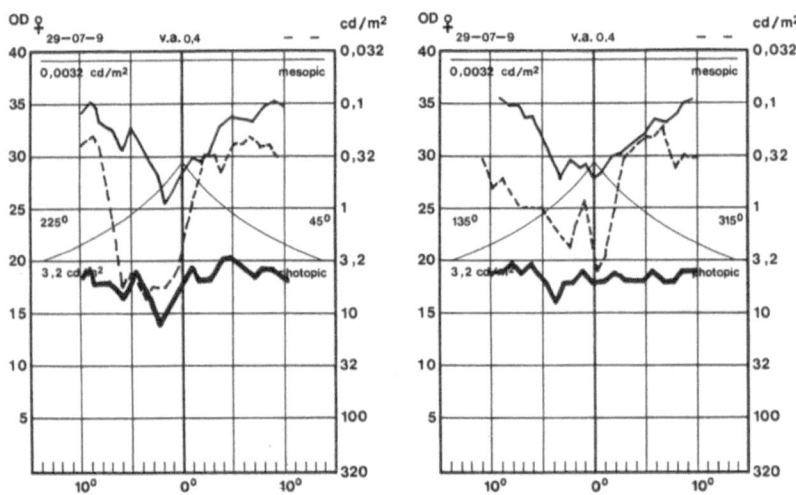

Fig. 2ᵇ ⁻ ᶜ. Results of DSP in 4 meridians. For explanation see legend fig. 1 and text.

374

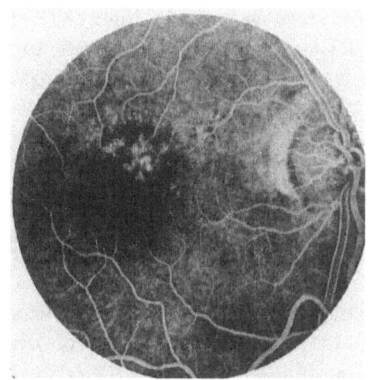

Fig. 3a. Results of FFA of case 3 (see text).

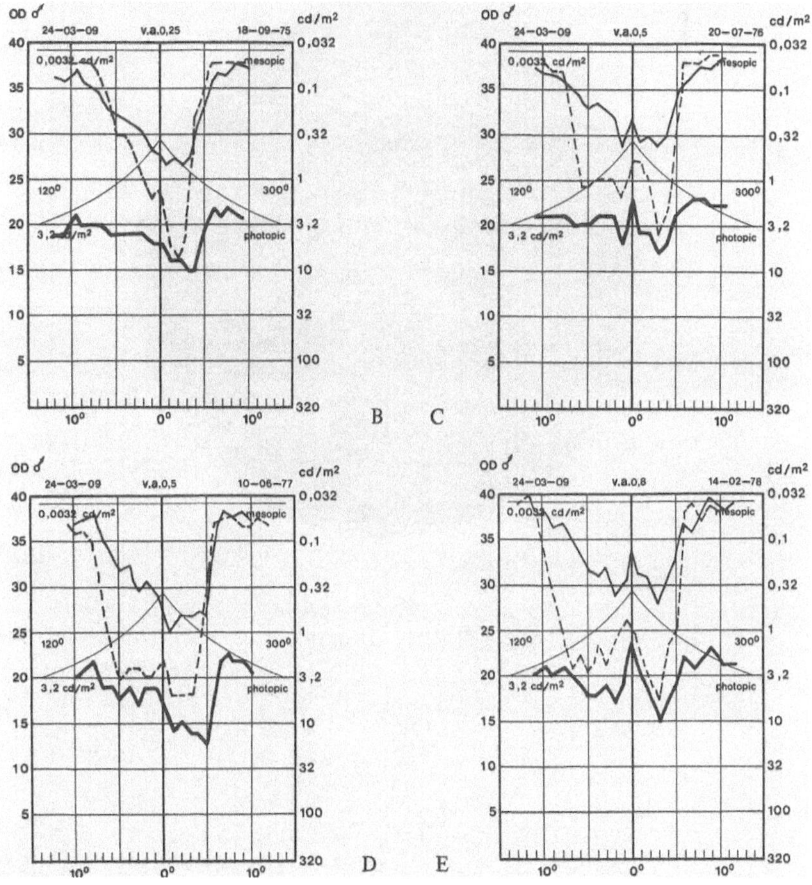

Fig. 3^b - e. Results of DSP in the 120° - 300° meridians, on four successive examinations (1975 - 1978). There is a spontaneous recovery of visual acuity and central sensitivity (see text).

Case 4: A woman of 68 years was seen in June 1977 (Fig. 4a - f). The visual acuity was 1.0 in the RE and 0.3 in the LE. Both fundi showed drusen. In the LE central edema was seen. FFA of the RE shows drusen while in the left eye a detachment of the RPE was seen.

The visual field of the RE showed a good central sensitivity with a deep (mesopic) paracentral defect for which no corresponding defect in the FFA was seen. The FP however shows an area of confluent drusen. The visual field of the LE shows a central and paracentral defect (M > P) (Fig. 4d). The paracentral defect corresponds with the RPE detachment, the central defect with the central edema.

The LE had lasercoagulation. The post-laser visual field shows a deep paracentral laser defect and an improvement of central sensitivity. The centre is almost 'dry' as indicated by an M/P ratio of almost one (Fig. 4e and f).

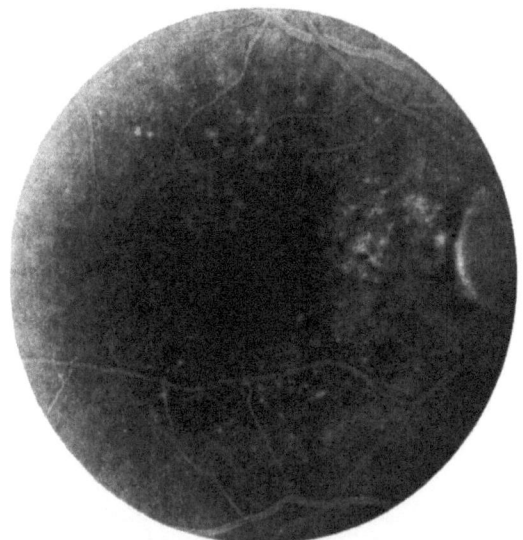

Fig. 4a. Results of FFA in the RE of case 4.

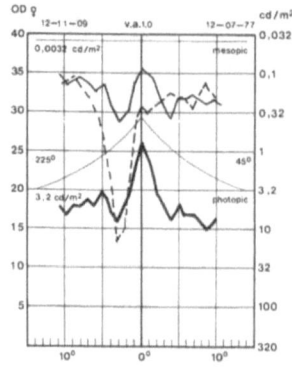

Fig. 4b. Results of DSP in the RE of case 4.

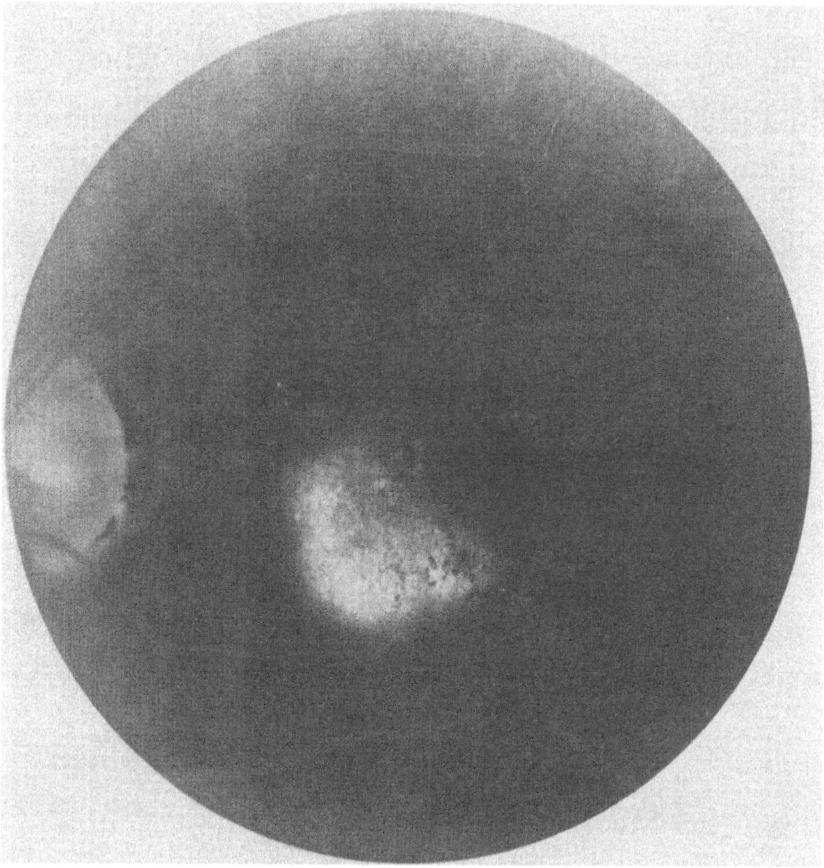

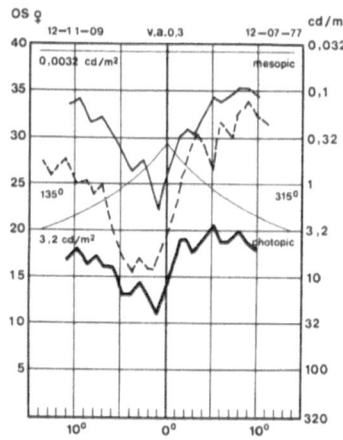

Fig. 4c. Results of FFA in the LE of case 4 before laser-coagulation.

Fig. 4d. Results of DSP in the LE of case 4 before laser-coagulation.

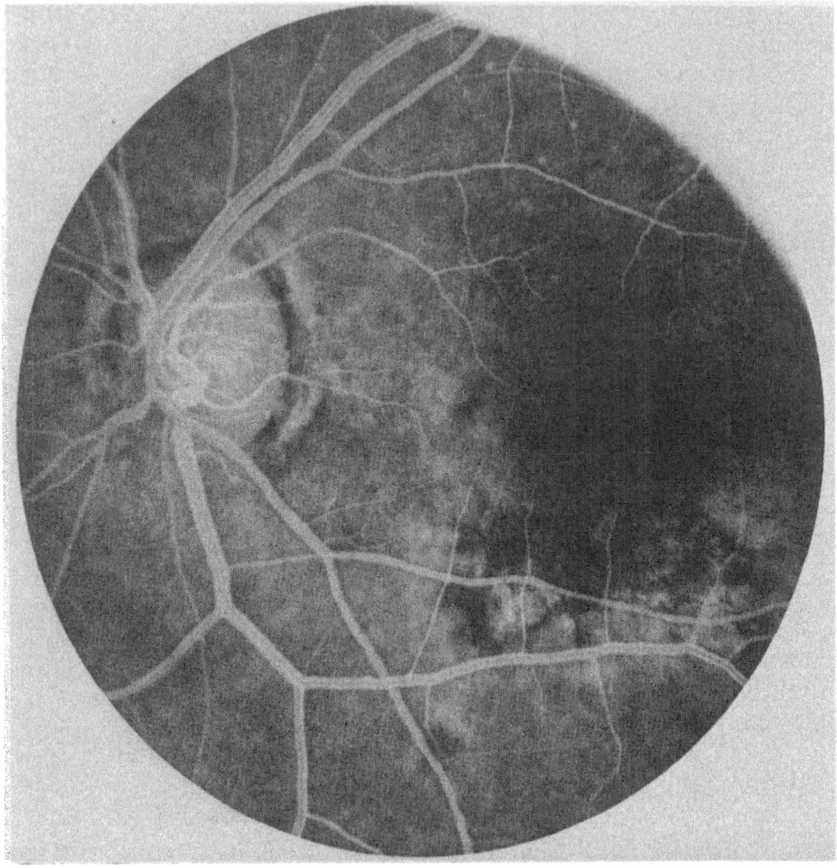

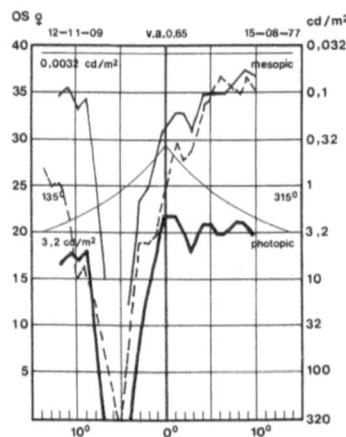

Fig. 4e. Results of FFA in the LE of case 4 after laser-coagulation.

Fig. 4f. Results of DSP in the LE of case 4 after laser-coagulation.

RESULTS AND DISCUSSION

At present (March '78) 99 eyes of 68 patients are being followed. The follow-up period ranges from 3 - 30 months with an average of 9 months.

Table I shows what happened during the follow-up period. In stage I and IIa there was a visual field deterioration in almost half of the cases. In stages IIb and III (usually with central edema and RPE detachment) approximately one quarter deteriorated. Improvement occured occasionally. The rate of deterioration is individually very different. Some patients went from stage I to stage III in 15 months and other remained stationary over 24 months in all stages.

We found that in general isolated drusen do not cause visual field defects. The static curve may show a kind of irregular course (Fig. 1) but defects of 0.5 log. unit do not occur. Confluent drusen may or may not show defects. If there are defects, the M-P ratio is always larger than one (mesopic intensity greater than photopic intensity). Macular (subneuro-epithelial) edema as well as a full RPE detachment present a defect in the visual field with a mesopic-photopic ratio greater than one. Sometimes lesions characterized by RPE dystrophy without evidence of sub−RPE fluid or subneuro-epithelial fluid can produce a visual field defect with an M−P ratio greater than one. Presumably in both cases the greater intensity of the mesopic defects is caused by a defect of the rod-system. In the follow-up period the mesopic defect almost always deteriorates before the photopic defect. Once the photopic defect is also deteriorating the disease seems to be in a more serious stage. If spontaneous resorption of fluid occurs or the RPE lesion is succesfully coagluted, the mesopic-photopic ratio returns to its normal value (as shown in case 4). This follow-up study showed that in the majority of cases the deterioration from drusen to SDMD indeed follows the pattern indicated by the stages I to III (Greve, Bos, de Jong & Bakker 1976; Greve, Bos & Bakker 1977).

Comparative mesopic-photopic central and paracentral static perimetry is an excellent way of:
1. establishing the degree of visual dysfunction and hereby;
2. establishing the stage of progress of the disease;

Table 1. Results of follow-up of 99 patients in the early stages of senile disciform macular degeneration.

Stages	Total number	Unchanged	Deterioration	Improvement
I	28	15	13	
IIa	25	11	10	4
IIIb	22	16	5	1
III	24	15	7	2
IV	37	No follow-up		

3. indicating very sensitively the presence of subretinal fluid and;
4. checking the results of laser-therapy. This method allows one to speak of a wet or a dry visual field.

REFERENCES

Greve, E.L., Bos, P.J.M., de Jong, P.T.V.M. & Bakker, D. Differential perimetric profiles in disciform macular degeneration; stages of development. *Docum. Ophthal. Proc. Series* 9: *327-337* (1976).

Greve, E.L., Bos, P.J.M., Bakker, D. Photopic and mesopic central static perimetry in maculopathies and central neuropathies. *Docum. Ophthal. Proc. Series* 14: *243-257* (1977).

Authors' address:
Eye Clinic of the University of Amsterdam
Wilhelmina Gasthuis
1e Helmerstraat 104
1054 EG Amsterdam
The Netherlands

THE RELATIONSHIP BETWEEN FUNDUS LESIONS
AND AREAS OF FUNCTIONAL CHANGE

JAY M. ENOCH, CONSTANCE RAMSEY FITZGERALD &
EMILIO C. CAMPOS

(Gainesville, Florida)

ABSTRACT

A simple scheme, applicable to central visual field studies, has been developed for
relating fundus photographs and fluorescein angiograms to visual field test position. As
interest in relating observed anatomical change with functional alterations evolves in
many laboratories, it becomes important to consider the degree of congruence between
observed lesions and functional changes. Evidence for disparity in area of involvement
using tests of visual function and observed retinal involvement will be presented. Actually both approaches complement each other as means of characterizing an anomaly.

In our efforts to relate visual field defects to anomalies observed by fundus
photography and fluorescein angiography, two separate questions arise, registration *and* identity of areas of involvement. Most recent manuscripts have
considered the problem of registration (Frisen & Schöldström 1977; Kani,
Eno, Abe & Ono 1977; Isayama & Tagami 1977; Enoch 1978). The registration technique used in this laboratory is shown in Figure 1 (Enoch 1978). In
this paper the question of identity of area or congruence between observed
lesions and measured functional changes will be considered.

Schloessler has made comparative measurements of a known scotoma,
the blind spot, using three different visual field test devices (Schloessler
1976). Measurement of any threshold is an estimate, and is subject to various types of error. Further the projective transformations of the tangent
screen versus the cupola lead to differences, especially if small angle assump-
tions are used in the analysis.

When one attempts to relate physical lesions observed by ophthalmoscopy or fluorescein angiography to functional changes revealed by visual field
testing, there are added sets of problems. In addition to the projective
transformation differences between tangent screen and cupola, there are
added projective transformations associated with the use of the camera and
the projector or other photographic or television viewing devices. Thus

* The research has been supported in part by National Eye Institute Research Grants
EY 01418 (to JME) and EY 01084 (to CRF), and Training Grant EY 07046 (to JME),
N.I.H., Bethesda, Md., U.S.A., and in part by a Fellowship supported by Fight-for-
Sight, Inc., New York City, in tribute to the memory of Hermann Burian, M.D. (to
ECC).

added distorting components are present. Stated simply, one must use care before carrying correlations too far.

We want to call attention to still another limiting factor which must be considered in such an analysis. Simply stated, many functional anomalies do not compare closely in terms of area and/or boundaries with visually observed changes which occur in the retina. The match is only approximate. Further, one psychophysical function may show hardly any change, while another function may be severely altered in the presence of a given lesion. The quality of the match is dependent in part on which function was tested, how reliable the determinations were, and whether the patient was cooperative; and in part on the degree of influence exercised by the affected part of the optical or neural chain upon the response sampled and the magnitude of the anomaly.

A visible lesion on the retina may be regarded as an indication of changes which are taking place currently, or which had occurred previously. In many conditions functional changes cover a much larger visual area than visible signs suggest. Similarly, marked alterations in appearance may be evident, but they may not be accompanied by concomitant functional alterations. For example, in senile macular degeneration, one often sees marked alterations of the pigment epithelium which may or may not be parallelled by meaningful functional changes. The particular functional changes encountered reflect the specific layers of the retina affected. In outer retinal disease, high luminance glare-type stimuli can delay recovery of sensitivity following exposure. If fluid forms under the retina either causing serous separation of the pigment epithelium or neural retina, receptor orientation will be altered and measures of the Stiles-Crawford effect will reveal anomalous response (Enoch 1978; Fankhauser & Enoch 1962; Smith, Pokorney & Diddie 1978; Campos, Bedell, Enoch & Fitzgerald 1978; Fitzgerald, Enoch, Campos & Bedell 1978). This, in turn, can alter resolution. If pathology extends to the inner retina then added complications are noted. Orderly change, apparently spreading vitread, first affects the outer plexiform layer, then the inner plexiform layer. (Enoch 1978) This could represent a differential sensitivity of cells to one (or more) particular substance(s) or an orderly program of change from outward vitread. Remissions do occur and there are relative quiet periods in the course of such anomalies resulting in surprisingly little apparent alteration in many response functions (Enoch 1978; Campos, Bedell, Enoch & Fitzgerald 1978; Fitzgerald, Enoch, Campos & Bedell 1978).

Another example of apparent discrepancy between direct observation and functional changes has been revealed in recent studies of diabetic retinopathy conducted in our laboratory (Enoch 1978; Enoch, Johnson & Fitzgerald 1977). In this disease the true extent of the functional anomaly may not be visible by ophthalmoscopy or fluorescein angiography (e.g., see Fig. 4 below). Further, in the case to be presented below (which is by no means unique) on one side of the visible anomaly there is more evidence of defect than the other (e.g., see Fig. 6 below). In addition, different functional tests are more or less affected by the underlying pathological processes (e.g., see Fig. 7 below).

When trying to analyze anomalies which are occurring in early diabetic retinopathy (not early diabetes), one finds dilated, tortuous capillaries, microaneurysms, and areas of capillary non-perfusion. There may be leaks from an anomalous retinal microvasculature as a result of the breakdown of the blood-retinal barrier, with the introdubtion of materials which are ordinarily foreign to the retina. Capillary non-perfusion creates local areas of relative ischemia. Also, so-called dot-and-blot hemorrhages are seen, and in some patients, hard yellow exudates are observed. Consulting Dr. L. Zimmerman on the location of the exudates, he points out that while foreign materials may diffuse in various directions through the retina, exudates may collect in the relatively avascular outer plexiform layer (Zimmerman pers. comm.) Histology has localized the hard exudates at that locus. Certainly in all cases observed here, they appear underneath capillaries. Dr. B. Fine points out that there is some form of effective limitation in the region of the outer plexiform layer (Fine pers. comm.) This has been termed the middle limiting membrane of the retina, although no true membrane is found. It is clear that the retinal vasculature does not penetrate beyond this level in the normal individual and that some barrier exists to the penetration of exudates past that region. These exudates take the shape of the anatomical features of the zone in which they are located. One might think of the visible areas of their deposition as the 'high water mark' of a leak — much in the same manner as the rim of sea weed and shells at the tidal high water mark found on the beach each morning.

In our studies we analyze a battery of visual function tests which include kinetic and static perimetry, a measure of a sustained- and a transient-like function, and the flashing repeat static test (Enoch 1978; Enoch, Lazarus & Johnson 1976; Johnson & Enoch 1977). In addition, where indicated, Stiles-Crawford functions, dark adaptation, increment threshold curves, interference acuity, etc. are measured in order to provide insight as to response at given retinal loci. By this means we have been attempting to develop quantitative layer-by-layer perimetry (Enoch 1978). If receptor orientation is altered, the Stiles-Crawford function is affected (Enoch 1978; Fankhauser & Enoch 1962; Smith, Pokorney & Diddie 1978; Campos, Bedell, Enoch & Fitzgerald 1978; Fitzgerald, Enoch, Campos & Bedell 1978). The sustained-like function may show an anomalous response when pathology is present in the inner or outer plexiform layer, while the transient-like function seems to show anomalous response only in the presence of anomalies of the inner plexiform layer (Enoch 1978). The flashing repeat static test reveals a fall-off in sensitivity in time when there are nerve conduction anomalies such as are present in retrobulbar optic neuritis and/or demyelinating disease, etc. (Enoch & Sunga 1969). A new test utilizing interference acuity measures provides added valuable information on this population (Enoch, Campos & Bedell 1978; Enoch, Campos, Greer & Trobe 1978). Thus through an analysis of these responses, local sites of anomaly can be described. The single case to be presented here for consideration was in-

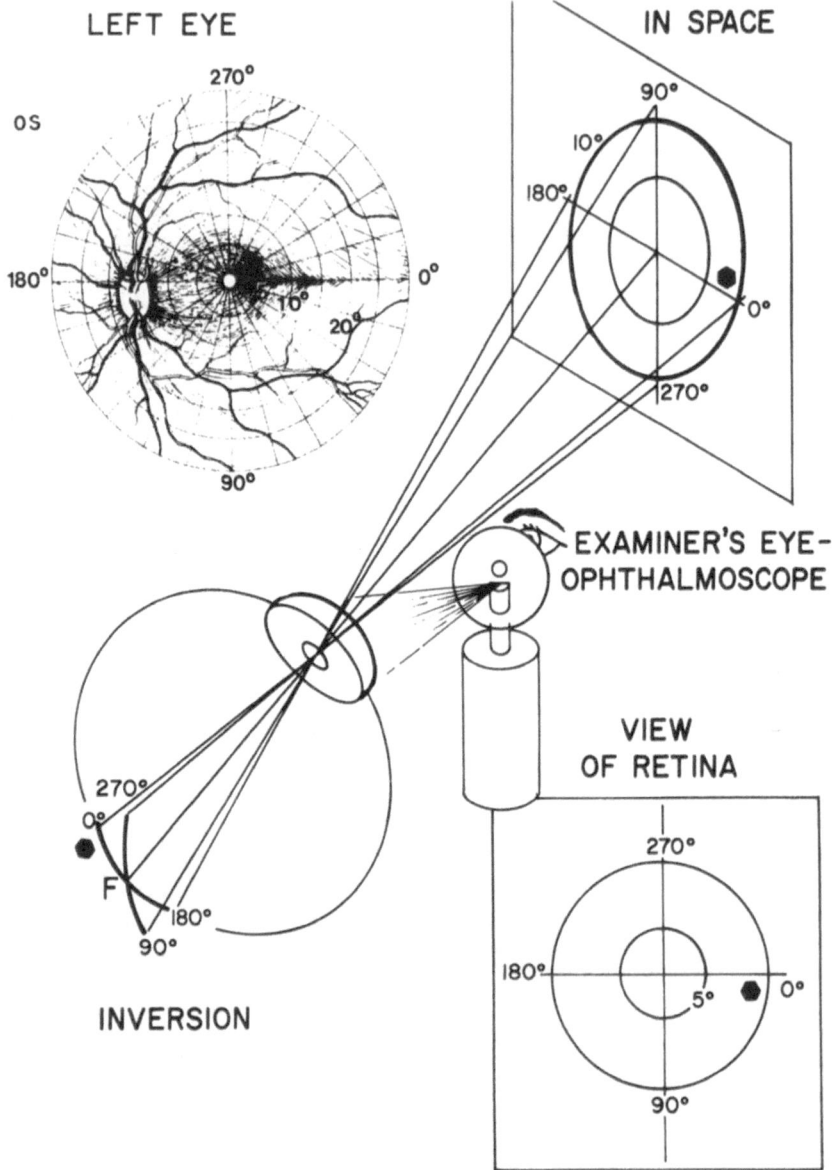

Fig. 1. A tangent screen grid or a test array projected onto a perimeter cupola is shown to the upper right. The nomenclature used for angle designation is that current-ly being employed on the Goldmann (Haag-Streit) and Harms-Aulhorn, Tübingen (Oculus) perimeters. The optical image of the tangent screen formed on the retina is inverted. That distribution as viewed by the clinician using a direct ophthalmoscope is seen to the lower right. Note the figure lying between 5° and 10° eccentricity on the 5° half meridian. The six-sided figure just *above* the 0° half meridian, (upper right) now appears *below* the 0° half meridian (lower right), this time to the observer's right (initially it was to the patient's right). Angles go counter-clockwise on the tangent screen, clockwise in the retinal view. The imaged display can be matched to anatomical retinal features by carefully relating the point of fixation and the *center* of the blind spot. Then one can project tested field points onto fundus pictures (upper left) of the retina or fluorescein angiograms. This figure has been reproduced from reference 4, courtesy the C.V. Mosby Co., Publishers, St. Louis, Mo., U.S.A.

cluded in the recent Proctor Lecture as an example of functional changes occurring in early diabetic retinopathy manifesting hard exudates (Enoch 1978). Comparable cases of the same type could be substituted. Other individuals with diabetic retinopathy revealed changes only in the transient-like function. Changes in the transient-like function are generally found in those cases with anomalies of the microvasculature but no retinal exudates in the region of study. Still other patients show changes in both functions, etc. If there is a local area of non-perfusion or advanced pathology, changes in both the sustained- and transient-like functions are noted. In this case receptor orientation was not altered nor was there evidence of anomalous response in the flashing repeat static test.

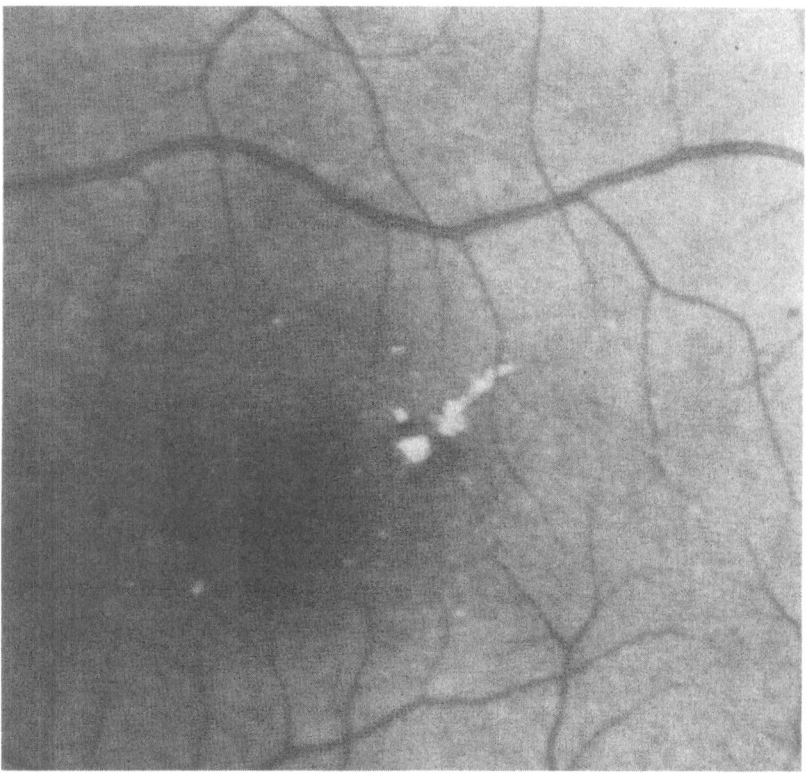

Fig. 2. Patient VC. Inner retinal pathology, early diabetic retinopathy, used as a model of microvascular changes in the inner retina, hard exudates are evident in this patient. This is an enlarged fundus photograph of the left macular region. Discrete point-like, hard, yellow exudates are seen with several coalescing to form a streak or comet-like exudate lying to the temporal side of the fovea. Four fine red points are seen about the largest (head-like) element (arrow), and a small arteriole is observed to bifurcate just above the tail-like portion of the exudate. This figure has been reproduced from reference 4, courtesy the C.V. Mosby Co., Publishers, St. Louis, Mo., U.S.A.

385

Case History

VC is a 42-year-old Caucasian male referred to this Clinic with a chief complaint of a spot in his vision O.S.

He has had diabetes for 12 years and is on insulin. He had a myocardial infarction at age 40 and has elevated triglycerides. There is a family history of diabetes.

His vision was found to be 20/20 O.U. Examination of the anterior segment was unremarkable. On funduscopic examination there was evidence of background retinopathy in both eyes. An exudate in the parafoveal area O.S. seemed to correspond with the visual field defect described by the patient.

Fluorescein angiography showed microaneurysms in the area of the hard exudate. The microvasculature was less altered elsewhere.

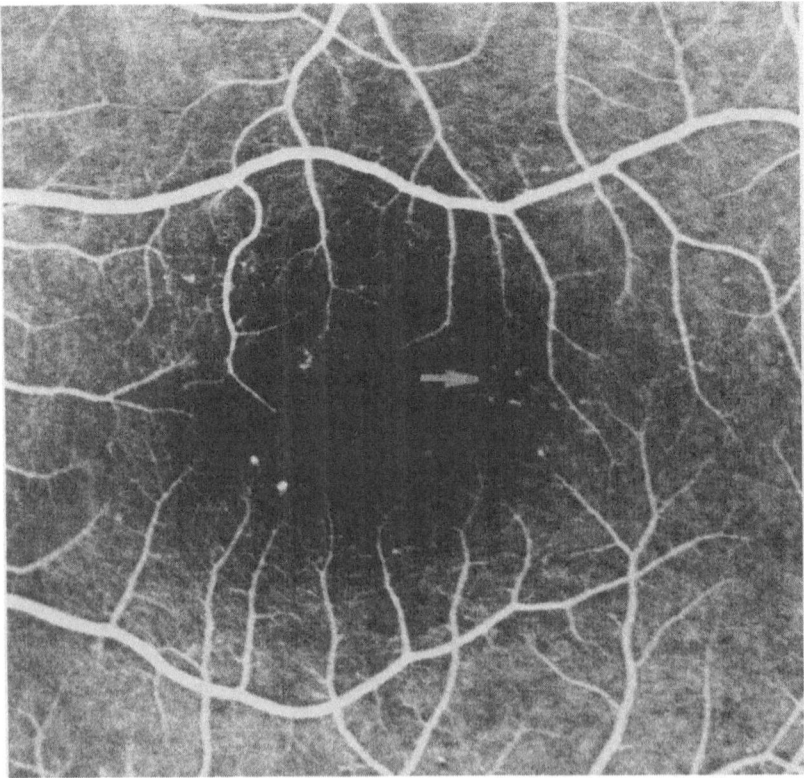

Fig. 3. This is a fluorescein angiogram of the same retinal area as that shown in Fig. 2. The exudate does not fluoresce. The four fine points (Fig. 2) surrounding the 'head' of the exudate turn out to be the microaneurysms which are visible on this fluorescein angiogram (arrow); similarly, the bifurcation of the small overlying arteriole is visible. This figure has been reproduced from reference 4, courtesy the C.V. Mosby Co., Publishers, St. Louis, Mo., U.S.A.

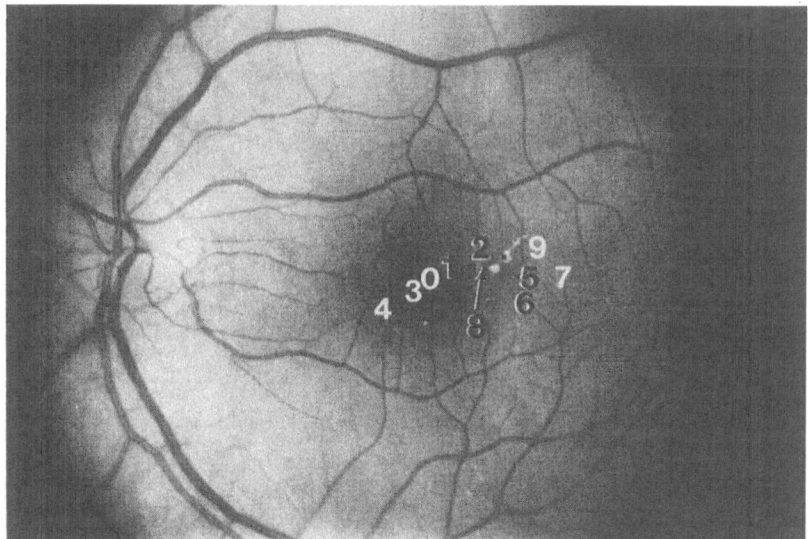

Fig. 4. This is a reproduction of a less maginified view of Fig. 2 with points tested superimposed upon the photograph. The location of these points is based on the scheme shown in Fig. 1. The points tested are replicated in Fig. 6 where added information is provided. Test point 10 is missing from this record. The sustained-like function was normal at the points indicated by white numbers, and it was markedly anomalous where the black numbers are presented, but only slightly anomalous at point 6. The small black dots represent the asterisks of Figs. 6 and 7. Zero is the point of fixation. The exudative streak is clearly seen. This figure has been reproduced from reference 4, courtesy the C.V. Mosby Co., Publishers, St. Louis, Mo., U.S.A.

SYMBOLS USED
SUSTAINED–LIKE FUNCTION

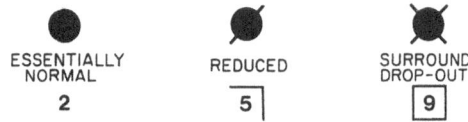

TRANSIENT – LIKE FUNCTION

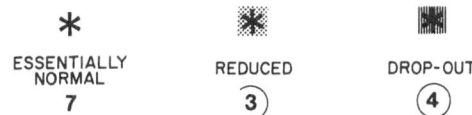

Fig. 5. , This is a simple scheme for categorizing normal and anomalous response to tests of the sustained- and transient-like functions. Two sets of symbols are shown for each function. The lower ones were used on visual field representations where crowding prevented use of the upper set of symbols. This figure has been reproduced from reference 4, courtesy the C.V. Mosby Co., Publishers, St. Louis, Mo., U.S.A.

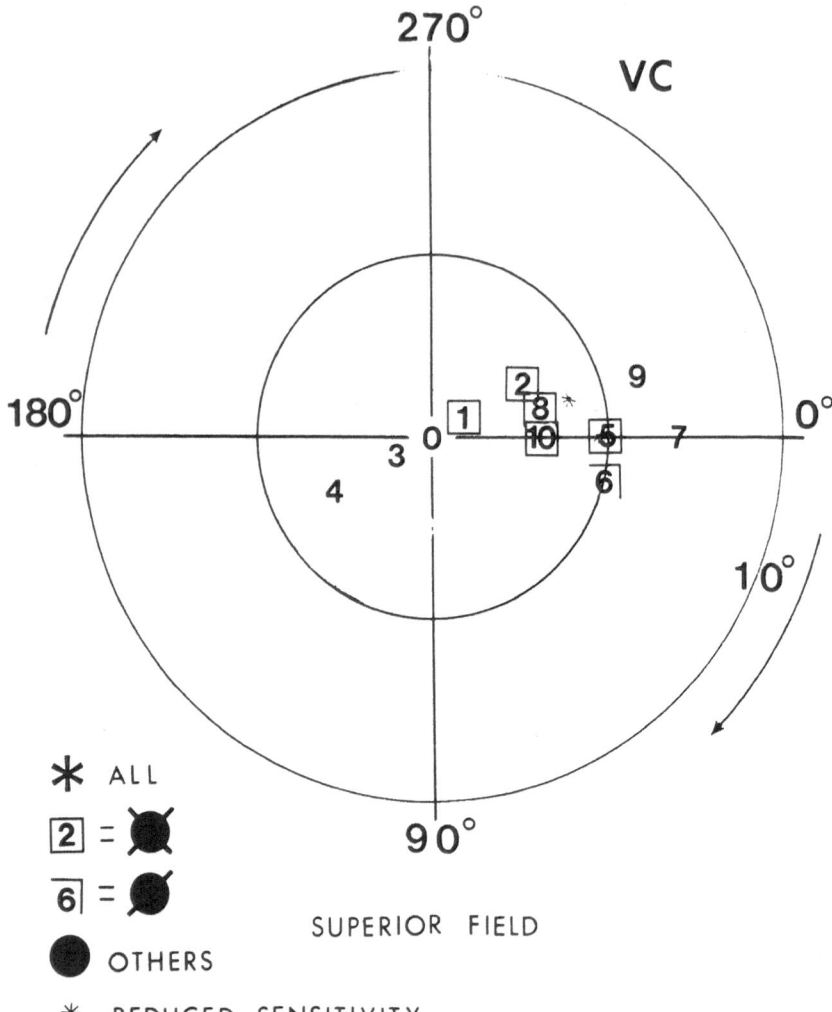

Fig. 6. This figure is based on the display shown in the lower right hand corner of Fig. 1. Here are shown the points at which the sustained- and transient-like functions were tested in Patient V.C. The symbols used are explained in Fig. 5. The second set of symbols, the numbers plus overlays, were used to prevent overcrowding. The fine asterisks appearing on the figure are explained in Fig. 7. At Points 1, 2, 5, 8, and 10 the surround-like portion of the sustained-like function had dropped out and it was reduced at Point 6. Sustained-like function data were normal at the fixation point (0) and Points 3, 4, 7 and 9. All transient-like functions and flashing repeat static test data were normal. This figure has been reproduced from reference 4, courtesy the C.V. Mosby Co., Publisher, St. Louis, Mo., U.S.A.

This patient exhibits a well defined region of exudates just temporal to the left fovea. Added fine exudates are scattered about the retina. Careful observation of the fundus photo and fluorescein angiogram reveals the presence of four microaneurysms lying about the 'head' of the exudative area.

Fine exudates, an exudative streak to the temporal side of the fovea, and occasional indications of either dot and blot hemorrhages or microaneurysms are observed in the fundus photograph seen in Fig. 2. Fluorescein angiography shows the latter to be microaneurysms (Fig. 3). Angiography also shows that early changes have occurred in the microcapillary structure, i.e., there is some tortuousity and dilation of capillaries. The location of the exudative streak can be inferred in Fig. 3 from the position of the four microaneurysms which surround the 'head' of the exudative streak and the bifurcating capillary which lies just above it. In some other cases exudative areas exhibit fluorescence. Using the technique described in Fig. 1, given points tested in the visual field can be associated with specific loci on the retina (Fig. 4). This scheme depends on the very careful plotting of the optic nerve head in order to locate the fovea relative to the optic nerve head. Since we only deal with the posterior pole, no correction for tan-

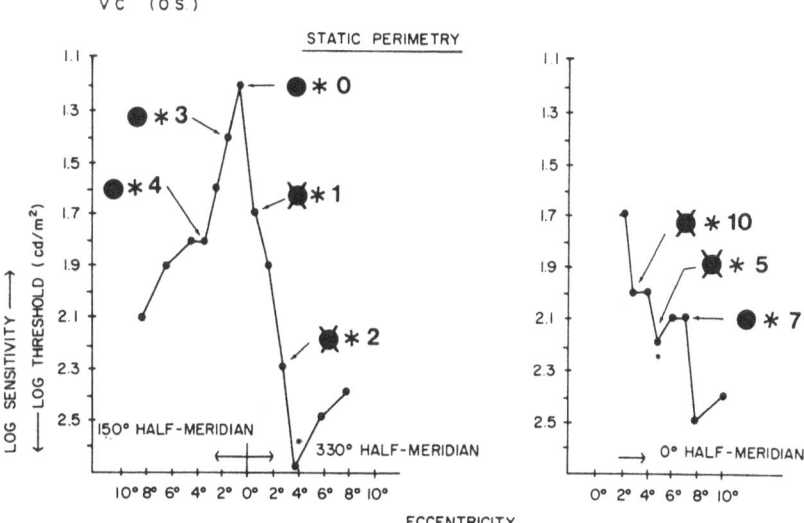

Fig. 7. These are static perimetric records made on patient V.C. The numbers indicate the points at which the sustained-like and transient-like functions, as well as the flashing repeat static test were determined. 0 represented the point of fixation. The disks with superimposed cross indicate where the surround-like portion of the sustained-like function dropped out (see Figs. 4-6, 8). The small asterisks indicate the possible location of the exudative streak, assuming it acts as a modest absorber of light, thus locally reducing sensitivity. Clearly, the static cuts do not provide adequate information to allow us to locate points where the sustained-like function is altered. They do signal the presence of an anomaly.

389

gential errors has been made. In essence we project from the line connecting the center of the optic nerve head to the point of fixation.

A simple scheme for describing the results of tests of the sustained-like and transient-like functions is indicated in Fig. 5. Because of the many points tested, points in the visual field which have been tested are indicated by numbers on Fig. 4 (and 6 and 7). In Figure 6, the field representation shown in the lower right hand corner of Fig. 1 has been used to display points tested and results of testing the sustained- and transient-like functions. A secondary coding system has been used to avoid crowding. The tiny asterisks on the field show the possible location of the exudative streak.

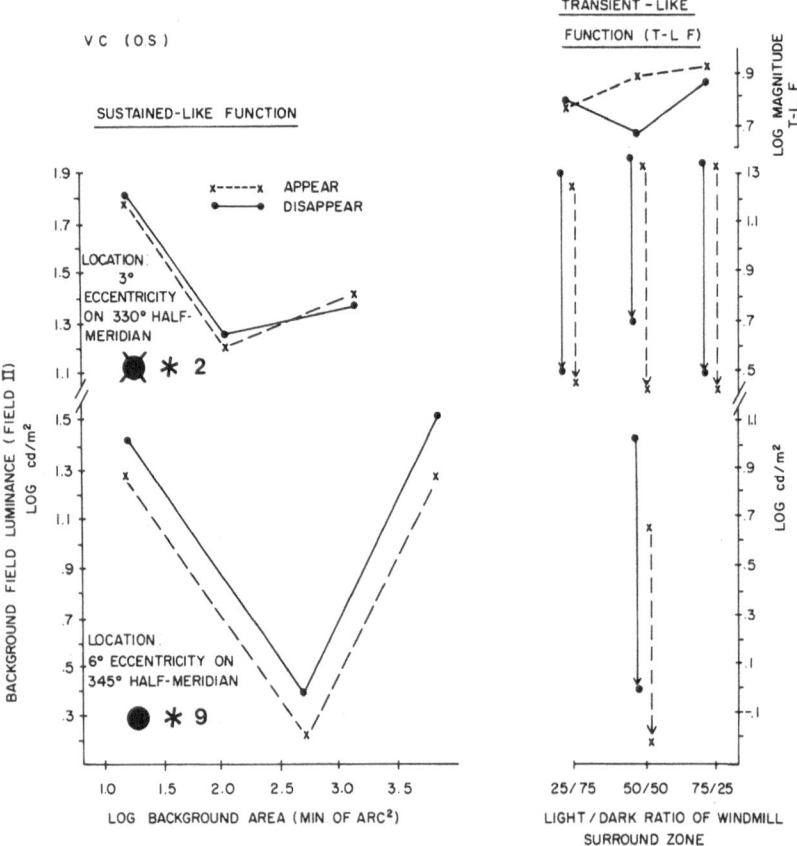

Fig. 8. These are sustained-like and transient-like function test data on patient V.C. at Test Points 2 and 9. Test Point 9 is normal. Test Point 2 shows a drop-out of the surround-like portion of the sustained-like function, i.e., the 'U' or 'V' shaped function is altered to form an 'L' shaped response curve. This is a major change in response. The transient-like function at both points is normal. These data are obtained at points just a few degrees apart (see Fig. 6). This figure has been reproduced from reference 4, courtesy the C.V. Mosby Co., Publisher, St. Louis, Mo., U.S.A.

These points have been deduced from the static cuts shown on Fig. 7 (see Fig. 4 also). The dips in the static cuts are believed to reflect the location of the exudative streak, i.e., it is assumed that the exudate acts as an absorber of light, thus locally reducing visual sensitivity.

In this patient it is obvious that only the sustained-like function is altered by the retinal pathology (Figs. 4, 6-8), that these changes are not symmetric relative to the exudative streak and that here the static cuts are really not predictive of the underlying changes in the sustained-like function. In Fig. 8, data from points 2 and 9 are presented. At point 9, normal sustained- and transient-like functions are recorded. At point 2, the surround-like zone of the sustained-like 'U' or 'V' function has dropped out. This is a *large effect* – compare data at points 2 and 9!

The sustained-like function alterations are more broadly distributed than the physical anomaly visible by ophthalmoscopy, i.e., the exudative streak. Further, these functional changes seem to be more concentrated on the foveal side of that streak – again suggesting a possible flow characteristic of an agent which influences response in the retina. The issue is not the presence of some material, but its concentration, the ability of the individual neurons to retain normal function, and how long that material is in the presence of those neurons. We believe that these changes in the sustained-like function have occurred in the outer plexiform layer (Enoch 1978). Functional recovery from alterations in sustained-like function anomalies have often been observed (Campos, Bedell, Enoch & Fitzgerald 1978; Fitzgerald, Enoch, Campos & Bedell 1978).

This gentleman has a history of high serum triglycerides. We hope to follow such cases further in time. It will be interesting to note how response relates to triglyceride concentration.

I've made no attempt here to explain how these tests are conducted and given limited time I must refer the interested reader to other documents to learn how the individual functional tests are conducted. (Enoch 1978; Fankhauser & Enoch 1962; Campos, Bedell, Enoch & Fitzgerald 1978; Fitzgerald, Enoch, Campos & Bedell 1978; Enoch, Johnson & Fitzgerald 1977; Enoch & Sunga 1969; Enoch, Lazarus & Johnson 1976; Johnson & Enoch 1977; Enoch, Campos & Bedell 1978; Enoch, Campos, Greer & Trobe 1978).

DISCUSSION & CONCLUSIONS

When attempting to relate functional lesions to observed physical landmarks in the retina, the argument can be carried just so far. Functional tests in certain instances may be more sensitive indicators and/or earlier indicators of change than observed ophthalmoscopic evidence. I strongly endorse the movement to try to relate the two forms of examination. On the other hand, attention is drawn to the limitations of such analyses. The one case above shows how we can deduce considerable information from the *combined consideration of functional and observed changes,* and available histological evidence. Clearly in the single case presented, there is no question that a functional anomaly is preferentially revealed by one test of function, that different vision test functions may provide different apparent areas of involvement, that the physically observed anomaly does not subtend the same retinal area as that revealed by functional testing, and that there need not be symmetry in functional changes on both sides of a physical anomaly. These data also point up the fact that we must look beyond development of kinetic and static perimetry, since other functional tests may provide greater or added information relative to local and system response. Perimetry must broaden its outlook. We are on the threshold of major new developments. (NIH guide).

REFERENCES

Campos, E., Bedell, H., Enoch, J., Fitzgerald, C. Retinal receptive field-like properties and Stiles-Crawford effect in a patient with traumatic choroidal rupture, *Documenta Ophthal.* 45: *381* (1978).

Enoch, J.M. and Sunga, R. Development of quantiative perimetric tests, *Documenta Ophthal.* 26: *215* (1969).

Enoch, J.M., Lazarus, J. and Johnson, C. Human psychophysical analysis of receptive field-like properties. I. A new transient-like visual response using a moving windmill (Werblin-type) target, *Sensory Processes* 1: *14* (1976).

Enoch, J.M. Quantitative layer-by-layer perimetry. The Francis I. Proctor Lecture, 1977, *Investigative Ophthal.* 17: *199* (1978).

Enoch, J., Johnson, C. and Fitzgerald, C. Human analysis of receptive field-like properties. VII. Initial clinical trials of the psychophysical transient-like function. *Documenta Ophthal. Proc. Series.* 14: *373* (1977).

Enoch, J.M., Campos, E. and Bedell, H. Visual resolution in a patient exhibiting a visual fatigue or saturation-like effect: Probably multiple sclerosis, *A.M.A. Arch. Ophthal.* (in press).

Enoch, J.M., Campos, E., Greer, M. and Trobe, J. Measurement of visual resolution at high luminance levels in patients with possible demyelinating disease, Proc. Internat. Ophthalmological Optics Symposium, Tokyo, May 8, 9, 1978.

Fankhauser, F. and Enoch, J.M. The effects of blur on perimetric thresholds, *A.M.A. Arch. Ophthal.* 86: *240* (1962).

Fine, B. Personal communication.

Fitzgerald, C., Enoch, J., Campos, E. and Bedell, H. Comparison of visual function studies in two cases of senile macular degeneration, The Harms Festschrift, *Klin. Monats. f. Augenheilkunde* (in press).

Frisen, L. and Schöldström. Relationship between perimetric eccentricity and locus in the human eye, *Acta Ophthal.* 55: *63* (1977).

Glaser, J., Savino, P., Sumero, K., McDonald, S. and Knighton, R. The photostress test in the clinical assessment of visual function. *Amer. J. Ophthal.* 83: *255* (1977).

Isayama, Y. and Tagami, Y. Quantitative maculometry using a new instrument in cases of optic neuropathies, *Documenta Ophthal. Proc. Series.* 14: *237* (1977).

Johnson, C. and Enoch, J.M. Human psychophysical analysis of receptive field-like properties. VI. Current summary and analysis of factors affecting the transient-like function, *Documenta Ophthal. Proc. Series.* 14: *367* (1977).

Kani, K., Eno, N., Abe, K. and Ono, T. Perimetry under television ophthalmoscopy, *Documenta Ophthal. Proc. Series.* 14: *231* (1977).

Research grant applications sought by the National Eye Institute on studies of the human visual system in health and disease using modern techniques of psychophysics and physiological optics: NIH Guide for Grants and Contracts, 7: No. 4, March 10, 1978, pp. 7-10.

Schloessler, J. The influence of visual field testing procedure on blind spot size, *J. Amer. Optom. Assn.* 47: *898* (1976).

Smith, V., Pokorney, J. and Diddie, K. Color matching and Stiles-Crawford effect in central serous choroidopathy, *Mod. Prob. Ophthal.* (in press).

Zimmerman, L. Personal communication.

Authors' address:
Dept of Ophthalmology
University of Florida
College of Medicine
Box J 284 JHMHC
Gainesville, Florida, J 2610
U.S.A.

Docum. Ophthal. Proc. Series, Vol. 19

VISUAL FIELD CHANGES AFTER PHOTOCOAGULATION IN RETINAL BRANCH VEIN OCCLUSION

KIMIKO MATSUDAIRA & RYUJIRO SUZUKI

(Tokyo, Japan)

ABSTRACT

Many studies on the visual acuity after photocoagulation (PC) in retinal branch vein occlusion (RBVO) have been reported. However, only few reports have been presented about the visual field changes before and after PC of venous occlusive diseases. We examined the visual field, using a Goldmann-perimeter, of 27 eyes (25 cases) with RBVO treated with a Xenon arc photocoagulator. The changes of the visual field after PC were divided into 4 groups as follows: 1. paracentral scotoma (pCS), 5 eyes 19%, 2. relative arcuate defect (rAD), 9 eyes 33%, 3. absolute arcuate defect (aAD), 11 eyes 41%, 4. peripheral defect (pD), 2 eyes 7%.

Visual field changes in RBVO are mainly represented by the pCS group and the rAD group.

The pCS group did not show aAD, but the rAD group showed a high incidence of aAD by PC.

The prognosis on visual field changes of these groups are different after PC.

INTRODUCTION

Photocoagulation is an important procedure for the treatment of retinal branch vein occlusion (RBVO). However, reports on the studies of its visual field changes, before and after PC, are rather scarce. Therefore, we analysed the visual field changes before and after PC.
py.

MATERIALS AND METHODS

The subjects were 27 eyes of 25 cases which were treated with the Xenon are photocoagulator for RBVO.

The kinetic visual fields were examined with a Goldmann perimeter. Also, in some of them, a Friedmann Visual Field Analyser (FVFA) was used for static perimetry. A Carl Zeiss photocoagulator made in West Germany was utilized in this study.

RESULTS AND CASES

Table 1 shows the distribution of the types of visual field changes before and after the PC. Among 8 eyes showing paracentral scotoma (pCS) before

PC, 5 eyes still remained in pCS but 3 eyes progressed to relative arcuate defect (rAD) with a normal v/4 isopter, after PC.

Among 18 eyes showing rAD before PC, 6 eyes remained in rAD, and after PC 10 eyes and 2 eyes progressed to absolute arcuate defect (aAD) and peripheral defect (pD) affected to v/4 isopter, respectively.

The peripheral visual field did not show any improvement, getting rather worse when PC was applied. The relation between the central area of the visual field by kinetic perimetry and the visual acuity after PC were analysed, as seen in Table 2.

In general when the central area of the visual field was improved, the visual acuity was also improved.

The changes of the visual field after PC were divided into 4 groups, and a typical case of each group will be presented here.

1. paracentral scotoma, 5 eyes (19%)

Table 1.

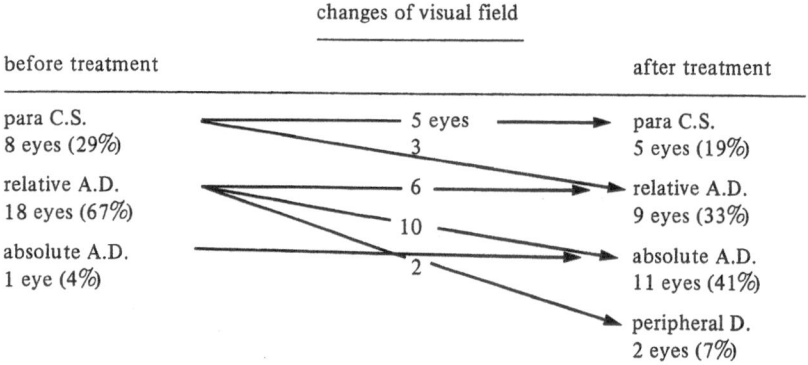

changes of visual field

before treatment   after treatment

before treatment	changes	after treatment
para C.S. 8 eyes (29%)	5 eyes / 3	para C.S. 5 eyes (19%)
relative A.D. 18 eyes (67%)	6 / 10	relative A.D. 9 eyes (33%)
absolute A.D. 1 eye (4%)	2	absolute A.D. 11 eyes (41%)
		peripheral D. 2 eyes (7%)

C.S.: central scotoma, A.D.: arcuate defect, D.: defect

Table 2.

visual field / visual acuity	improved	unchanged or deteriorated
improved	22 eyes	5 eyes
unchanged or deteriorated	5 eyes	3 eyes

In the cases of this group, hemorragic foci were small in size. Even visual field changes became enlarged after PC; aAD was not seen (Fig. 1).
(Fig. 1).
2. relative arcuate defect, 9 eyes (33%)
The hemorrhagic foci were extensive in the cases of this group and many of them showed pathological changes to a severe degree (Fig. 2).
3. absolute arcuate defect, 11 eyes (41%)
It is a characteristic of the group that all the cases had AD before the treatment (Fig. 3).
4. peripheral defect, 2 eyes (7%)

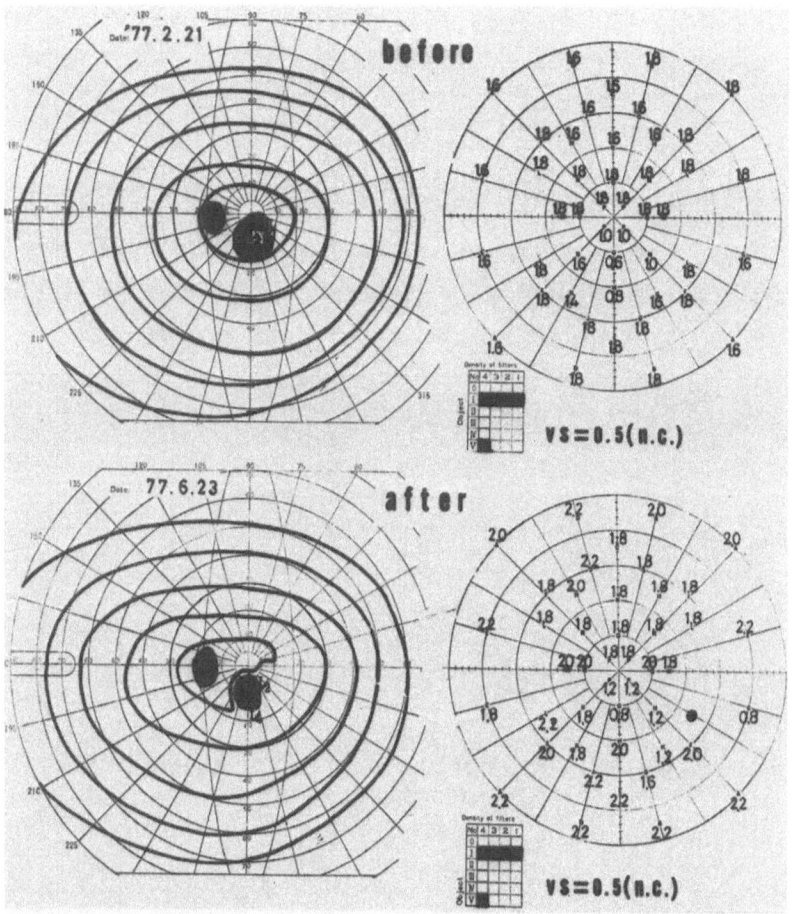

Fig. 1. Patient with superior temporal branch retinal vascular occlusion showing paracentral scotoma. Partial defect of I/1 isoptor and reduction in size of scotoma were seen after PC.

In this group pathological foci were present in the periphery therefore the visual acuity had not decreased. For preventing vitreous hemorrhage the PC was employed in this group (Fig. 4).

In order to see the occurrence of rAD of the RBVO, (Aulhorn 1963; Birchall, Harris, Drance & Begg 1976), data of 59 patients' visual field were analysed.

According to the result shown in the Table 3, rAD was found in 26 cases 44% and occupied a large part of the cases together with pCS.

DISCUSSION

The patients with RBVO have usually some subjective symptoms of visual field disturbance from the onset.

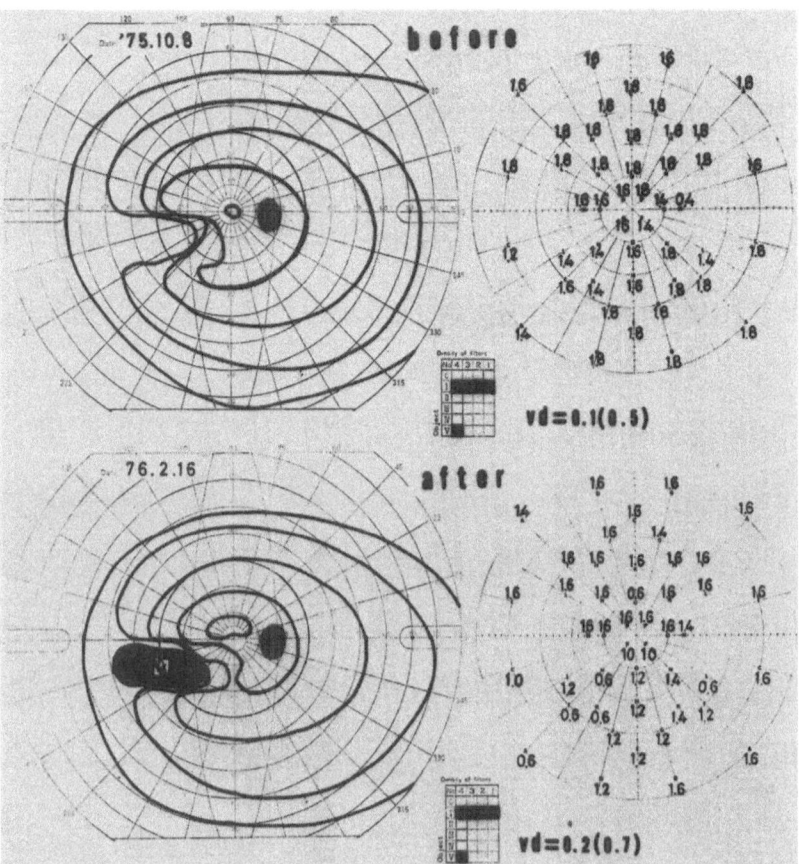

Fig. 2. Patient with superior temporal branch retinal vascular occlusion showing relative arcuate defect. Relative arcuate defect of I/4 isoptor become very deep and widened, and a scotoma of V/4 isoptor appeared.

398

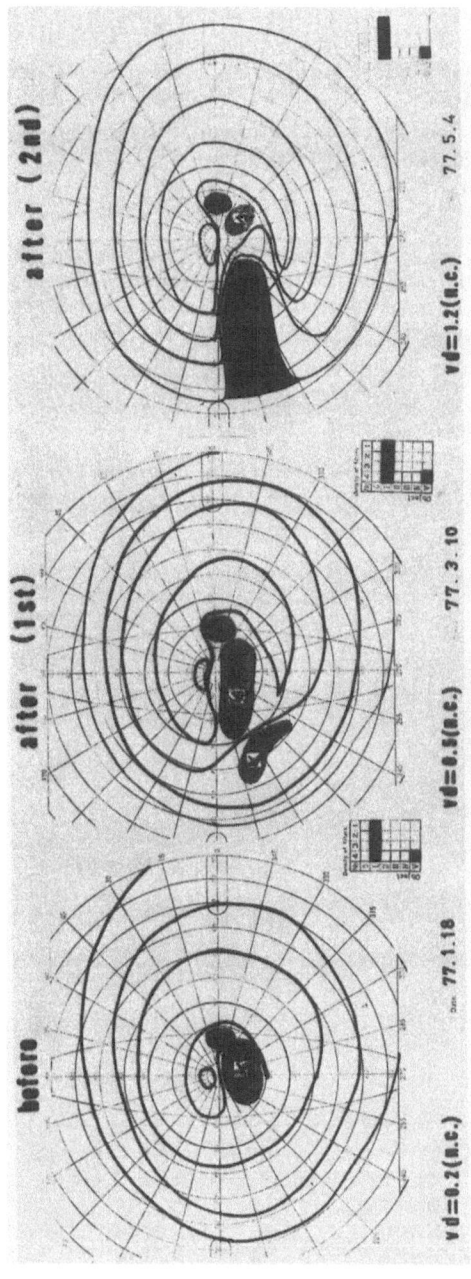

Fig. 3. Patient with superior temporal branch retinal vascular occlusion. The visual field changed from paracentral scotoma to relative arcuate defect by the 1st PC. The visual field deteriorated to an absolute arcuate defect after 2nd PC. However the visual acuity gradually improved.

399

However, only two cases complained of enlargement of the visual field defected after PC, and in these cases the visual acuity had not been recovered. recovered.

The other patients did not recognize the change, in spite of deterioration of the visual field after PC. In 1973 Campbell (1973) studied the changes the visual fields with small scotomata after PC, but reported that he did not find any sector defect at all.

In 1975 Oosterhuis (1975) reported a case of development of a paracentral nerve fibre bundle defect after PC.

In 1977 Laatikainen (1977) reported that no deterioration of visual field could be found PC.

As described above, according to the reports the visual field disturbances after PC were varied, ranging from neglogible to moderate in degree.

However, in our cases, aAD appeared in 11 eyes (41%) after the PC, and they all showed rAD before PC.

Considering the results of this study, visual field changes in this disease

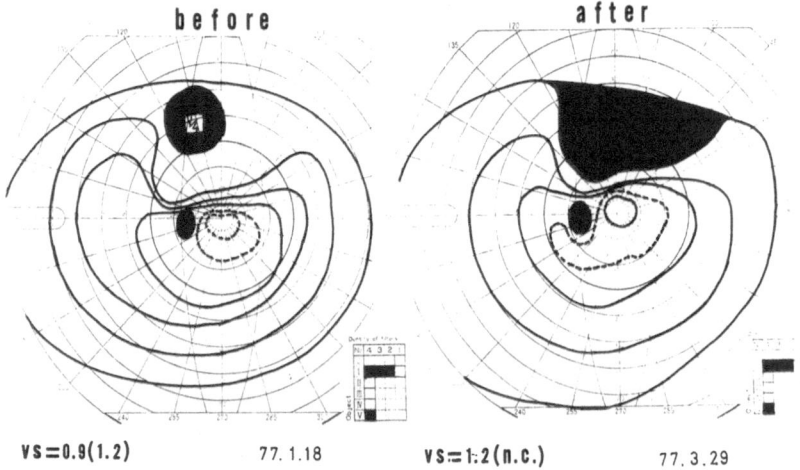

Fig. 4. Patient with inferior temporal branch retinal vascular occlusion. Peripheral defect was seen after PC.

Table 3.

visual field changes	eyes	%
paracentral scotoma	25	42
relative arcuate defect	26	44
peripheral constriction	8	14
total	59	100

are mainly represented by the pCS group and the rAD group. The pCS group did not show aAD, but the rAD group showed a high incidence of aAD by PC.

Clearly, the prognosis on visual field changes in these groups were different after PC.

Therefore, the prognosis of the visual field may be evaluated by performing perimetry before the coagulation therapy.

CONCLUSION

1. Visual field changes in RBVO are mainly represented by the pCS group and the rAD group.
2. Among 8 eyes showing pCS before PC, 5 eyes showed pCS and 3 eyes progressed to rAD after PC.
3. Among 18 eyes showing rAD before the treatment, 6 eyes remained in rAD, 10 eyes progressed to aAD and 2 eyes showed pD.
4. The peripheral visual field never improved after PC.
5. In general when the central area of the visual field was improved, the visual acuity was also improved.

REFERENCES

Aulhorn, E. Gesichtsfeldveränderungen bei Netzhautgefässverschlüssen. *Klin. Monatsbl. Augenheilkd.* 143: *234-247* (1963).

Birchall, C.H., Harris, G.S., Drance, S.M. & Begg, I.S. Visual field changes in branch retinal vein occlusion. *Arch. Ophthalmol.* 94: *747-754* (1976).

Campbell, C.J. & Wise, G.N. Photocoagulation therapy of branch vein obstructions. *Am. J. Ophthalmol.* 75: *28-31* (1973).

Laatikainen, L. Photocoagulation in retinal venous occlusion. *Acta Ophthalm.* 55: *478-488* (1977).

Oosterhuis, J.A. & Sedney, S.C. Photocoagulation in retinal vein thrombosis. *Ophthalmologica, Basel.* 171: *365-379* (1975).

Authors' address:
Department of Ophthalmology
Tokyo Medical College Hospital
6-7-1 Nishi-shinjuku, Shinjuku-ku
Tokyo 160, Japan

Docum. Ophthal. Proc. Series, Vol. 19

VISUAL FIELD CHANGES IN MESOPIC AND SCOTOPIC CONDITIONS USING FRIEDMANN VISUAL FIELD ANALYSER

TAKAKO HARA

(Tokyo, Japan)

ABSTRACT

By attaching a central fixation target to Friedmann Visual Field Analyser (FVFA), the author recorded a central visual field under scotopic condition (SC) in addition to routine mesopic condition (MC) on 30 normal eyes, 60 eyes with pigmentary retinal degeneration (PRD) and 4 eyes with acquired PRD-like diseases. Normal profile under SC was flat from 5° to 25°. It was similar to MC. The central area showed a depression of 1.2 log unit. PRD was divided into two types based on the FVFA profile and the mode of progression of PRD was discussed. In acquired chorioretinal diseases, local and steep depression coinciding with lesions in ocular fundus was observed. That was different from PRD which usually showed general depression.

INTRODUCTION

The visual field change in pigmentary retinal degeneration (PRD) becomes prominent under reduced background luminance. The central visual field change within 25° has special meaning for the following two reasons.

(1) The central visual field as well as the central visual acuity is the most important visual function in daily life.

(2) In many cases of PRD, the width of the central visual field is preserved until late stage. However, the preserved areas are not always normal and there are many differences in the height and shape of the central visual field island. Therefore, it is significant to reveal the state of the central visual field of PRD under three kinds of conditions, photopic (PC), mesopic (MC) and scotopic (SC).

Experiments were carried out to investigate the following three matters.

(1) The normal threshold under SC.

(2) Visual field change of PRD under the above mentioned three conditions.

(3) The difference in the visual fields between PRD and acquired PRD-like diseases.

MATERIALS AND METHODS

30 normal eyes of 30 persons were used as control. As PRD 60 eyes of 30 persons were used. In addition 4 eyes of 2 cases of congenital stationary nightblindness were examined. As acquired PRD-like diseases 4 eyes of chlo-

roquine retinopathy, 2 eyes of central retinal venous thrombosis and 4 eyes of simple glaucoma were examined. For campimetry the modified FVFA was used. The author attached a simple fixation target to FVFA 1,2 to perform the static quantitative perimetry easily under SC.

First, the change under MC was measured and following 30 minutes dark-adaptation the change under SC was measured by using FVFA. Goldmann perimeter and Goldmann-Weeker's adaptometer were used for photopic-kinetic perimetry and dark-adaptation respectively.

RESULTS

1. Normal. Normal threshold under SC was flat from A to N point resembling MC. At the fovea it sunk to 2.35 log unit showing a reduction of sensitivity of 1.2 comparing to the flat area (Tab. 1).

2. PRD. At the stage of wide visual field by kinetic perimetry PRD could be divided into two types of FVFA and was tentatively named M = S and M < S types respectively.

M = S type: The threshold under MC was similar to that of SC and the rod system did not function (Fig. 1a). Most of all typical PRD cases were included in this type and the average age was younger than the other type.

Table 1. Mesopic and scotopic thresholds of normal eyes
(Mean and standard deviations of 30 eyes).

Pattern	Mesopic Condition		Scotopic Condition	
	M	S.D	M	S.D
A	1.71	0.17	3.56	0.28
B	1.74	0.15	3.56	0.23
C	1.74	0.16	3.54	0.25
D	1.76	0.16	3.57	0.23
E	1.73	0.17	3.56	0.29
F	1.74	0.14	3.53	0.29
G	1.72	0.14	3.53	0.25
H	1.73	0.13	3.54	0.27
J	1.72	0.12	3.55	0.35
K	1.71	0.14	3.57	0.27
L	1.72	0.14	3.54	0.26
M	1.73	0.12	3.54	0.29
N	1.73	0.13	3.55	0.26
O	1.76	0.12	3.47	0.32
P	1.72	0.13	3.11	0.30
Macula	2.17	0.20	2.35	0.22

M < S type: The thresholds under MC and SC were separated. Rod function under SC was active (Fig. 1b). Most of all cases of non-pigmented PRD were included in this type.

Central field (5° radius) was always preserved in spite of various changes outside this area. Thus changes inside of 5° radius were studied and divided into two types which were tentatively named A and M types respectively (Table 2).

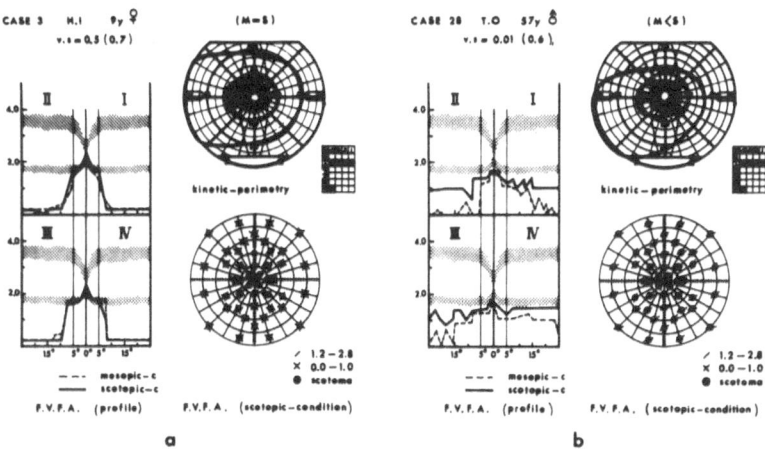

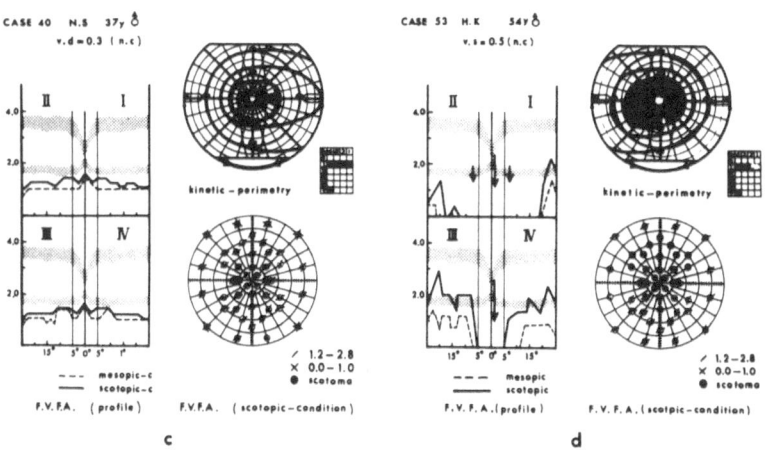

Fig. 1. FVFA chart and profiles. (a) M = S type of PRD. (b) M < S types of PRD. (c) Congenital stationary nightblindness. (d) Chloroquine retinopathy.

Two shadows of each profile indicate the normal range under scotopic (top) and mesopic (bottom) conditions.

405

Table 2. FVFA Profiles of PRD.

	Case	Age	Sex	D–A Curve
A TYPE	3*	9	F	10^{-3}
	4*	22	F	10^{-3}
	22(R)	27	F	10^{-2}
	26	10	M	10^{-2}
	27*	8	F	10^{-3}
	30*	9	M	10^{-2}
11 eyes				
M TYPE	1(L)	26	F	10^{-4}
	10*	28	M	10^{-3}
	20*	49	F	10^{-3}
	28*	57	M	10^{-2}
7 eyes				

Case	Age	Sex	D–A Curve
15	18	F	10^{-2}
16	32	M	10^{-4}
17*	34	F	10^{-2}
22(L)	27	F	10^{-2}
24	38	F	10^{-2}
29(L)	12	F	10^{-2}
10 eyes			
2*	22	M	10^{-4}
5(R)	59	F	10^{-3}
8	65	F	10^{-3}
12(R)	48	M	10^{-3}
14	59	F	10^{-4}
18	52	M	10^{-5}
21(R)	48	F	10^{-4}
25	23	F	10^{-2}
29(R)	12	F	10^{-3}
13 eyes			

Case	Age	Sex	D–A Curve
6	32	F	10^{-2}
7	8	M	10^{-2}
9*	20	F	10^{-2}
12(L)	48	M	10^{-3}
19	27	M	10^{-2}
21(L)	48	F	10^{-2}
23	29	M	10^{-2}
12 eyes			
1(R)	26	F	10^{-4}
5(L)	59	F	10^{-3}
11*	19	M	10^{-3}
13	69	F	10^{-4}
6 eyes			

※ Wide visual field by kinetic perimetry

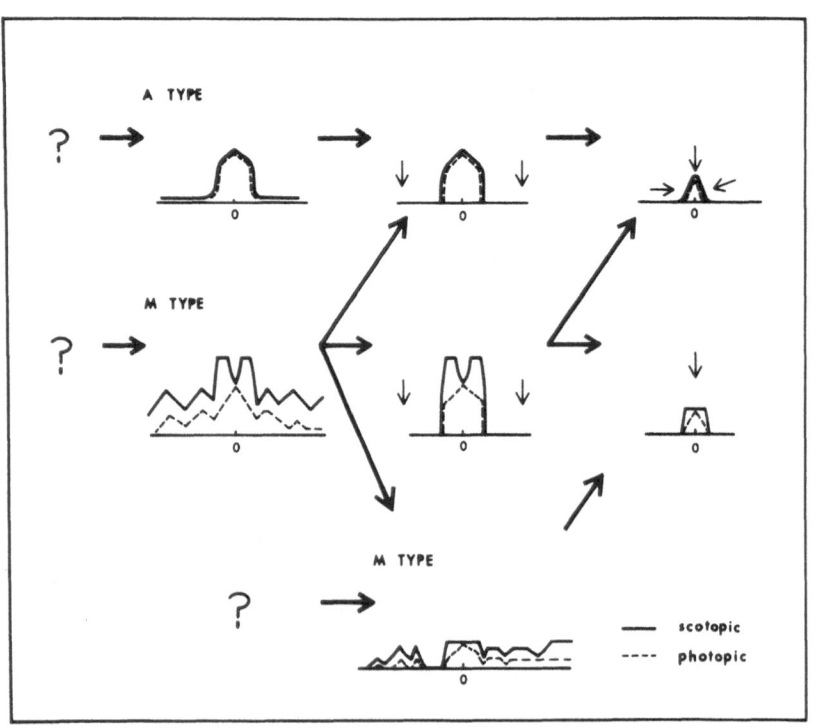

Fig. 2. Schematic drawing of the progress in PRD.

A-type: The threshold under MC was similar to that of SC and the rod system did not function.

M-type: Rod function in the central area remained almost normal, and was then generally depressed.

3. Congenital stationary nightblindness. Profile showed an almost flat curve with 1.0 log unit and the thresholds of MC and SC were almost similar (Fig. 1c). It was quite different from PRD. Dark-adaptation curve was monophasic.

4. Acquired PRD-like diseases. At the quadrantes where severe damages were detected by kinetic perimetry, FVFA profiles showed steep depressions under MC and SC. At the quadrantes where damages were slight, thresholds under MC and SC separated (Fig. 1d).

DISCUSSION

Like MC FVFA profile of the normal threshold the SC profile was almost flat in the areas outside the central part of 5° radius, making the detection of pathological changes easier.

In RPD present results revealed the remarkable increase of the threshold with FVFA in the area outside of the central part of 5° radius even at the stage of wide visual field with kinetic perimetry. As for the central part the threshold was normal in some cases and not in other. Based on the results mentioned above, the author tried to discuss the mode of the progression of PRD (Fig. 2); At the stage where the kinetic visual field is still intact, PRD was divided into two types based on FVFA, A and M which had areas of paracentral sensitivity of various grades (outside 5°). At the advanced stage, these areas disappeared and at the late stage, also the central part was lost.

Concerning the peripheral field, similar tendency was reported (4). The author confirmed that the same procession was going on in the central area even at the stage of wide visual field and the collapse of the central part of the visual field followed the same pattern as the periphery.

CONCLUSION

By using FVFA in PRD various changes were detected in the central visual field even at the stage of wide visual field by kinetic perimetry. These changes were identical to those occurring in the periphery. The mode of the progression of these changes was also discussed.

ACKNOWLEDGEMENT

The author expresses deep thanks to Professor H. Matsuo for his guidance in this research.

REFERENCES

Friedmann, A.I. The assesment of the efficacy of the glaucoma control by static perimetry or point analysis of clinical visual thresholds. *Trans. Ophthalmol. Soc. U.K.* 82: *381-358* (1962).

Friedmann, A.I. Serial analysis of changes in visual field defects employing a new instrument to determine the activity of diseases involving the visual pathways. *Ophthalmol.* 152: *1-12* (1966).

Matsuo, H., Endo, N., Suzuki, K. & Tasaki, S. Quantitative visual field in retinitis pigmentosa. *Jpn. J. Clin. Ophthalmol.* 22: *281-292* (1968).

Mizukawa, T., Otori, T. & Fujita, N. Recent advances in quantitative perimetry. *Jpn. J. Ophthalmol.* 15: *1109-1119* (1961).

Author's address:
Department of Ophthalmology,
Tokyo Medical College,
6-7-1 Nishishinjuku, Shinjuku-ku,
Tokyo, Japan 160

408

RELATIONSHIP BETWEEN PERIMETRIC ECCENTRICITY AND RETINAL LOCUS IN A HUMAN EYE

LARS FRISÉN & GUNILLA SCHÖLDSTRÖM

(Göteborg, Sweden)

A patient with unilateral blindness and optic atrophy due to a spheno-orbital meningioma requested removal of the blind eye because of pain and disfiguring proptosis. With the patient's consent, photo-coagulation markers were placed along the horizontal meridian of the retina prior to surgery. The angular coordinates in visual space of the markers were measured with an ophthalmoscopic procedure. The loci of the markers were also determined in a flat preparation following removal of the eye. The relationship between retinal arc and perimetric eccentricity was found to be approximately linear up to at least 50 degrees of angle, as predicted from previous model eye analyses. Full details have been presented elsewhere (Frisén & Schöldström 1977).

REFERENCE

Frisén, L. & Schöldström, G. Relationship between perimetric eccentricity and retinal locus in a human eye. Comparison with theoretical calculations. *Acta Ophthalmol.* 55: *63-68* (1977).

Author's address:
Dept. of Ophthalmology
University of Göteborg
Sahlgren's Hospital
S - 413 45 Göteborg
Sweden

A NEW INTERPRETATION OF THE RELATIVE CENTRAL SCOTOMA FOR BLUE STIMULI UNDER PHOTOPIC CONDITIONS

R. LAKOWSKI & P. DUNN

(Vancouver, Canada)

ABSTRACT

In an earlier paper a relative central scotoma for a blue stimulus as reported by Verriest and Israel and others was not found. The reason was thought to be a combination of luminance and target size differences between the experimenters, involving the phenomenon of summation.

A Goldmann perimeter identical to Verriest's was used to examine six subjects on the Goldmann targets at three different target sizes and at the luminances used by Verriest.

Results show duplication of Verriest's results when his method is followed, however this involves changing both size and maximum target luminance from colour to colour. When photometrically equated targets are used, and only target size is varied, from colour to colour, it becomes apparent that the foveal sensitivity for the blue target is no different than for the other targets, and in fact it is the parafoveal thresholds which are higher for the blue target. These results show an increase in sensitivity to a short wavelength stimulus with a dominant wavelength λD 454 nm, outside the fovea, the effect being maximal at the parafovea. This effect was absent in our study using a target of λD 474 nm, at a higher luminance value and a smaller target size.

A relative central scotoma for 'blue' stimulus presented under photopic conditions was reported by Verriest and Israel (1965) and confirmed by others (Hansen, 1974; Greve et al., 1974; Ronchi & Galassi, 1976). However, Lakowski (1977), using a high luminance chromatic Goldmann perimeter showed that chromatic targets (red, green, and blue) with a maximum luminance of 318 cdm^{-2} and size of 0.25 mm^2 in diameter gave retinal thresholds (for 0-180 meridian and 10 cdm^{-2} background luminance) within the range of thresholds for observers tested with our achromatic target of equivalent size and luminance. An apparent relative scotoma was found for the blue target only when Verriest's equivalent brightness method was used (i.e., using different sizes of targets for different colours and when this was presented in a graphic form based on the actual instrumental (lettered) values. It was considered that the relative scotoma might be due in part to the experimental design in which low luminance was used for the blue target (6.0 cdm^{-2}) or to the fact that a larger target had to be used (to achieve

* This work was supported by MRC grant No. 4342

equivalent brightness) or even for both reasons, and that the phenomenon of summation was involved.

This paper involves further investigation of the central scotoma for a blue target. Here the luminances of the chromatic targets (red, green and white) are kept constant and equivalent to the blue, but sizes of targets have been varied.

METHOD

To duplicate Verriest and Israel's results as accurately as possible, measurements were made with a Pritchard photometer (Model 197 OPR) on a standard (unmodified) perimeter at UBC's Department of Ophthalmology. Luminance levels of the achromatic target and background were set to 1000 asb and 31.5 asb with a A.G. Metrawatt Luxmeter in the manner described in the Users Manual. This was done several times using two Luxmeters, and each time luminance levels were measured with the Pritchard photometer, and then an average value was calculated, giving luminances in each case corresponding to the nominal values indicated by the Luxmeter. In addition, the Goldmann three-coloured filters (as used by Verriest & Israel) were mounted, the achromatic luminance set at 1000 asb with the Luxmeter, and resulting luminances measured with the photometer (corrected by the $V\lambda$ characteristics of the standard CIE observer). Again average values were obtained.

The actual luminances given by the Goldmann perimeter are shown in Table 1, and were used to duplicate the experiment of Verriest and Israel (1965). Similarity between the two experiments is limited by any differences between the particular Goldmann instruments used. (It is interesting to note that 42 asb is within the 40-45 asb range suggested by Goldmann (1946) originally as the adaptation luminance for this perimeter).

Six subjects between 16-22 with normal colour vision (as determined by a battery of colour vision tests including the Picford-Nicholson anomaloscope) were tested using the right eyes only. All subjects had unaided normal acuity of 1.0. Three target sizes were used: Goldmann I (6.4'), II (12.9'), and III (25.9'). The luminance of the red, green, and white targets were photometrically equated at the fovea to the luminances of the blue

Table 1. Actual Goldmann perimeter luminances.

	Nominal asb.	$cd\bar{m}^2$	Actual asb.	$cd\bar{m}^2$
Background Luminance	31.5	10	42.0	13.33
Stimulus Luminance				
Achromatic	1000.0	315	1500.0	476.19
Blue			10.8	3.43
Blue/Green			204.0	64.76
Red			81.3	25.81

stimulus used by Verriest and Israel, that is, 10.8 asb. With this modification the threshold gradients were investigated to duplicate their experiment. Table 2 gives the test conditions, which were randomized across subjects.

Table 2. Test conditions with Goldmann perimeter.

	Colour	Size (Goldmann Perimeter)	Maximal Luminance (asb)
Brightness equivalence	White	1	1500.0
	Green	1	204.0
	Red	2	81.2
	Blue	3	10.8
Photometric equivalence	White	1.2.3.	10.8
	Green	1.2.3.	10.8
	Red	1.2.3.	10.8
	Blue	1.2.3.	10.8

Note: All tests with adaption luminance of 42 asb, CIE Illuminant 'A'.

RESULTS AND DISCUSSION

Figure 1 shows the results we obtained under these conditions. The resulting gradients are essentially similar to those obtained by the above authors,

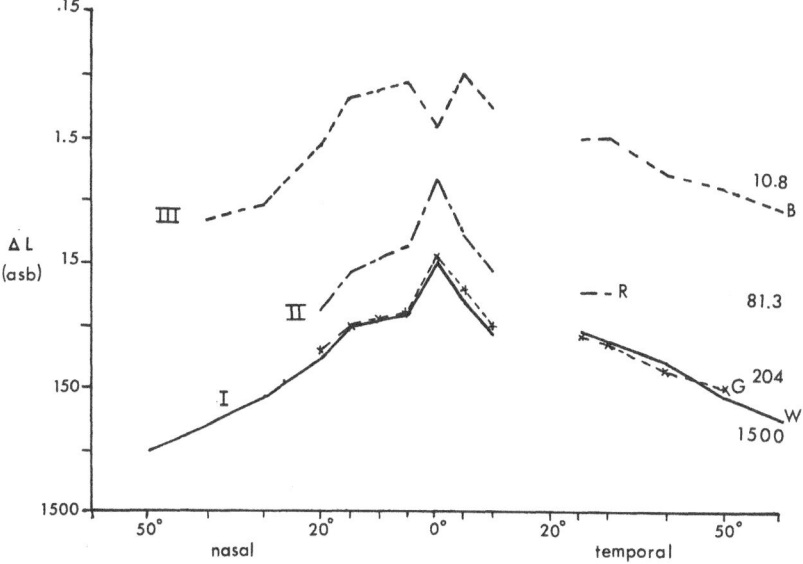

Fig. 1. Retinal threshold for 4 colour stimuli using the *equivalent brightness* method.

although the spread of foveal thresholds from white to blue is greater in our experiments. It is difficult to interpret the 'dip' in the blue gradient curve under these conditions, as the thresholds were obtained not only with different coloured stimuli and luminances, but also with targets of varying diameters.

Figure 2 shows threshold gradients obtained for four photometrically equated colour stimuli (red, green, blue, and white) with a maximal value of $\Delta L = 10.8$ asb, which is the maximal luminance obtained with the unmodified Goldmann instrument and its blue filter (dominant wavelength equivalent to λD 454 nm). Only target sizes were varied. It can be seen that no responses were recorded for size I except for the blue filter at 10-15° eccentricities on the nasal side. Target size II gave responses for green and blue, and only target size III produced gradients for all colours. Note that the 'dip' for the blue stimulus appears for both size targets (II and III).

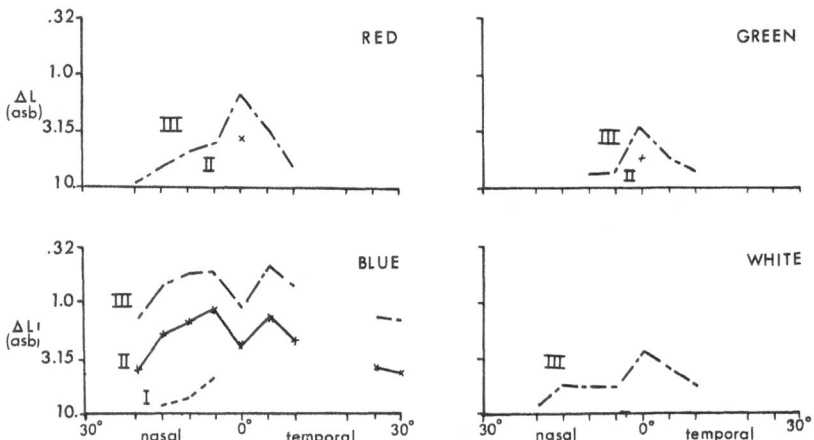

Fig. 2. Retinal threshold gradients observed for *photometrically equated* colour targets.

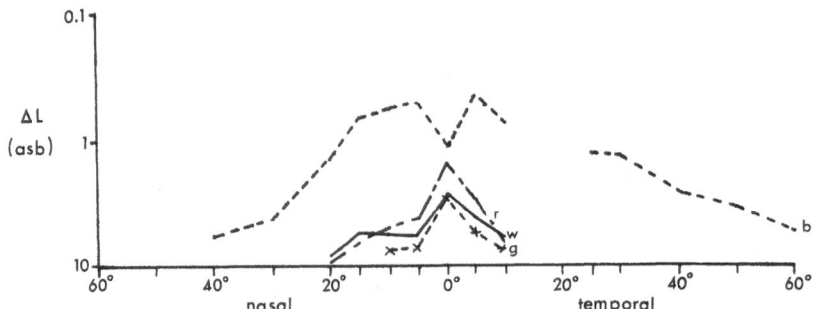

Fig. 3. Retinal thresholds for size III targets, equivalent luminance.

414

In Figure 3, threshold gradients are given for size III only in each of the colours used. These thresholds are placed on a common scale of intensities (ΔI) for all colours to facilitate comparisons. This figure shows clearly that the 'dip' or the 'relative central scotoma' for blue in fact reflects *increased parafoveal sensitivity*. The foveal threshold is slightly higher than that for red, green, and white targets, as is the entire gradient. What these results indicate is that there is an increase in sensitivity to a short wavelength stimulus with dominant wavelength λD 454 nm outside the fovea, the effect being maximal in the parafovea.

Such extrafoveal increases in sensitivity are well known to characterize the dark-adapted retina for achromatic as well as for most chromatic stimuli, excepting long-wavelength targets (Sloan 1939; 1950; Wentworth 1930; Nolte 1962). However, in this experimental setup only the short wavelength stimulus λD 454 nm seems to give this type of gradient under photopic conditions. No such effects were noted by Lakowski (1977) with a blue of dominant wavelength OD 474 nm and high luminance values for the targets. Further work is in progress to elucidate the effect of background luminance, its energy distribution, test object, sizes, and wavelength of target on the retinal thresholds.

REFERENCES

Goldmann, H. Demonstration unseres neuen Projektionskogel perimeters samt theoretischen und klinischen Bemerkungen über Perimetrie. *Ophthalmologica* 111: *187-192* (1946).

Greve, E.L., Verduin, W.M. & Ledeboer, M. Two-colour threshold in static perimetry. *Mod. Probl. Ophthal.* 13: *113-118* (1974).

Hansen, E. The colour receptors studied by increment threshold measurements during chromatic adaptation in the Goldmann perimeter. *Acta Ophthal.* 52: *490-500* (1974).

Lakowski, R., Wright, W.D. & Oliver, K. A Goldmann perimeter with high luminance chromatic targets. *Canad. J. Ophthal.* 12: *203-210* (1977).

Nolte, W. Bestimmung achromatischer Schwellen für verschiedene Spectrallichter. Inaugural Dissertation, Universitätsaugenklinik Tübingen (1962).

Ronchi, L. & Galassi, R. Absolute thresholds for monochromatic stimuli of various sizes and duration across the visual field. *Doc. Ophthal. Proceedings Series* 14: *423-426* (1976).

Sloan, L.L. Instruments and techniques for the clinical testing of light sense. III. An apparatus for studying regional differences in light sense. *Arch. of Ophthal.* 22: *233-251* (1939).

Sloan, L.L. The threshold gradients of the rods and the cones; In the dark-adapted and in the partially light-adapted eye. *Am. J. Ophthal.* 33: *1077-1088* (1950).

Verriest, G. & Israel, A. Application due perimetre statique de Goldmann au releve topographique des senils differentiels de luminance pour petits objects colores projectes sur un fond blanc. *Vision Res.* 5: *151-174, 341-359* (1965).

Wentworth, H.A. A quantitative study of achromatic and chromatic sensitivity from center to periphery of the visual field. *Psychol. Monogr.* 40: (3) Nr 183 (Dissertation). (1930).

Author's address:
Visual Laboratory
Department of Psychology
The University of British Columbia
2075 Wesbrook Place
Vancouver, B.C.
V6T 1W5

Docum. Ophthal. Proc. Series, Vol. 19

DISCUSSION OF THE SESSION ON METHODOLOGY

CHAIRMAN: H. MATSUO

Matsuo: First the presentation of Dr. Kani will be discussed by Dr. Ohta.

Ohta: Dr. Kani, congratulations for your splendid work. Question 1: Is it possible to register the results of the tests, and how do you register the records? Question 2: Is it possible to use colour T.V.?

Greve: As this is such a fascinating subject I should like to ask Dr. Kani whether he could explain to us what the differences are between the apparatuses that have been demonstrated and also what the difficulties are. I can imagine that one of the difficulties is the standardization. What type of stimulus and background has been used exactly?

Werner: I'd like to ask if you had the opportunity of using this machine for patients demonstrating the localized slit-like deficiencies in the retinal nerve fiber layer which has been described.

Kani: To Dr. Ohta. First Question: at present we sketch the results directly from the television screen by hand. We have no method for good registration. We hope to handcopy the images on the monitor television screen by using computer memory. The second question, colour TV: this is still under investigation. To Dr. Greve: in the first model a natural view system is used. In the second model we use Maxwellian view. We make photometry using a phantom eye and also subjective measurement with artifical pupil was made. I have no idea how to measure the amount of light with the Maxwellian view system.

Because we use infrared television, some lesions are not detectable on monitor TV. screen.

To Dr. Werner: I have no experience with nerve fiber bundle defects and its measurements. Some results will be presented by Dr. Tagami of the Kobe university.

Greve: Dr. Kani, is the method now in a stage were we, who are not familiar with the method could apply it, or are the difficulties such that we wait till you have solved them? Do you understand what I mean? The pictures are beautiful both of Dr. Ohta and you and the other people who are working with this type of system but I like to know how difficult it is to work with these apparatus? Could we now start using them?

Kani: It is very difficult because we use infrared rays. The fundus is not so clearly demonstrated. This is the biggest problem for us.

Ernest: I would think that the infrared image and the target would be out of the focus. Is that a problem?

Kani: In the first model with the natural visual system we used a correction lens before the eye. In the second model the focussing is separately made by the focussing system of the fundus camera.

Frisen: I would like to ask two questions about the registration of the fundus image and the test-spot. I have not been able to understand if you can view the test-spot on the fundus-image or if you see two super imposed images that perhaps are not perfectly registred. The only possibility I know of getting in to this was the slide of by Dr. Enoch, where he showed that his fundus picture is transformed into a central tangential projection and the central tangential projection is not equidistant as our usual perimetric projection is. The other question is, if you can view the fundus image and the image of the test-spot at the same time, I guess they cannot be in focus both of them at the same time.

Matsuo: Next Dr. Matsudaira's paper.

Ernest: You reported a 41 percent incidence of arcuate defects after photocoagulation. Might the use of Laser coagulation decrease involvement of the inner retina? Did the patients complain of scotomas after photocoagulation?

Matsudaira: We cannot compare both Xenon and argon laser photocoagulation, because we didn't use laser coagulation at that time. And second: a few patients complained about scotomas after treatment.

Matsuo: Then the next paper is of Dr. Greve. Any comment? Please Dr. Aulhorn.

Aulhorn: I think it may be a little dangerous to super-impose the picture of the fundus on the perimetric chart in cases of macular damages. Because in these cases, most of the time, there is an excentric fixation and then we don't know were we are if we do so. The other danger is that in cases of ametropy, the magnification is very different in myopia and hyperopia. I think it seems to be a very exact method because if looks so, if you superimpose but in my opinion it is not.

Greve: I think that certainly in early stages of drusen the problem of fixation is not there. Of course, for out type of investigation the most interesting stages are these early stages. Patients with a visual acuity of 0.75 or 0.5 usually have a good central fixation. If you have large disciform lesions you loose your central fixation, but then it is not so interesting any more for this kind of comparative investigation. As for the magnification, I don't think that the effect is that large that it seriously influenced the measurements and of course you can search around the position on the photograph to find the particular lesion.

418

Matsuo: I would like to proceed to Dr. Ohta's paper.

Kani: Dr. Ohta, one question: with your method of testing, how do you measure the visual fields of patients with poor fixation or central scotoma?

Ohta: We have much difficulty with the patients who have poor fixation. In these cases we control the position of the optic disc on the T.V. screen.

Matsuo: Dr. Inatomi's paper will be discussed. Dr. Enoch?

Enoch: A recent study published by Dr. Lewis Harvey (university of Colorado) supports the findings of the overlap of the two visual fields.

Friedmann: We also found that in homonymous hemianopia the field defects are not necessarily confined to the vertical meridian.

Matsuo: Comments on Dr. Enoch's paper.

Enoch: Since questions by Frisen and Aulhorn refer to our efforts as well, I should like to comment. The projective transformation error that we encounter is probably limited because, as you saw in those two cases, we were well in the central 8 or 9°. When we get outside of that we recognize that there must be errors and you noticed we don't use fine points to indicate the areas of correspondance but rather indicate approximate areas of correspondance. In response to Dr. Aulhorn's question, in our case we, at least at this point, have limited all studies to patients with visual acuity of 20/50 or better, much in the same way as Dr. Greve. To handle the magnification question related to refraction error I also had an contactlens on the eye and that minimises that particular problem. And lastly I think it is terribly important in keeping with Dr. Frisen's question, to point out that we have a compounding of errors here and we must be very careful not to try to carry these arguments of registration too far. The one advantage of the new camera type devices, if I have understood their optics, is that the stimulus distortion and the camera distortion may be equal but please realize that this is a distorted view.

Aulhorn: Let me say something to the refractive error. It is wonderful if you have a contactlens but if you have a long eye, than you have an other magnification in the perimetric correlation than if you have a shorter eye. This contactlens helps only in cases of afakia or if the refractive error is in the anterior part of the eye.

Enoch: Yes and no. We use the same correction-modality both for the field and the fundus picture. But the camera has a different distortion than the perimeter. This is the whole point I was just making.

Matsuo: Then I would like to proceed to the discussion of the non-read papers.

Friedmann: Dr. Hara's paper succeeds in showing that visual field analysis in diseases affecting dark adaptation can be very effective. They employed a visual field analyser with special fixation device for dark adapted perimetry, Goldmann photopic kinetic perimetry and also Goldmann-Weekers dark adaptometer for assessing dark adaptation. They also had the photopic and scotopic E.R.G. It is an extremely well done paper and they found interesting results in that the real pigmentary degenerations show completely different visual fields from acquired diseases which end up by being the socalled pseudo retinitis pigmentosa type of disease and they found completely different results in stationary night blindness. The paper interests me because I find that global dark adaptation is a very inaccurate test and they confirm that it is very difficult to differentiate from the dark adaptation curve between these different types of diseases and I think that their technique goes a long way to help us in this direction.

Verriest: The paper of Lakowski and Dunn 'A new interpretation of the relative central scotoma for blue stimuli under photopic conditions.' Is an extension of the investigation of the phenomenon that I described with Israel in 1965, namely the central scotoma which is evidenced in static profile perimetry when one uses a blue target against the white background of about $10\,cd.m^{-2}$ of the Goldmann perimeter (or this of about $3.18\,cd.m^{-2}$ of the Tübingen perimeter). Later on Verriest and Kandemir (1974) and Lakwoski, Wright and Oliver (1977) showed that this central scotoma for a blue objects disappears at higher background luminances.

In their actual paper, Lakowski and Dunn studied further parameters as target luminance and size in order to elucidate the origin of the scotoma, that is ascribed to parafoveal sensitivity to lights of shorter wavelenghts. This is in complete agreement with the conclusion of the 1977 paper of Verriest and Uvyls published in Documenta Ophthalmologica and in which we studied another factor, namely age, the central scotoma for blue being less deep after the age of 15 years.

Furthermore, we showed that this developmental feature is not due to the preceptoral factors, but to an improvement which age of the foveal functions.

I should be pleased to hear Lakowski's comments about this new aspect of the problem.

SUMMARY OF SESSION IV: METHODOLOGY

CHAIRMAN: H. MATSUO

At the 2nd IPS Symposium, Dr. Kani presented his new method, namely, the fundus-controlled perimetry, which attracted a good deal of our attention. This time, he showed us his instrument which has been developed into an advanced stage. I would like to express my sincere appreciation for his streneous efforts. The advantages of this method are already given in the summary made by Prof. Aulhorn at the previous symposium. Some of the Japanese investigators have happened to come up with the similar ideas to Dr. Kani's method. Prof. Inatomi, who had published the results of the experiments based upon this idea in 1967, reported today his latest studies.

Prof. Isayama's plan has also been published. At the scientific exhibition of this symposium, in addition to these instruments, Prof. Ohta's new fundus photo-perimeter is displayed. This responds to the suggestion made by Prof. Goldmann at the 2nd symposium. That is to say, Prof. Ohta's instrument has an advantage of displaying the results of perimetry on the fundus photograph by one step of procedure.

As the chairman of the Research Group on Methodology, I have asked for the members' opinion on the following three points as regards the development of perimetry.

1) Necessity of studies on basic visual functions related the development of perimetry. 2) Development of new perimetric methods and its possibilities by means of studying perimetric conditions and relevant factors. 3) New methods of techniques of more economical, simplified and effective examination of perimetry from the practical point of view.

So far I have received several answers and some of them are very beneficial. Collecting these opinions, I am going to readjust and inform the RG members of them so that they will serve usefully as the data for development of method. Thank you.

THE ENLARGEMENT OF THE BLIND SPOT IN BINOCULAR VISION

A. DUBOIS-POULSEN

(Paris, France)

ABSTRACT

With a polarising system it is demonstrated that the size of the blind spot is considerably larger in dichoptic than in monoptic vision. The temporal and photometric modalities of the phenomenon are studied and discussed.

INTRODUCTION

In 1952 we described with C1. Magis a phenomenon upon which we subsequently came back in several publications (Dubois-Poulsen, 1952). It is worthy of development, for it has not been studied in full. The blind spot of which the dimensions are statistically well known, when measured in monocular conditions, considerably widens in binocular ones. It is an example of inhibition in the normal visual field which deserves full attention.

The present study endeavours to consider the variations of the phenomenon according to the type and to the photometrical conditions of the experiences performed. It is known that four investigations are available for the analysis of binocular vision, the polarized light, the complementarily coloured glasses, (red and green in general) the synchronization of flickering lights. We did not use the fourth one, the stereoscopy which seems more simple but is highly disadvantageous because of its narrow field limited to macular and paramacular vision.

PRINCIPLES

The polarized light is the simpler available method. The patient is fitted with a spectacle, each glass of which is a polarizing filter. One is polarized at 90° and the other one at 180°. The luminous target is supplied with a polarizing filter orientated at 90° or 180°. The eye which is covered by the filter polarized perpendiculary with the axis of the test cannot see it, whereas the other eye sees it perfectly well. The advantage of this is in working with white light.

Apart from the pair of glasses, the patient has not the impression undergoing a sophisticated instrumentation. In no condition, is the conscious of the separation artifically created between each eye. He perceives the totality of the perimetric background and all details in the surrounding and therefore

423

puts in work all the processus inherent with this binocular situation.

There is another classical method using coloured glasses. If a red glass is put before an eye and a green one is front of the other and if the target is green, it will not be perceived by the eye viewing with the red glass and will be seen as identical with the background. Only one eye is therefore tested. This method is worse than the proceeding one, for the colour difference between the two eyes gives to the patient an artificial feeling which is unlike the normal vision.

The third method uses the flickering light. If each eye is successively occluded during half the time with a frequency exceeding the critical fusion frequency the background seems to be uniformely lighted under the Talbot level.

If the luminous target is also flickering, one can find a given frequency when it will be perceived during the period ascribed to one eye and not during the period assigned to the other one. The subject seems to see binocularly except for the target which is seen monocularly.

INSTRUMENTATION

We work with a black Bjerrum screen situated at I meter from the patient's eye. The fixation point was a phosphorescent white. The lighting of the screen was 30 lux, its luminance 0,6 nits as measured with a nitometer.

The test presentator was designed by Magis in 1952. It is constituted by a bulb having a linear filament (6V-0,5 A) by a condenser which focused the light on the posterior extremity of a plexiglass bar, 50 cm in lenght, with a rectangular section (IOmmX 25 mm). The light is transmitted to the other extremity of the bar and is uniformerly spread over an opaque and white plexiglass plate which is perfectly responding to the Lambert's law and the constancy of which has been verified with a precision of circa 2° until 50° in excentrically. A housing situated between the two lenses of the condenser allows the insertion of neutral grey Kodak Filters to modify the luminance, of coloured filters or of polarizing filters (Polaroid HN.42 Transmission 42%).

At the extremity of the bar is arranged a cat's eye allowing variations in the linear dimensions of the square target with sides varying from 5/IOmm to 22 millimeters.

The luminance without grey filters is equal to 26,5 cd.m2. The apparatus has a black coating, the reflexion coefficient of which is equal to that of the perimetric screen.

The patient's head is resting on a head support. He wears polarizing or coloured spectacles. When the experimentation was done by us we used a dental stent print so that the head was strictly immobile. We did not use such a device for ordinary subjects. Secondly we placed a compur obturator before one eye of our patients. It was occluded and was only open to give binocular vision during a short and measurable time.

The apparatus for successive occlusions has been very simply built with a black rotating disk of large dimensions (diameter 0,50 m) extending beyond the patient's face, and situated in front of his eyes it was perforated by two opposite sectors of 90° through which the patient could see the Bjerrum screen. The rotation axis was put before his nose. The speed was 30 cycles/sec. giving 60 flashes/sec. for each eye.

The speed of the motor could be variated from IO cycles/sec. to IOOO cycles/sec.

In this way each eye was occluded during the time the other was seeing and vice versa. A. Magitot's test projector was placed along the patient's temple and projected tests on the screen through the disk. The tests could therefore be seen only by the eye from the same side. The speed gave the sensation of binocular vision.

EXPERIMENTS

We examined 20 patient's all emmetropic to avoid the variations in position and dimensions of the blind spot. We began by measuring the spot in monocular vision and then in binocular vision by the three methods, with a test of 4,2 mm and 6cd/m2. The spot was constantly larger in binocular vision.

In a second series of experiments we placed the test in a point in the zone of enlargement of the spot on the vertical meridian or on the horizontal one. When the non examined eye was occluded the test was perceived because it was seen monocularly.

But when the second eye was open, it suddenly disappeared and we tried to measure the speed of this reflex

A

The blind spot when measured with the dimensions and the luminance of tests as above mentioned gave an average of 7° in width in the vertical meridian and 6° for the horizontal meridian. The distance from its internal side to the fixation point varied from 12° to 13°30'. The average may be calculated at 12°45'. On the vertical meridian the average numbers I/3 above the horizontal line and 2/3 under may be considered as correct.

The average width of the spot in binocular vision is approximately of 9° on the horizontal meridian and of 8°30' on the vertical meridian. There is thus a rounding effect of the spot by enlargement of its horizontal axis.

If the spot is measured monocularly using smaller tests with weaker contrasts i.e. I mm2 with 3cd/m2 luminance its dimensions can exactly be superimposed on the binocular ones. The zone which is called the amblyopic zone of Sinclair has been put in evidence and it seems that the binocular enlargement takes a similar place. If the experiment is done again monocularly with the same small tests, the spot widens again in binocular vision but not in such an extent (circa I/2°). In total darkness with a phosphorescent point of fixation the spot measured with a test of 4 mm2 in width, and under a luminance of 0,06 cd/m2 is very wide and it does not widen in binocular vision.

In conclusion we can say that the spot widens in binocular vision by a quantity which is equal to the extent of the Sinclair zone which corresponds to the luminous conditions of background and test stimulation.

The results are the same whatever the experimental conditions. Polarization, coloured filters, temporal alternative.

B

The reflex of enlargement is very rapid. We so endeavour to measure its speed.

With the polarization it is almost instantaneous. The minimum duration of the obturator aperture was of I/50 sec. (average).

Under I/50 the test was not seen. We verified that it remained still visible if situated at IO° on the vertical meridian passing through the fixation point.

With the alternative method it is as rapid. There is a temporal summation because of the speed of the light flicker.

With the coloured filters it is very slow; the test needs a longer time to disappear in binocular vision (I/IO Sec.). It is certainly due to the hesitation of the eye between the vision in green or in red before the fusion.

CONCLUSIONS

The use of the binocular vision induces in the visual field some inhibition effects which become prominent with the phenomenon of widening of the blind spot. The inhibition takes place at the site of the zone of less sensibility surrounding the spot which was called the amblyopic zone by Sinclair.

It is worthy of attention because the principal inhibition reactions, already known in the visual field are consecutive to steady monocular fixation and cease with binocular vision. They are described within the sphere of local adaptation or Troxler phenomenon. It is here the inverse for the inhibition takes places in binocular conditions. Whereas the Troxler phenomenon is peripheral in nature the second one must be central.

These phenomena are without doubt of great importance in strabismus especially, in Swann's syndrome where the blind spot of an eye is substituted to the fixation point.

REFERENCES

Dubois-Poulsen, A. Le champ visuel. Topographie normale et pathologique de ses sensibilités-1952-I Vol. 1175 p. Masson et Cie edit. Paris. pp 313, 314 et 315.
Magis, Cl. In Dubois-Poulsen -Le champ visuel -Masson et Cie Edit. pp 477, 478.

Author's address:
8 Avenue Daniel — Lesueur
Paris VII
France

426

EVALUATION OF PERIMETRIC PROCEDURES
A STATISTICAL APPROACH

MARIANNE FRISÉN

(Göteborg, Sweden)

ABSTRACT

A very precise formulation of the purposes of the visual field examination and proper handling of the time factor are important for any evaluation and comparison of perimetric procedures. If information about the predictive value of a procedure is desired, it is also necessary to involve the prevalence of abnormal cases in a well-defined population. A probabilistic approach to the measurement of performance is recommended. Some common measures, e.g. sensitivity and predictive value, are described as they apply to clinical perimetry. Some new measures are proposed for the evaluation of follow-up examinations.

INTRODUCTION

Evaluation of perimetric procedures is necessary for several purposes. One purpose may be to choose the 'best' among a number of procedures. Another is to obtain information on where efforts for improvement should be concentrated. A third purpose may be to gain knowledge about limitations and possibilities of a procedure in use. A comprehensive evaluation must include many different aspects. Only aspects which can be analysed statistically will be discussed here.

When evaluating how good a given procedure of perimetry is, the first problem is to decide what the word 'good' is to mean, exactly. In some way the meaning has to be associated with a specific purpose. There is no procedure which is best for all purposes, as will be demonstrated by some examples.

The procedure which is optimal to detect an absolute scotoma in the area of 5° around the fovea would concentrate all observations to this area and use a stimulus which is clearly supraliminal in this area. The procedure can thus not be the same as that which is optimal to detect a relative scotoma in a specified area in the periphery. This extreme example demonstrates that a universally optimal procedure is inconceivable. There are less extreme examples of the implications of the goal of the procedure. The best procedure to detect a relative quadratic depression will not be the same as that which is optimal to detect absolute scotomata of unknown number and location. Also, the best screening procedure will hardly be the best procedure for follow-up of a known defect.

MEASURES OF HOW WELL A PROCEDURE DISCRIMINATES
BETWEEN NORMALS AND ABNORMALS

The terms 'normal' and 'abnormal' are convenient but have to be exactly defined for each study. For example, 'normal' could be defined as 'cases which do not have a specified visual field defect' or 'cases where the utility of further examination of the patient is less than a specified value'. 'Abnormals' will be defined as the complement to 'normal'. However, to discuss measures of discrimination between two states 'normal' and 'abnormal', it is not necessary to know the precise definition of the two states. The following are some commonly used measures of diagnostic performance:

The *sensitivity* of a diagnostic procedure is the proportion of abnormals which are detected and thus correctly classified.

The *specificity* is the proportion of the normals which are correctly classified.

The *predictive value of the diagnosis 'normal'* is the proportion of those classed as 'normal' who in reality are normal.

The *predictive value of the diagnosis 'abnormal'* is the proportion of those classed as 'abnormal' who in reality are abnormal.

In order to compute the sensitivity and specificity it is necessary to know not only the diagnosis but also the true state of a number of cases. This can be obtained by more extensive examination of the patients or by using simulated visual fields with known properties. The latter approach has been used in a comparison of subjective and objective judgements of the shape of visual field isopters (Frisén & Frisén 1975). Examples of the results are given in Table 1. While the sensitivity is about the same for the two types of judgements, the specificity is better for the objective one.

In order to compute the predictive values it is also necessary to specify the prevalence of 'abnormals'. The predictive values are calculated directly or by a formula based also on the sensitivity and specificity. The prevalence and thus the predictive values are of course dependent on the characteristics of the population. Prevalences, and predictive values, are different in e.g. a

Table 1. Comparison between subjective judgements and a simple objective method for discrimination between normal and abnormal isopters. Central normal (elliptic) isopters and corresponding isopters with a small quadrant defect were tested. 25 isopters of each type were judged. For each isopter there were 25 simulated observations.

| Isopter | Fraction of isopters judged as defective by | | | | | |
| | Subjective judge No. | | | | Average subjective judgment | Objective method |
	I	II	III	IV		
Normal	0.44	0.24	0.20	0.12	0.25	0.12
Defective	0.80	0.76	0.44	0.82	0.71	0.72

presumably healthy population attending a health control, and a population of patients referred to a specialized diagnostic unit.

When more than two states (e.g. 'normal', 'disease A' and 'disease B') are of interest, the formulas are more complicated but the principles of analysis are the same.

In perimetry there is a limiting factor of great importance, namely time. Nearly every perimetric procedure will have a very good capacity for discrimination if just the patient and the perimetrist were willing and able to spend a long time together without deteriorating quality of the examination. On the other hand, if just very short time is available, all methods will have a poor performance and only very extensive defects can be detected with a reasonable probability.

It is therefore necessary to introduce the element of time (and other 'costs') in the measurements of performance. One simple way of taking care of the time variable is to state the sensitivity etc. for a standard period of examination e.g. 15 minutes. The measures of performance can also be expressed as functions of time.

In some cases 'time' might be replaced by e.g. 'number of observations'. This is not so when two methods of different characters, such as kinetic and static perimetry, are compared.

THE USE OF THEORETICAL MODELS TO IMPROVE THE DIAGNOSTIC PROCEDURE

Even with the same practical performance (i.e. collection of information) the discriminating ability could be quite different dependent on the way of handling the data. In order to discriminate it is necessary to have some idea of what is characteristic of a normal case in contrast to an abnormal one. This idea could be more or less detailed and useful. The knowledge can be quite general in nature (e.g. normal isopters are elliptical in shape) or specific for a given patient (e.g. the appearance of the retinal nerve fiber layer suggests the presence of a nasal visual field defect). To illustrate the effect of knowledge about whether e.g. temporal or nasal defects are suspected, results from a simulation study are illustrated in Table 2.

Table 2. Comparison between judgements with and without knowledge about the probable location of a defect. Normal (elliptic) isopters and corresponding isopters with a slight quadrant defect were tested. For each isopter there were 25 simulated observations. The figures are based on the simulation of 2000 isopters of each kind.

Isopter	Fraction judged as defective by the objective test procedure	
	No a priori knowledge	Knowledge of suspected side
Normal	0.107	0.036
Defective	0.83	0.82

A general idea or model about the characteristics of normals and abnormals is a knowledge which might improve the efficiency of the diagnostic procedure in the same way as the information about a specific patient. However all new models have to be tested. If the new model of what is characteristic of normal and abnormal cases is quite wrong, it will be of no use. It is not necessary, however, that the model is exactly true in order to be useful. A sufficient approximation of the true conditions can be the base of a valuable diagnostic method. The statistical way of determining what is a 'sufficiently good approximation' has been described (Frisén 1974) in the context of whether or not the model of an ellipse would be sufficiently accurate approximation for normal isopters to be the basis for a diagnostic method.

ANALYSIS OF SOURCES OF VARIATION

An analysis of the sources of measurement errors is of considerable use when attempting to improve methods. It is also of value to guide which method would be preferable for different purposes where different measurement errors play different roles.

An analysis of the relative importance of different sources of unwanted variation of measurement can be made experimentally by repeated measurements under different conditions. A crude analysis can also be made by comparing the different components of two methods.

FOLLOW-UP STUDIES

When the purpose of a perimetric examination is not to classify a visual field as 'normal' or 'abnormal' but to follow a patient with serial examinations, the measurements of performance are more complicated. It is possible to characterize the ability to *describe* the visual field by 'accuracy' and 'precision', but the pure description is seldom the ultimate purpose. The question is often whether or not there has been a change over the time.

The problem of comparing visual fields from *two* occasions and to determine whether or not there are differences apart from the inevitable random variations is a minor problem. Measures of performance can easily be calculated in the same way as for the discrimination discussed above. The error rates also have a direct correspondance to the well-known errors (of type I and type II) of statistical tests.

However, when an individual is followed over several occasions, the problem of describing performance is quite different. The sensitivity will now depend on the number of examinations performed and has to be evaluated as a function of time. New special measures, such as 'the ability to detect a slowly progressing change before it becomes irreversible' and 'average waiting time until a slowly progressing change is detected' are of interest.

REFERENCES

Frisén, L. & Frisén, M. Objective recognition of abnormal isopters. *Acta Ophthalmol.* 53: *378-392* (1975).

Frisén, M. Stochastic deviation from elliptical shape. An applied study. Almqvist & Wiksell, Stockholm (1974).

Author's address:
Department of Statistics
Viktoriagatan 13
S-411 25 Göteborg
Sweden

EYE MOVEMENTS DURING PERIPHERAL FIELD TESTS MONITORED BY ELECTRO-OCULOGRAM

YOSHIHITO HONDA, AKIRA NEGI & MASAKI MIKI

(Kyoto, Japan)

ABSTRACT

EOGs of twenty patients (forty eyes) were recorded as an indicator of gross eye movements during peripheral field tests. Poor fixation was found among cases of non-cooperative children and older patients with senile dementia. EOGs of such patients showed prominent square-wave potentials, indicating eye movements and probability of low reliability of fields measured. Poor fixation was also noted for patients with large central scotomas or very poor vision. Gaze shifts appeared to the same extent on both eyes of normal subjects and were independent of the size of the targets.

INTRODUCTION

Kinetic visual fields are affected by several factors, for example, size, color and movement of the test object as well as psychophysiological conditions of both subject and examiner. Test object parameters can now be precisely controlled by employing a Goldmann perimeter (Goldmann 1945, 1946). However, human factors are not constant, and sometimes induce errors in measured fields (Honda 1978). In this study, the gaze shifts of normal and diseased eyes during peripheral field tests were monitored by the electro-oculogram (EOG) and were shown to be important factors inducing errors in measured fields.

METHODS

EOGs were recorded during peripheral field tests of both normal and diseased eyes of 20 patients (40 eyes) who had no oculomotor anomalies. A Goldmann perimeter (Haag Streit AG) was used to determine isopters for V-4 and V-1. EOG electrodes were affixed at the inner and outer canthi of the tested eye. The signals were amplified (time constant: 2.0 sec) and continuously recorded on a pen-writing oscillograph. A deviation to the right of the eye under test produced an upward deflection on the oscillograph. The subject was instructed to signal the appearance of the target and this response produced a square-wave deflection on the second (lower) trace of the recorder. The system was calibrated by inducing 10-30 degree horizontal eye movements before and after the EOG recordings.

The non-tested eye was shielded from light by a black eye-patch.

433

RESULTS

Fig. 1 shows EOGs of a myopic patient who had no ocular disease and had shown good reproducibility in field tests. Biphasic spike-waves on the EOG recording are artifacts due to blinking. Square-waves of longer time course (arrows) indicate eye movements. Gaze shifts of this degree were observed in the other patients with good reproducibility of measured fields and were considered to be normal.

In several exceptional cases poor fixation was observed. These were found among non-cooperative children and older patients with senile dementia. EOGs of such subjects showed numerous, prominent square-wave potentials, indicating frequent gaze deviations, and low reliability and validity of measured fields. Within the limits of available space, examples of EOGs of a few representative cases are presented.

Fig. 2 presents EOGs from an eight-year-old girl whose fixation on the central target was quite poor in spite of her otherwise good visual function. Poor fixation resulted from incomplete understanding of the test and lack of cooperation with the examiner. The degree of gaze shifting in this subject was the same for both the V-4 and V-1 isopters for either eye (both eyes normal).

Poor fixation was also found among patients who had large central scotomas or quite poor vision even when they were cooperative and intelligent

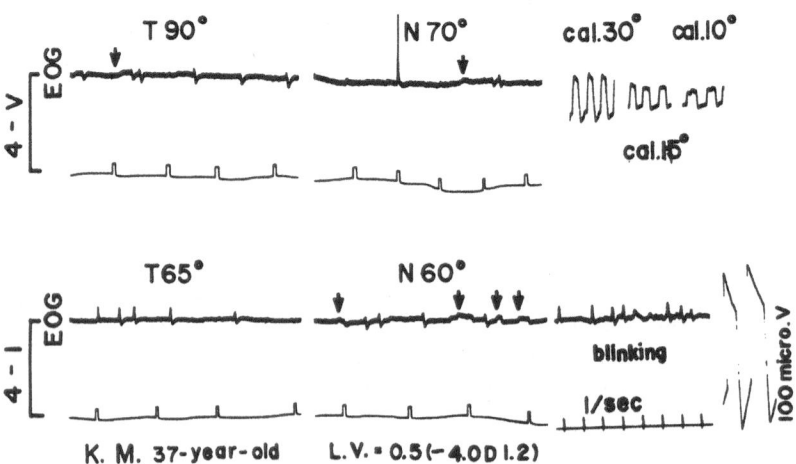

Fig. 1. Recordings of EOGs (upper traces) and square-wave response pulses (lower traces) from a 37-year-old woman. She had no ocular disease but was myopic. V-4 and V-1 isopters were determined. T 90° indicates that responses were recorded during measurement of the temporal field and the measured field was approximately 90°. N 70° indicates that responses were recorded during measurement of the nasal side and the field was 70°. Arrows indicate eye movements. Calibration records indicate EOG trace excursions for horizontal eye movements of 30°, 15° and 10°.

enough to understand the test. Fig. 3 shows examples of EOGs from a patient who had a retinal detachment in the inferior-temporal quadrant. Her fixation on the central target during the temporal measurements was good but was incomplete during measurements on the nasal side. Fig. 4 presents EOGs of a patient who had poor vision due to excessive myopia (−20D) with myopic degeneration of the macula. His gaze continually shifted throughout the measurements although he completely understood the test.

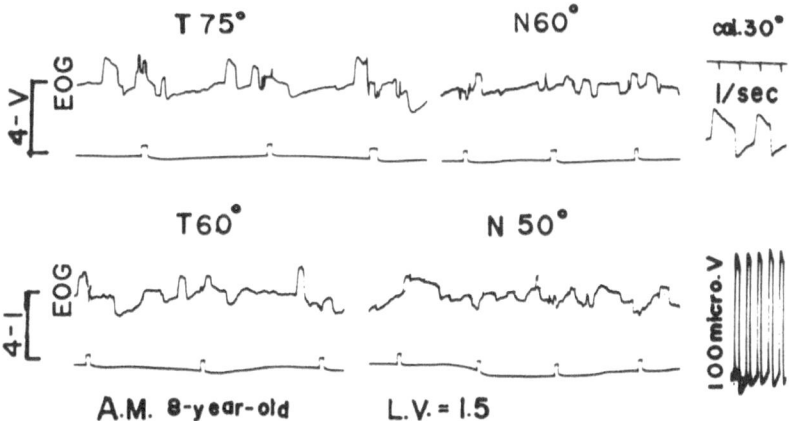

Fig. 2. Excerpts of recordings from an eight-year-old girl with no ocular disease but very poor gaze fixation. Details as for Fig. 1.

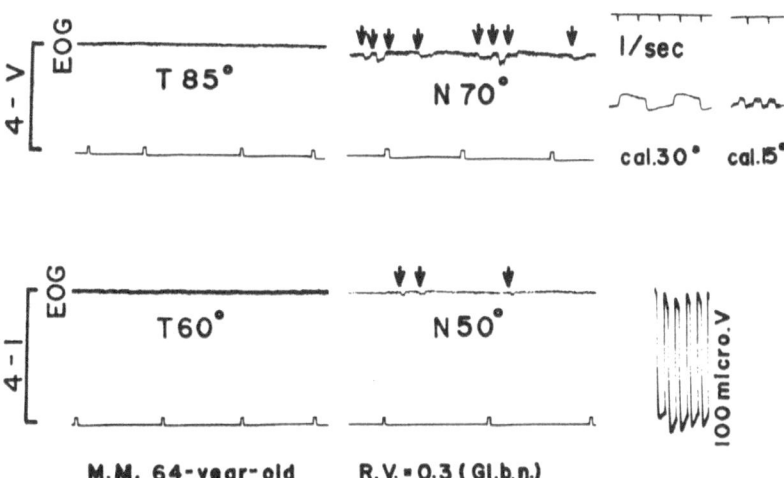

Fig. 3. Excerpts of recordings from a 64-year-old woman hospitalized because of retinal detachment in the lower-temporal quadrant of her right eye. These are from a post-operative field test of the right eye. Fixation was poor during field tests on the nasal side. Details as for Fig. 1.

435

DISCUSSION

The EOG is a measure of the retinal standing potential. Therefore, monitoring of eye movements by EOG techniques is applicable only for patients who have a relatively high standing potential. A very fine movement such as a flick is difficult to detect, even from an intact eye having a high standing potential, and only gross eye movements can be followed by the EOG. However, EOG recordings during field tests provide important objective data on fixation and can be an aid in determining the validity of the measured field. In this investigation, poor fixation was found among non-cooperative children, older patients with senile dementia and among diseased eyes with large central scotomas or very poor vision. The EOG provides an electrophysiological representation of phenomena frequently observed through the monitoring system of the Goldmann perimeter. Continuous recordings of eye movements during field tests illustrate how difficult it is to measure valid fields on these patients and to detect brief changes of central fixation through the monitoring system. Gaze shifts of such patients are continuous and irregular.

In this study only horizontal eye movements were described and discussed. EOG recordings for vertical movements during upper and lower field tests were observed to show the same tendencies as seen for horizontal deviations. The ability to adequately fixate is a complex function of higher brain centers, intelligence, character and cooperation of the subject, even when

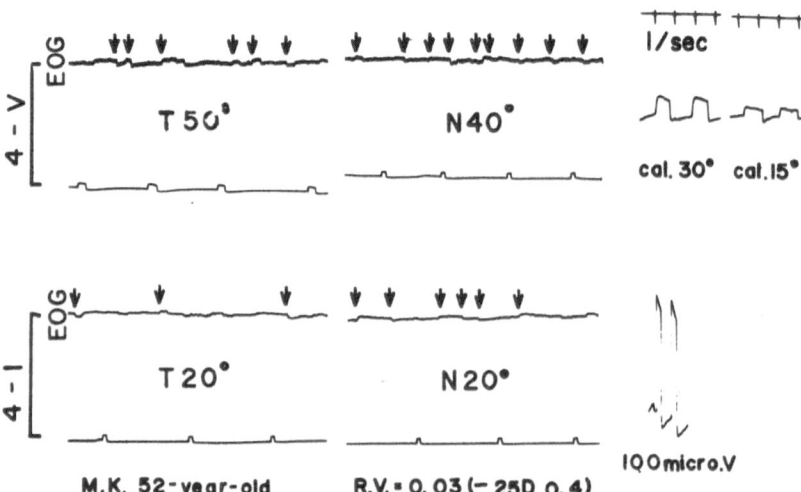

Fig. 4. A 52-year-old man was hospitalized because of total retinal detachment from the macular hole on his left eye. His right eye has a high myopia and myopic chorioretinal atrophy but no retinal detachment. Recordings are from his right eye. The refractive state is not corrected. Details as for Fig. 1.

436

visual function is normal. Therefore, flutter of gaze appeared in normal eyes independently of the size of targets.

In studying the two dimensional record of EOGs, it might be possible in future to estimate the extent of gaze shift by comparing the recording to the calibrations, and to add or subtract the size of the eye movement to or from the measurement, giving a more valid estimate of that point on the isopter.

The timing of the eye movement was sometimes critical for the accuracy of the responses. An eye movement immediately preceding the response might suggest that the subject was cheating, that is, looking at the target. One immediately following or during the response, on the other hand, might indicate that the subject was simply verifying that the response was accurate. This might be used for the field test of feeble-minded children.

REFERENCES

Goldmann, H. Ein selbstregistrierendes Projektionskugelperimeter. *Ophthalmologica* 109: *71-79* (1945).

Goldmann, H. Demonstration unseres neuen Projektionskugelperimeters samt theoretischen und klinischen Bemerkungen über Perimetrie. *Ophthalmologica* 111: *187-192* (1946).

Honda, Y. The standard errors of peripheral visual fields measured at a long interval. *Jap. J. clin. Ophthalm.* (in the press).

Author's address:
Department of Ophthalmology
Kyoto University Faculty of Medicine
Sakyo-ku, Kyoto 606
Japan

TRIAL OF A COLOR PERIMETER

HIROSHI KITAHARA, KENJI KITAHARA & HIROSHI MATSUZAKI

(Tokyo, Japan)

ABSTRACT

The 500 watts xenon lamp was used as a light source. The maximum luminance of the white object was set up to be 25,000 cd/m² at 59' visual angle and the maximum white background luminance was 2,200 cd/m² at 10°.

INTRODUCTION

The study of visual field using painted color objects was initiated by Aubert in 1857, and it was extensively applied in the clinic until the Goldmann perimeter was introduced. However, intensive colorimetrical studies with color perimeter, especially with monochromatic color objects, were reported by Hansen (1974), Greve (1974), Lakowski (1977), Verriest (1977) and others. Particularly, Hansen (1974) tried to measure the static perimetry with improved Goldmann perimeter and suggested that higher luminance for adaptation was necessary in order to isolate the green-sensitive mechanism from the red one. Our color perimeter was constructed in order to determine the characteristics of wavelength on the retinal area and to investigate visual function and thus practical use in the clinic (Fig. 1).

Fig. 2 shows the optical diagram of this color perimeter. Light for the test object and for the background field was provided from the same light source (XeL). The test object was projected on the inner surface of the bowl guided by the optical glassfiber (OF). The object light could be filtered through 16 interference filters (half height width of their spectral transmission curves ranged from 7 nm to 14 nm). The dominant wavelengths of these filters were within 400 nm to 700 nm with the intervals of 20 nm. The radiance values of each object light on the cornea are shown in Fig. 3. The color filters for background light were exchangeable freely for a particular purpose, like the color filters for the test object. As for the chromatic background light for the isolation of the three color mechanisms by Wald's selective adaptation method, the following color filters were applied; the yellow light Corning 3-67, the purple with Wratten No. 35, and the blue with Corning 5-57. The luminance value was 1,300 cd/m² for the yellow background, 51 cd/m² for the purple and 170 cd/m² for the blue one. The luminance of object or background light was continuously adjustable with optical wedges (W₁ and W₂) and ND filters (ND₁ and ND₂). Enlargement of background field up to 50° of visual angle was also possible. The test light irradiation was controlled from 10 msec. to 9,999 msec. by a time regulator. Remote control system was applied for selecting the test object and background light and also for adjusting luminance, duration and interval of irradiation.

RESULTS

With this perimeter static color perimetry was performed under two conditions, one was Stiles's two-color threshold technique and the other was under high luminance white background.

The subjects with fully dilated pupil after the instillation of tropicamide were asked to wear the 4 mm diameter artificial pupil for this measurement. All measurements were expressed as log relative sensitivity in the relative numbers of quanta per second incident on the cornea. The duration of the object light irradiation in the present experiment was set up in 0.25 sec. and the interval of each stimulation was 2 sec. The results obtained under the condition of yellow, purple or blue background and the results obtained from the white background of 1,000 trolands are presented in this paper.

The spectral sensitivity curves at the fovea of normal subject (J.I.) are shown in Fig. 4. Three color mechanisms of blue, green, and red could be

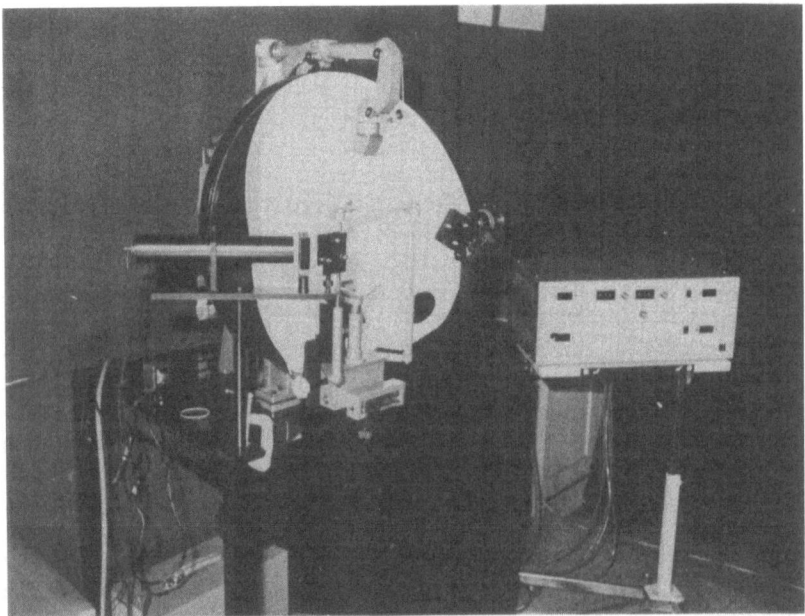

Fig. 1. Photograph of our original color perimeter with the remote control system. Optical system was fixed on the right foot side.

440

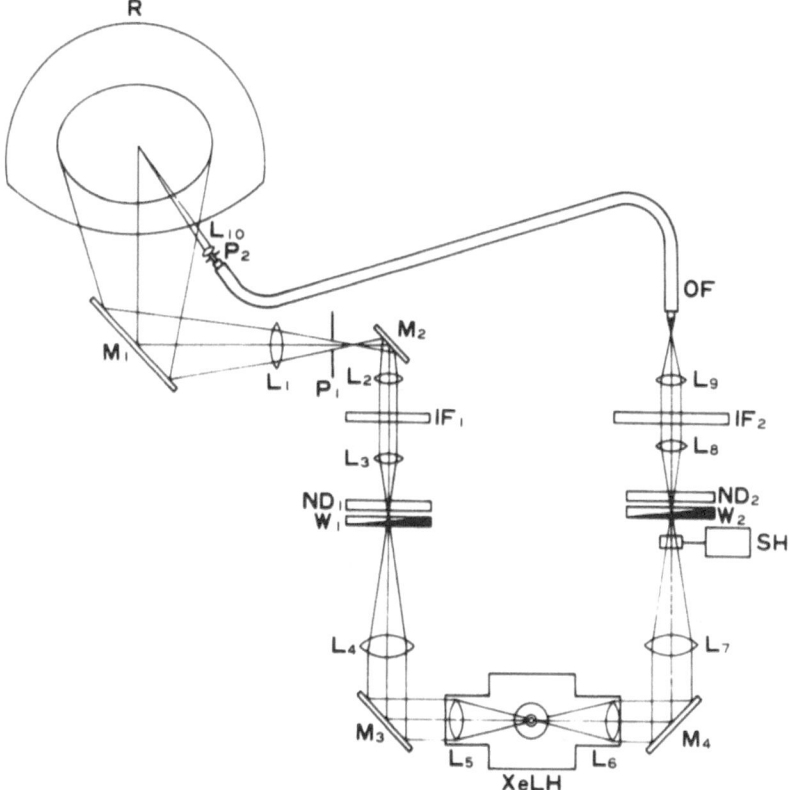

Fig. 2. Diagram of the optical system of the color perimeter. Light path of the test object on the right side, that of the background on the left. Both were supplied from the same light source (XeL).

M_{1-4}: Mirror, L_{1-10}: Lens (Convex lens), P_{1-2}: Pattern, I.F.$_{1-2}$: Interference filter, ND_{1-2}: Neutral density filter, W_{1-2}: Optical Wedge, XeL: 500 watts Xenon lamp, SH: Shutter, OF: Optical glassfiber, R: Refrecteve surface of the bowl.

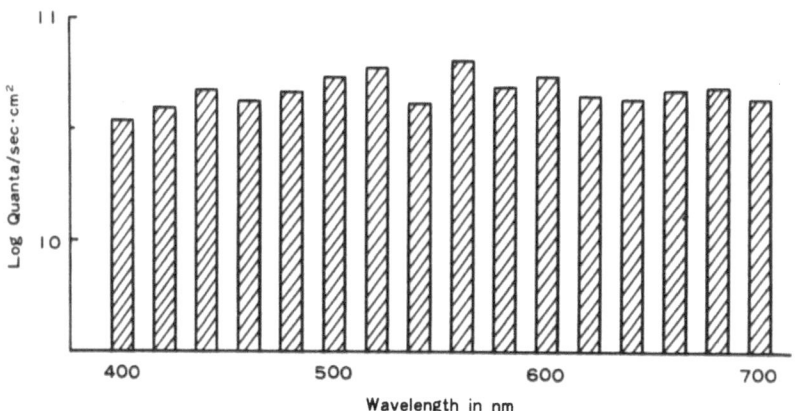

Fig. 3. Quantity of radiation light incident of each object light on the cornea.

clearly isolated with this perimeter. In order to investigate the distribution of each color mechanism on the retinal area, the sensitivity curves were measured on the basis of the static perimetry with the test light of the peak wavelength of each color mechanism. Fig. 5 indicates the sensitivity curves of normal individual (J.I.) measured on 45° − 225° meridian line under the following conditions: on the yellow background with the test light of 440 nm (the approximate peak wavelength of the blue-sensitive mechanism), on the purple background with the test light of 539 nm (the approximate peak wavelength of the green sensitive mechanism) and on the blue background with that of 582 nm (the approximate peak wavelength of the red sensitive mechanism). On the yellow background, the sensitivity curve shows marked decline at the fovea and reaches the maximum sensitivity at 1° - 2° with its gradual fall toward the periphery. On the contrary, on the purple or on the blue background, the sensitivity curve shows the sharpest rise at the fovea with its abrupt drop toward the periphery but the sensitivity curve on the blue background has slightly sharper decline than that on the

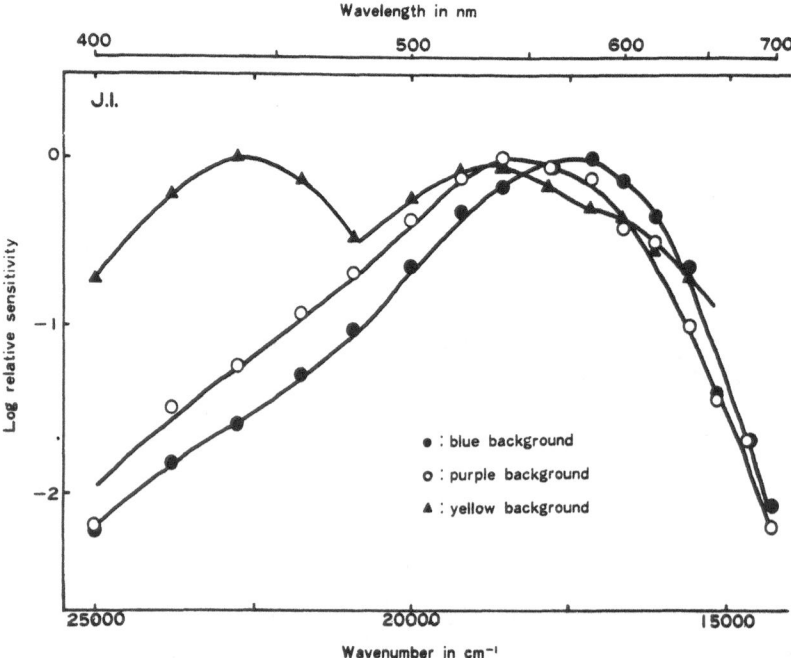

Fig. 4. The spectral sensitivities of the three color mechanisms in normal trichromats J.I. measured in the fovea. Log relative sensitivities in the relative numbers of quanta per second on the cornea. All peak rensitivites have been brought arbitrarily to the same height. Filled triangles: the blue-sensitive mechanism, measured on the yellow background; Open circles: the green-sensitive mechanism, measured on the purple; Filled circles: the red-sensitive mechanism, measured on the blue one.

442

purple one. Fig. 6 shows the sensitivity curve of the normal subject (A.S.) measured on the basis of the static perimetry under the condition of the white background of 1,000 trolands with the test light of 440 nm, 539 nm, and 600 nm (the approximate peak wavelengths of the three color mechanisms under this condition). The sensitivity curves indicate the same tendency as those under the condition of the colored background but further investigations will be advisable.

Our color perimeter was designed as follows: white maximum luminance of test object was 25,000 cd/m^2 at 59' of visual angle and that of the background was 2,200 cd/m^2 at 10°. The three color mechanisms could be isolated using the two-color threshold technique with this color perimeter. Moreover, the static color perimetry was tried on colored background and it was also performed on a high luminance white background. A higher luminance for adaptation than that adapted in this experiment is preferable for investigating the Stiles's $\pi\,3^-$ mechanism.

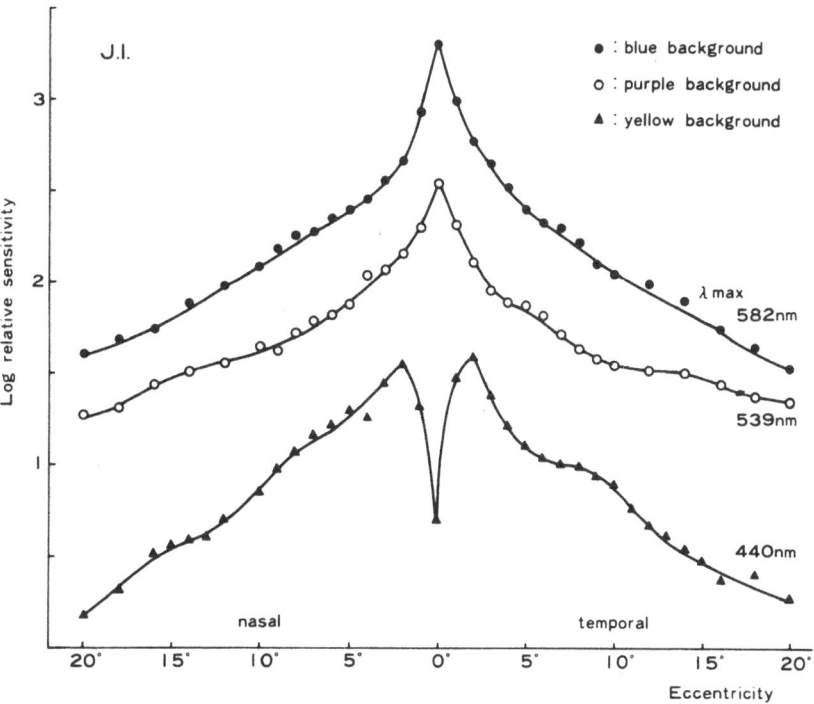

Fig. 5. The sensitivity curves measured on the basis of the static perimetry on the colored backgrounds. Filled triangles: on the yellow background with the test light of 440 nm; Open circles: on the purple background with the light of 539 nm; Filled circles: on the blue background with that of 582 nm. All curves have been given the arbitrary height for comparison.

443

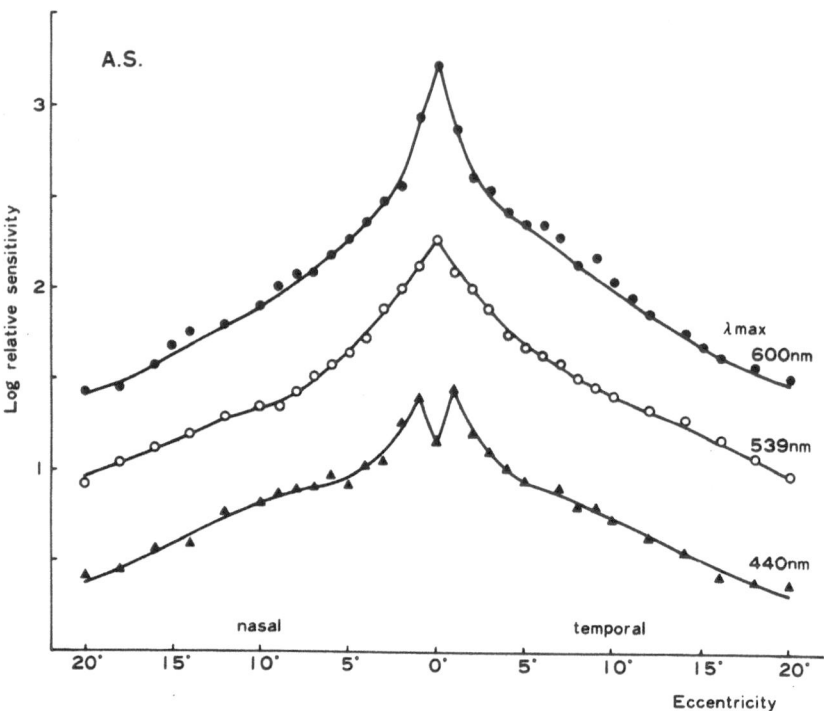

Fig. 6. The sensitivity curves measured by the method based on static perimetry on the white background of 1,000 trolands. Filled circles: with the test light of 440 nm; the peak wavelength of the blue-sensitive mechanism, Open circle: with the test light of 539 nm: the peak wavelength of the green-sensitive mechanism; Filled circles; with that of 600 nm, the peak wavelength of the red-sensitive mechanism under this condition. All curves have been given the arbitrary height for comparison.

ACKNOWLEDGEMENTS

The authors deeply appreciate Prof. Tomoya Funahashi's guidance in our study and his reviewing of it. Mr. Yoshitaka Kanda of Sanso Co. Ltd. has been of invaluable help to us by his cooperation in manufacturing the apparatus.

REFERENCES

Greve, E.L., Verduin, W.M. & Ledeboer, M. Two-color threshold in static perimetry. *Mod. Probl. Ophthal.* 13: *113-118* (1974).

Hansen, E. The color reseptors studied by increment threshold measurements during chromatic adaptation in the Goldmann perimeter. *Acta Ophthal.* 52: *490-500* (1974).

King-Smith, P.E. Visual detection analysed in terms of luminance and chromatic signals. *Nature* 255: *69-70* (1975).

Kitahara, K. Measurement of spectral sensitivity of retinal receptors *Acta Soc. Ophthal. jap.* 81: *1549-1562* (1977).

Lakowski, R., Wright, W.D. & Oliver, K. A Goldmann perimeter with high luminance chromatic targets. *Canad. J. Ophthal.* 12: *203* (1977).

Stiles, W.S. Color vision; The approach through increment threshold sensitivity. *Proc. Natl. Acad. Sci.* 75: *100* (1959).

Tamaki, R. Visual functions in open-angle glaucoma. A study on sensitivity-duration curve. *Jap. J. Clin. Ophthal.* 32: *17-22* (1978).

Verriest, G. & Kandemir, H. Normal spectral increment thresholds on a white background. *Die Farbe* 23: *3-16* (1974).

Verriest, G. & Uvijls A. Spectral increment thresholds on a white background in different age groups of normal subjects and in acquired ocular diseases. *Doc. Ophthal.* 43, 2: *217-248* (1977).

Wald, G. The receptors of human color vision. *Science* 145: *1007* (1964).

Author's address:
Department of Ophthalmology
Jikei University School of Medicine
3-19-18, Nishishinbashi, Minato-ku
Tokyo, Japan

Docum. Ophthal. Proc. Series, Vol. 19

VIDEOPUPILLOGRAPHIC PERIMETRY
PERIMETRIC FINDINGS WITH RABBIT EYES

SATORU KUBOTA

(Tokyo, Japan)

ABSTRACT

The videopupillographic perimetry of the normal colored rabbits was examined. An improvement was effected of the test target of the videopupillographic perimeter originated by Narasaki et al., and a central visual field to 7° could be obtained with this apparatus. The results of videopupillographic perimetry in the colored rabbits were as follows:
1) For the measurement of the central visual field, the sensitive area of pupillary light reflex on the retina was a band of 10° to 20° degrees wide extended horizontally below the disc and medullary nerve fiber. This area was observed approximately congruent to the so-called visual streak.
2) For the measurement of peripheral visual field, the threshold of light reflex on the ventral side was lower than that on the dorsal side of the retina and of the disc and/or of the medullary nerve fiber.

INTRODUCTION

Objective measuring of the visual field has been important in experimental animals for study of visual function in drug intoxication etc.. The measurements of the visual field in rabbits using videopupillographic perimeter by Narasaki et al. (1973) and by Tokuda (1974) revealed that the sensitive area of pupillary light reflex existed in the lower area of the visual field.

In the present study, the comparison between videopupillographic perimetry and fundus in the normal colored rabbit was examined to make clear the relation between the sensitive area of pupillary light reflex and visual streak using videopupillographic perimeter originated by Narasaki et al..

MATERIAL AND METHOD

1. The apparatus: The videopupillographic perimeter used for this study is diagrammed in Fig. 1. In the original apparatus, its target could move from 75° to 17° on every meridian, but additional 17° to 7° can be measured using this new attachment showed in Fig. 2. This attachment is composed of

* This investigation was supported in part by a grant from the Japanese Ministry of Labor.

the two prisms through which 67% of the luminosity of the target is allowed to pass.

2. Subject: Two adult normal colored male rabbits weighing approximately 2.5 kg with reflexions of + 1.25D. and + 1.75D. respectively.

3. Methods of pupillographic perimetry: The unanesthetized rabbits were fixed as in Fig. 1 and measuremnt was performed under the following conditions: time 18:00 pm; room temperature 25°C.; and after dark-adaptation of one hour. The localizations of the disc center and of both ends of the medullary nerve fibers were accurately measured ophthalmoscopically at every examination of the visual field. Fig. 3 is a fundus photograph at the time of measurements in this videopupillographic perimetry.

a) Peripheral visual field measurements: The background luminosity was 0.04 asb. (but that of the movable round area alongside the target was 0.004 asb.). The luminosity of the test target was from 2000 to 34000 asb. in rabbit No. 1 and from 600 to 6000 asb. No. 2. The meridians were in 8 positions from 0° to 315°, and thresholds of pupillary light reflex at intervals of 5° and/or 10° were obtained from 75° at periphery to 17° at center.

b) Central visual field measurement: The background luminosity was 0.2 asb. (under 0.02 asb.) The luminosity of the test target using the new attachment was from 1300 asb. to 23000 asb.; the thresholds of pupillary light reflex were measured at every 5°.

RESULTS

To check the accuracy of the attachment, detection of the human blind spot was performed. The pupillary light reflex was not obtained at 13° and at 15° on the left eye meridian of 185° under the conditions of background luminosity 1.0 asb. (under 0.1 asb.) and of target luminosity 600 asb.

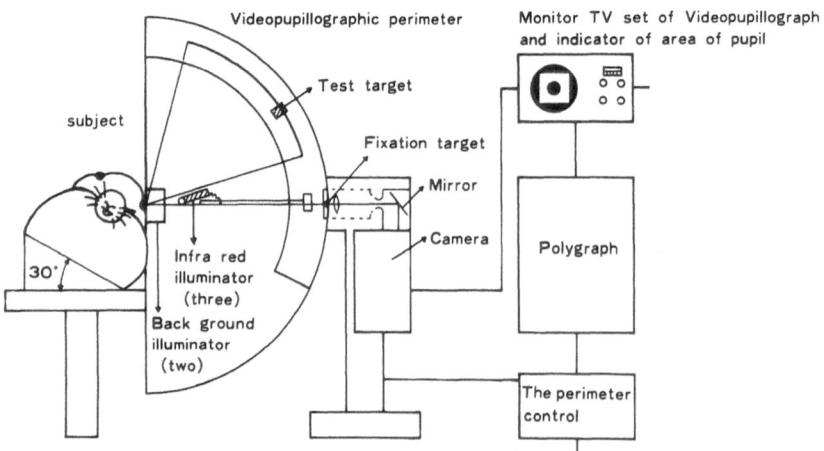

Fig. 1. Diagram of the videopupillographic perimetry apparatus.

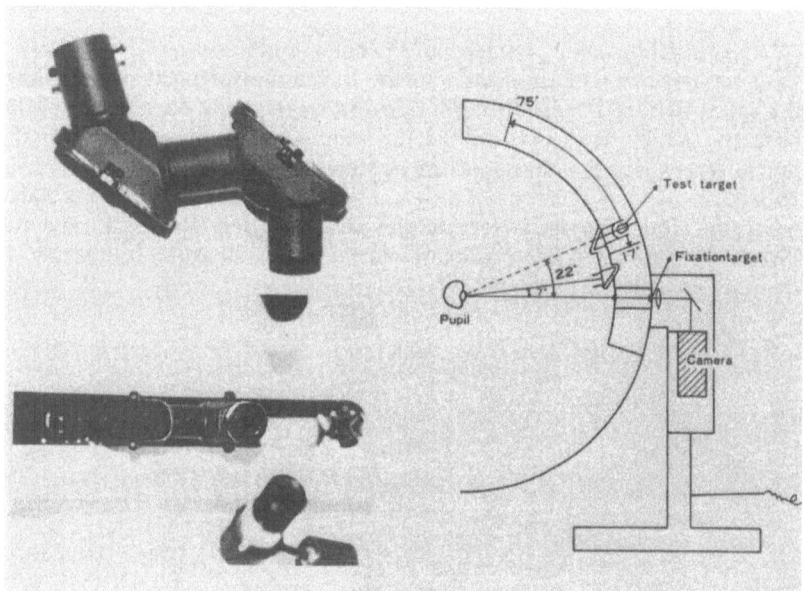

Fig. 2. A new attachment (left) and diagram of the videopupillographic perimeter with the attachment mounted on the original target (right).

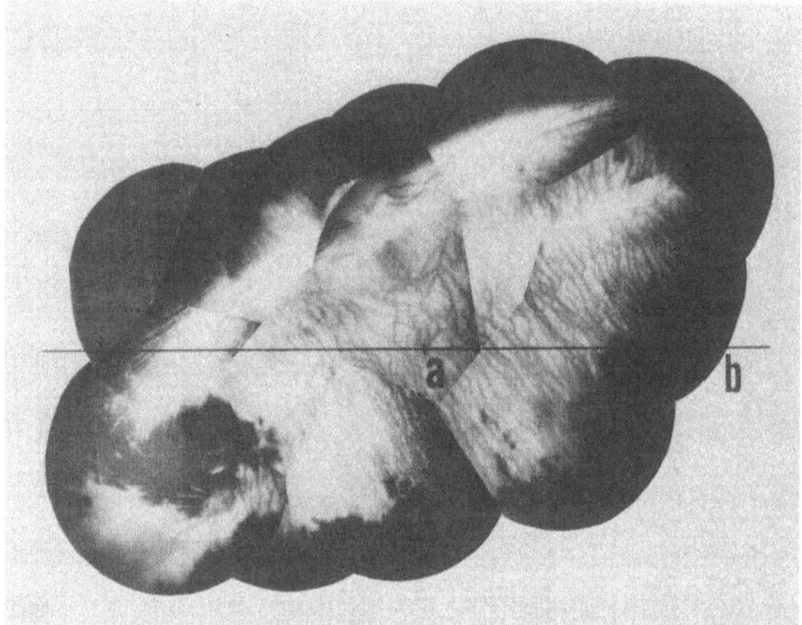

Fig. 3. The fundus photograph of No 1 rabbit (right eye).
Point a; assumed posterior pole.
Straight line b; horizontal line.

Videopupillographic perimetry of the colored rabbits:
1) Peripheral visual field measurement: In the measurement of periphery, the visual field of the rabbit was influenced by the body position, by eyelid position and by the length of the fur when the animal was fixed in the rabbit box. Also, the thresholds of pupillary light reflex were different in both subjects, and after many measurements were taken, the most stable point was found to be 40° from the center at meridian 135° and the thresholds were changed to relative value 1 at 19000 asb. in rabbit No. 1,

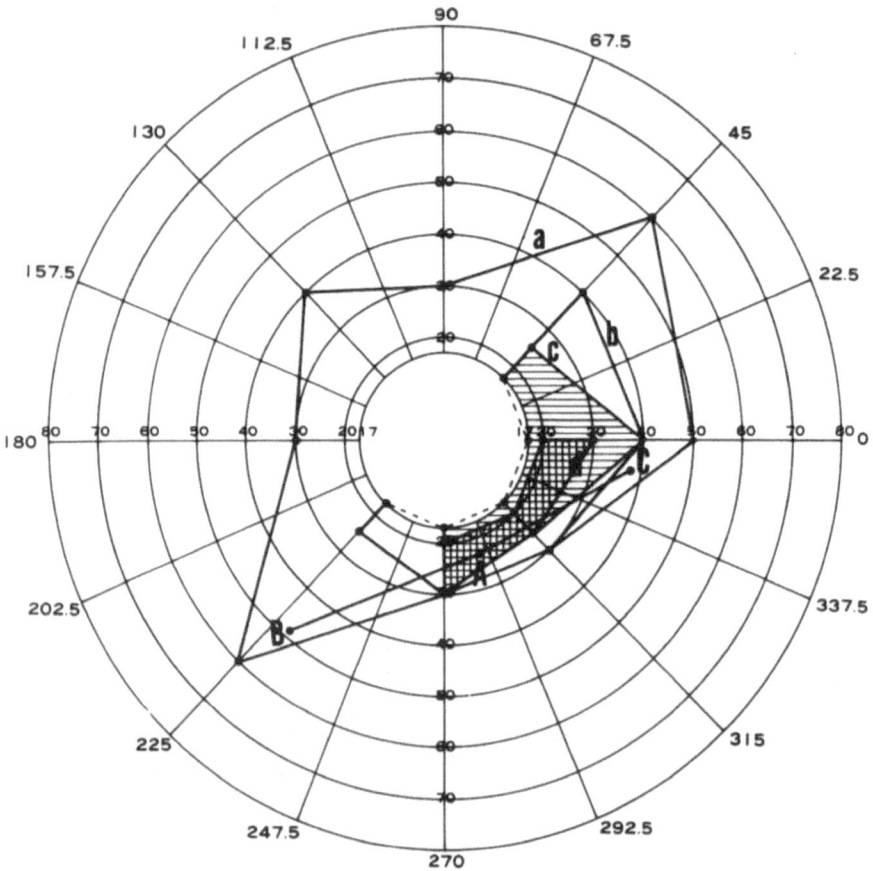

Fig. 4. The peripheral visual field measured on rabbit No. 1 (right eye).
The threshold of the pupillary light reflex.
Background luminosity; 0.04 (under 0.004 asb. in the area alongside the target) Target luminosity; 2000-34000 asb. (19000 asb. = relative value 1).
The area within the connected line a; under the threshold of relative value 1.
The area within the connected line b; under the threshold of relative value 0.63.
The area within the connected line c (   ); under the threshold of relative value 0.5.
he area within the connected line d (   ); under the threshold of relative value 0.32.
A; the center of the disc. B, C; the peripheries of the medullary nerve fibers.

450

and 6000 asb. in rabbit No. 2. Fig. 4 indicates the thresholds of rabbit No. 1 in the right eye. The area of the threshold within the relative value 1.0 was recognized from 225° to 0° meridian, and was obtained only near to the disc and to the medullary nerve fibers. Proportionate to lower thresholds, the area became localized near to the disc and to the medullary nerve fibers.

The results for rabbit No. 2 were similar to those of rabbit No. 1.

2) Central visual field measurement: In measurement of the peripheral visual field, the area of the lower threshold was found at the central portion of the disc and of the medullary nerve fibers on meridians from 225° to 0°; however, expansion of the area was accurately examined in more detail to 7° of the center using the new attachment. The thresholds of light reflex in rabbit No. 1, right eyes on meridians were measured from 225° to 0° at every 22.5° and at every 5° from the center. Five measurements were performed on different dates. The pupillary light reactive area was as indicated in Fig. 5, included within the closed line, consequently it was a band shape area with 10° to 20° wide extending horizontally near to the central side of the disc and of the medullary nerve fibers. Furthermore, the area of the thresholds lower than that of the band area was not localized.

DISCUSSION

Videopupillographic perimetry plays a large role in objective measurements of visual field because pupillary light reflex as studied by Lowenstein et al.

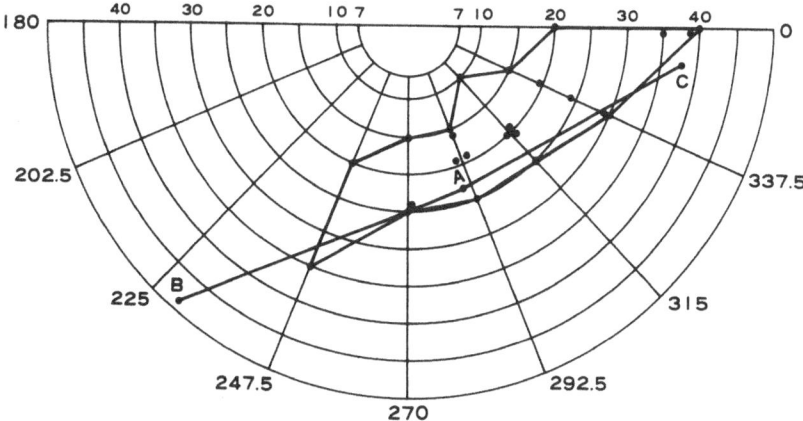

Fig. 5. The central visual field measured on rabbit No. 1 (right eye).
Background luminosity; 0.2 asb. (under 0.02 asb. in the area alongside the target).
Target luminosity; 1300-23000 asb.
The area within the connected line; the pupillary light reactive area of 5 times measurements under the threshold relative value 1 (= 23000 asb.).
The dotts; the pupillary light reactive points under the threshold relative value 0.32.
A; the center of the disc. B, C; the peripheries of the medullary nerve fibers.

(1964) is significant as an indicator of retinal activity, and because it can also tell us the condition of the visual pathway from lateral geniculate body.

In the measurements of videopupillographic perimetry, pupillary light reflex of rabbits was considered to be especially related to the autonomic nervous system, and therefore the conditions of time of measurement, of room temperature, etc. were taken into consideration, and thus the results were reproducable in each rabbit. The sensitive area of pupillary light reflex on the rabbit retina by this perimetry approximately agreed with the so-called visual streak, which existence was also proved histologically by Yonemura et al. (1970). The data obtained from this experiment show the possibility to examine the visual field of the animals with videopupillographic perimeter, and to study the visual field impairment in experimental animals.

ACKNOWLEDGEMENTS

The author gratefully acknowledges the kind support in the preparation of this manuscript by Prof. Tomoya Funahashi and Shiro Narasaki (formerly Associate Professor at Jikei University School of Medicine).

REFERENCES

Lowenstein, O., et al. The pupil as indicator of retinal activity. *Amer. J. Ophthalmol.* 57: *569-596* (1964).

Narasaki, S., et al. Videopupillographic perimetry. Findings and its method used in human and rabbits eyes. *Acta Soc. Ophthalmol. Jap.* 77: *1278-1310* (1973).

Narasaki, S. et al. Videopupillographic perimetry reformed perimeter. *Acta Soc. Ophthalmol. Jap.* 79: *1765-1769* (1975).

Tokuda, K. Experimental study of chloroquine retinopathy influence of chloroquine intravenous injection to the visual fields and to the threshold of light reflex. *Acta Soc. Ophthalmol. Jap.* 78: *1031-1044* (1974).

Yonemura, D. & Masuda, Y. Visual streak and distribution of ganglion cells in rabbits retina *Acta Soc. Ophthalmol. Jap.* 74: *1-5* (1970).

Author's address:
Department of Ophthalmology, Jikei University
School of Medicine, 25-8, Nishi-shinbashi
3-chome, Minato-ku, Tokyo 105, Japan

Docum. Ophthal. Proc. Series, Vol. 19

CLINICAL EXPERIENCES WITH A NEW MULTIPLE DOT PLATE

ETSURO SHINZATO & HARUTAKE MATSUO

(Tokyo, Japan)

ABSTRACT

We developed a new meridian multiple dot plate, the procedure of which is explained. Visual field changes detected by kinetic perimetry with Goldmann perimeter, when assessed by the new meridian multiple dot plate showed as high grade depression. The differences between the results of meridian multiple dot plate and Tübinger perimeter were pointed out. In normal subjects, the profile of both values were parallel with a discrepancy within 1.3 log units. In glaucomatous visual field changes, the discrepancy of profile showed extreme separation. The reason for the separation of the two values is regarded as the result of abnormal temporal summation.

TEXT

We have developed two new front plates for the Friedmann Visual Field Analyser, of which one is a standard plate, the other a meridian multiple dot plate (MDP) (Matsuo et al. 1975). The normal threshold of the standard plate was reported in 1977 (Shinzato 1978) and another report about early glaucomatous visual field changes detected by the standard plate is submitted for publication (Shinzato). In this report, visual field changes, including those due to retinal disease, disturbance of visual pathway and glaucoma, detected with the Goldmann perimeter (GP) are assessed and results compared with those obtained using the MDP. In addition, some differences in the results of profile perimetry between Tübinger perimeter (TP) and the MDP in case of glaucomatous visual field changes are discussed.

MATERIALS AND METHOD

The MDP consists of 14 pairs of targets, with a member of each pair located on either side of the fixation point in a straight line. The first five pairs are situated at one degree intervals, from $2°-6°$ on either side of the fixation point, the next eight are at two degree intervals from $9°-22°$ and the last is at $25°$ from the fixation point. The size of targets is increased to maintain a 10 minute visual angle. As the MDP can be revolved through $360°$, examination of the entire central visual field up to $25°$ is performed easily. Target presentation time is one millisecond, against a background luminance of 0.03 asb (0.01 cd/m^2).

Nine eyes in 5 patients, including Harada's disease, ciloretinal occlusion, craniopharyngioma, arteriovenous malformation of the posterior lobe and glaucoma were studied. First, the visual field changes were detected by kinetic perimetry with GP, second, the visual field defects were assessed by MDP.

RESULTS

Case 1. Harada's disease. Male, 41. Visual acuity, vd = 0.04 (0.8), vs = 0.04 (0.7). Chief complaint: bilateral central scotoma and metamorphopsia. Slit-microscopic finding showed a slightly warm current in the anterior chamber and vitreous opacities. Ophthalmoscopic finding showed dense edematic lesions at the posterior pole of the fundus of both eyes. Fig. 1 shows the results of kinetic and profile perimetry.

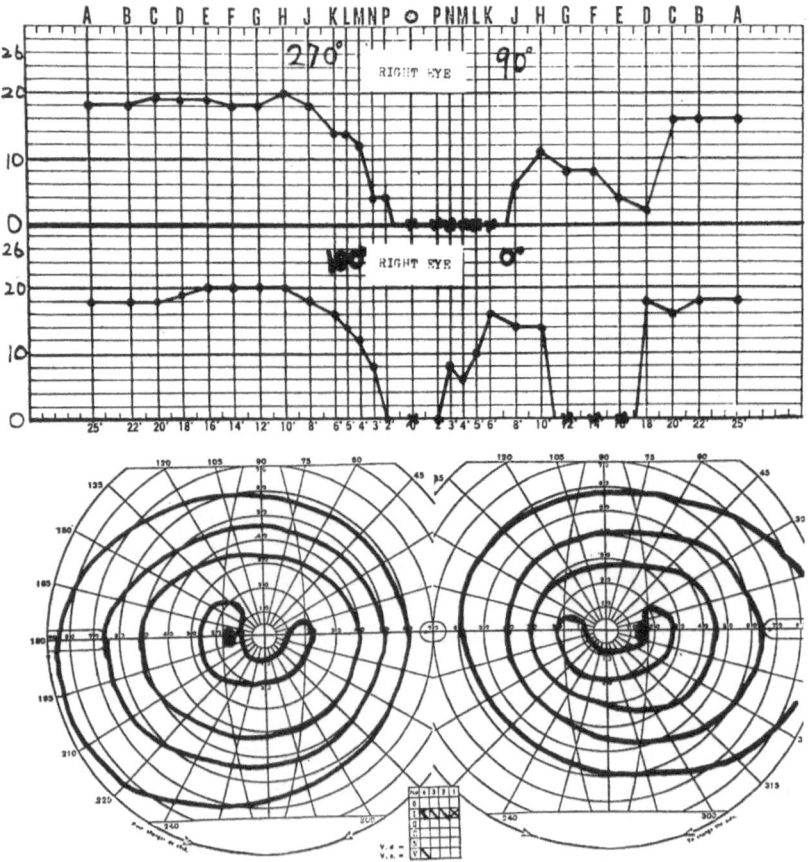

Fig. 1. Visual field changes in case 1. Central depression with I/2 was detected by kinetic perimetry. High grade depression beyond maximum luminance was detected by profile perimetry with MDP.

454

Case 2. Cilioretinal occlusion. Male, 58. Chief complaint: right central sco-toma. Vd = 0.1 (nc), vs = 0.9 (nc). Ophthalmoscopic finding showed an edematic lesion in the macular area and hypertensive fundus corresponding to Keith-Wegner two in grade. Fig. 2 shows the results of kinetic and profile perimetry.

Case 3. Craniopharyngioma. Female, 28. Chief complaint: temporal foggy vision of both eyes. Vd = 1.2 (nc), vs = 0.5 (nc). Media and fundi of both eyes showed no abnormal findings. Fig. 3 shows the results with both kinds of perimetry. Bitemporal hemianopic scotomas were detected by kinetic perimetry.

Case 4. Arteriovenous malformation of the posterior lobe. Female, 48. No complaint. She was admitted to the Department of Neural Surgery. Vd = 0.7 (1.2), vs = 0.7 (1.2). Media and fundi of both eyes showed nothing in

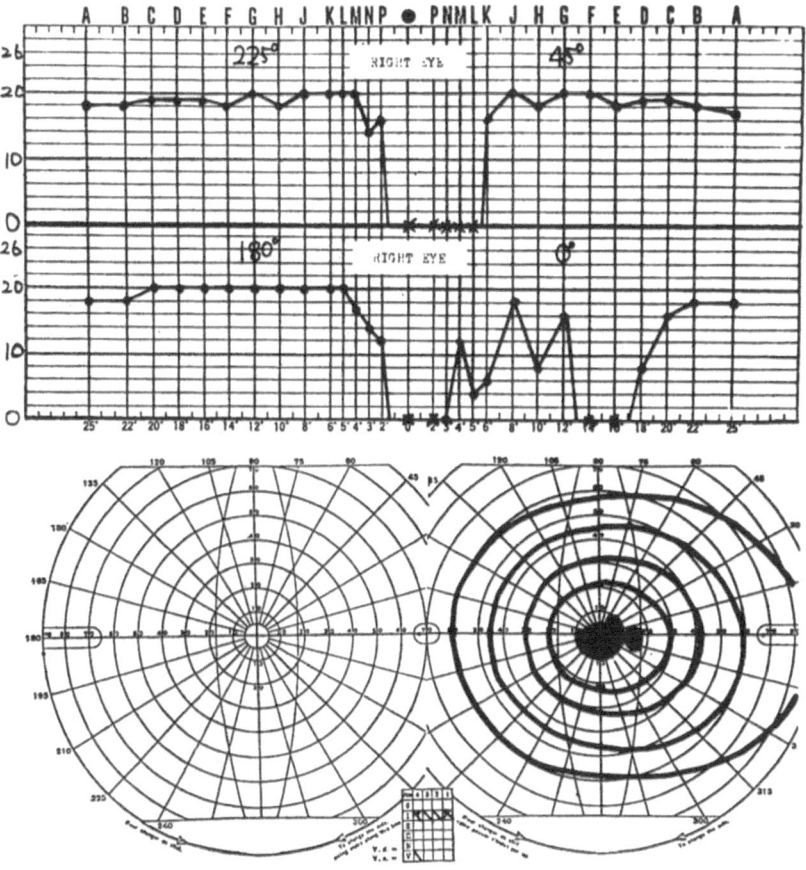

Fig. 2. Visual field changes in the right eye of case 2. Central depression with I/4 was detected by kinetic perimetry. No perception by MDP on the central field.

455

particular. The results of both types of perimetry are showed in Fig. 4. Right homonymous quadrantanopic defect of both eyes were detected.

Case 5. Glaucoma. Female, 30. Chief complaints: headache and bilateral ocular pain. $Vd = 0.03$ (1.2), $vs = 0.04$ (1.2). Intraocular pressure was 22 mm.Hg. in the right eye and 24 mm.Hg. in the left eye. C value was 0.21 in the right eye and 0.14 in the left eye. Gonioscopic finding showed open angle 4 in grade. Ophthalmoscopic findings showed large cupping in both eyes. Fig. 5 shows the results of both types of perimetry.

DISCUSSION

1. Results of kinetic perimetry and static perimetry.

From the results of case reports, it is evident that the visual field defects

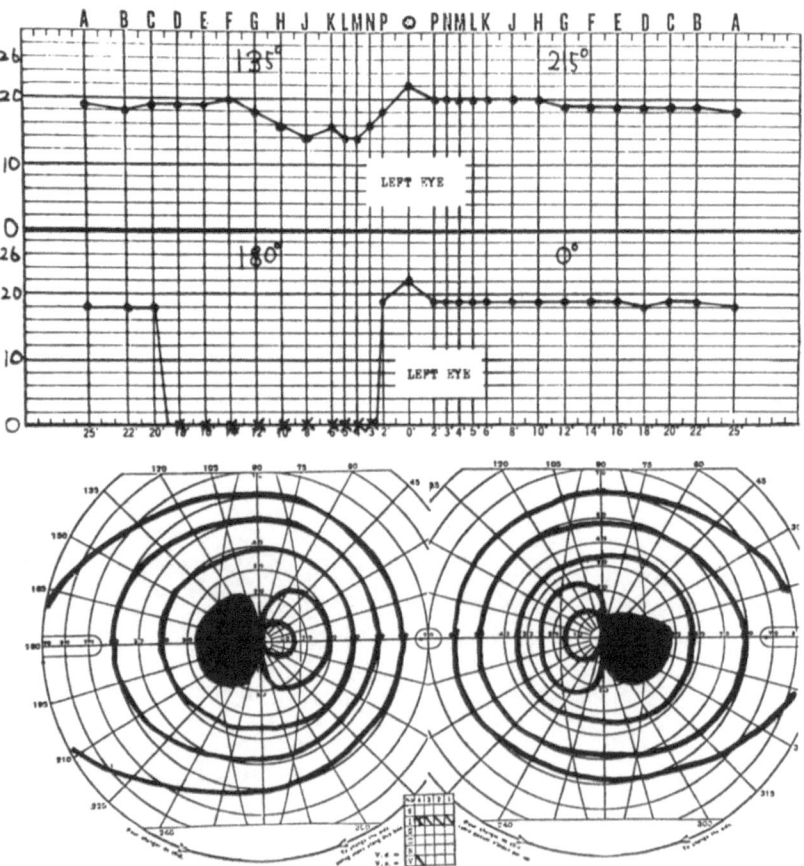

Fig. 3. Visual field changes of case 3. Bitemporal hemianopsic scotoma was detected by kinetic perimetry with I/4. No perception was detected on the 180° meridian of left eye by profile perimetry with MDP.

detected by kinetic perimetry were demonstrated as high grade depression by static perimetry with MDP.

2. Some differences in results between MDP and TP.

The normal MDP and TP profiles shows parallel sensitivity curves. The discrepancy between the profiles is limited to within 1.3 log units. Figs. 6 show glaucomatous visual field changes assessed by MDP and TP. By MDP, no response was obtained at maximum luminance in certain targets, but TP showed a measurable value. The differences in response between the two methods require explanation. In both methods, the conditions of measurement are identical apart from presentation time. The presentation time of MDP is one milisecond and that of TP is 1000 millisecond. Temporal summation (Bloch's law) regulates short presentation time such as one millisecond and has no effect of temporal summation for the long presentation

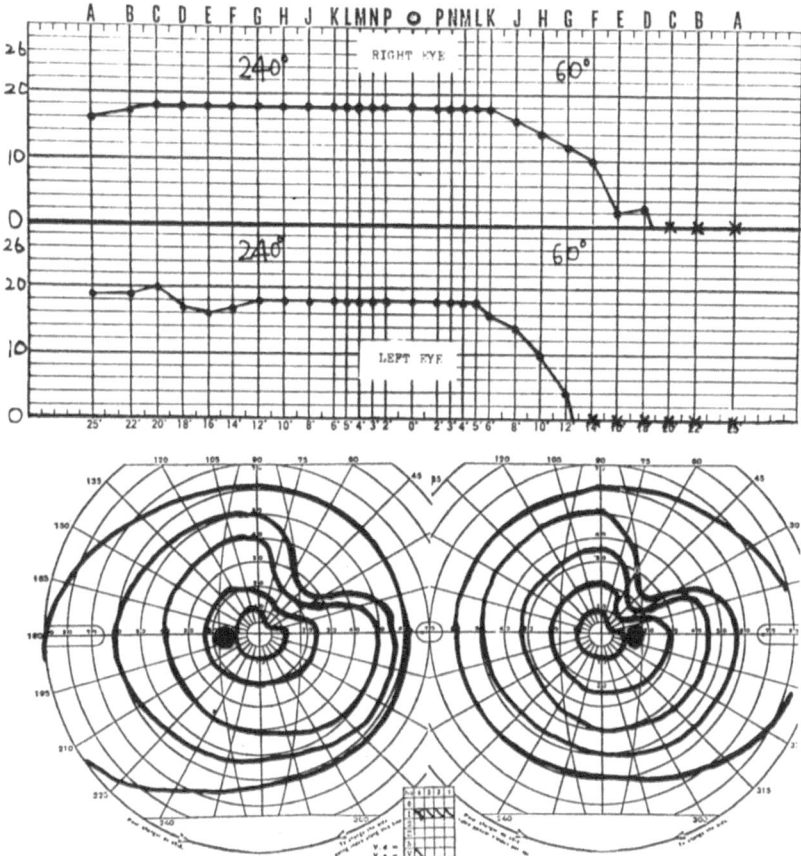

Fig. 4. Visual field changes of case 4. Right homonymous quadrantanopic defect was detected in both eyes. MDP detected high grade depression beyond maximum luminance on the 60° meridian.

457

time such as 1000 millisecond. If temporal summation were to take place more slowly in a visual field defect (if more time were needed to reach the threshold) it is theoretically possible that abnormal summation would be compensated for the surplus time of the long presentation time (Greve 1973). According to this hypothesis, the discrepancy between the two methods on the visual field defect showed abnormal temporal summation. From the results of Figs. 6 and 7, abnormal temporal summation would be compensated for by a long presentation time such as 1000 millisecond. Shinzato, one of the present authors, reported on the relationship of abnormal temporal summation in early glaucomatous visual field changes in 9 eyes of 6 people (Shinzato 1978). In the future, abnormal temporal summation must be investigated in variouss cases.

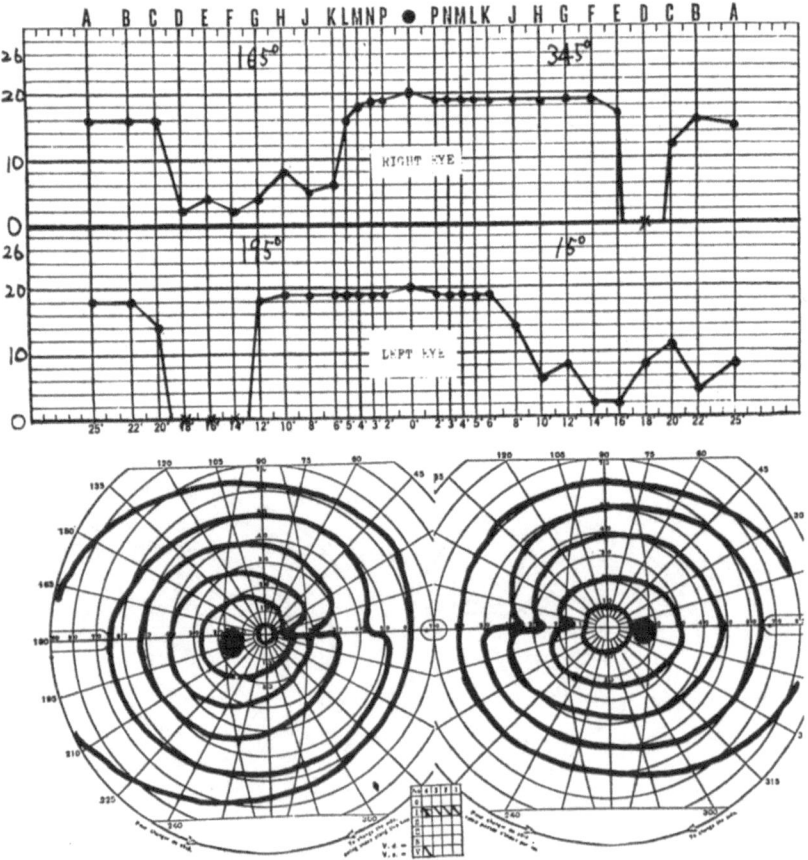

Fig. 5. Visual field changes of case 5. Typical nasal step was detected by kinetic perimetry with I/4, I/3, I/2. High grade depression was detected by MDP on the meridian of 165° in the right eye and 15° in left eye.

458

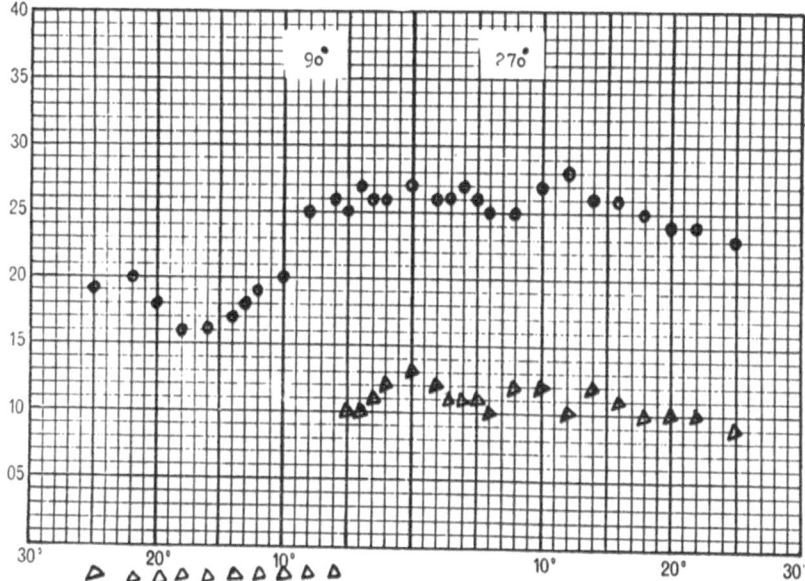

Fig. 6. The thresholds of two presentation times in glaucomatous visual field changes. No parallel depression was obtained but the discrepancy of profile showed extreme separation on the 90° meridian.

△ shows responses to 1 millisecond

o shows responses to 1000 milliseconds

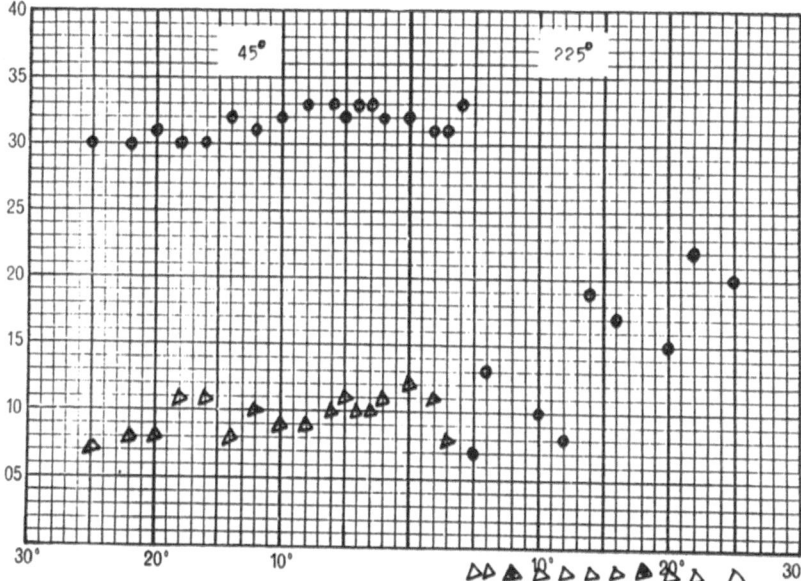

Fig. 7. The thresholds of two presentation times in glaucomatous visual field changes. General depression was obtained with short presentation time. On the 225° meridian, no perception was detected by presentation time of 1 millisecond but measureable values were detected by presentation time of 1000 millisecond.

REFERENCES

Greve, E.L. Single and multiple stimulus static perimetry in glaucoma; the two phases of perimetry. *Documenta Ophthal.* 36: *91-93* (1973).

Matsuo, H. et al. Trial manufacture of a new central quantitative perimeter. The 11 th. Ophthalmologic Optics meeting at Kanazawa, September, 1975.

Shinzato, E. Quantitative perimetry using new developed static campimeter, discussion on normal subjects. *Acta. Ophthal. Jap.* 82: *167-174* (1978).

Shinzato, E. Quantitative perimetry using new developed static campimeter, discussion on early glaucomatous visual field changes. *Acta. Ophthal. Jap.* being submitted for publication.

Author's address:
Department of Ophthalmology
Tokyo Medical College Hospital
6-7-1 Nishishinjuku, Shinjuku-ku
Tokyo, 160, Japan

ELECTROENCEPHALOGRAPHIC PERIMETRY
CLINICAL APPLICATIONS OF VERTEX POTENTIALS ELICITED BY FOCAL RETINAL STIMULATION

TOHRU MARUO

(Kobe, Japan)

ABSTRACT

For the determination of an objective measurement of human visual field, an averaged Vertex Potential was measured instead of occipital VER. The spot of the stimulus was used from Goldman's perimeter with the intensity of 1000 asb, the target size of 64 mm² and the background intensity of 10 asb. The random stimuli from 2 to 6 sec were given to a test subject with the duration of 1000 msec. The objective perimetry by using this procedure almost correlated with the subjective perimetry under the same conditions. Namely, Vertex Potentials could be elicited even by focal stimuli at peripheral parts of a retina such as temporal 70° or nasal 50°. And reproductibility of the responses were least stable during the measurement from 4 or 5 parts of a visual field. This method seems to be available for the measurement of visual field both in normal and pathological cases who have an abnormal visual field.

INTRODUCTION

An application of Visual Evoked Responses (VER) for the objective measurement of the human visual fields has been done by various researchers. The first trial was made by Copenhaver in 1963 (Copenhaver & Beinhocker 1963). Various reports have been made afterwards, however, there were many discrepancies among the researchers. There were possible due to following reasons: e.g. 1. The use only of occipital VERs, 2. The effect of stray light, 3. The interference of unsteady fixation.

If ordinary equipment of the perimeter such as Goldmann's could applied for presentation of a stimulus on the retina in objective perimetry, the results from both objective and subjective measurements could be compared. For the application using Goldmann's perimeter as a stimulus there is one report available, which measures occipital VER (Adachi 1977). It was well known that occipital VERs picked up foveal functions dominantly and the stimulus given at the peripheral portion of the retina could not elicit occipital VER. Therefore it is necessary to have another procedure established.

The Vertex potential, which was first reported by Davis in 1939, is a non specific component and it has a relatively stable wave to any given stimuli from the outside such as light, tone or touch (Davis, Davis, Loomis, Harvey & Hobart 1939, Davis, Mast, Yoshie & Zerlin 1966).

In this study, the Vertex Potential has been used to measure Electroencephalographic-perimetry (EEG perimetry) as the objective perimetry. The stimulus was obtained from a modified Goldmann's perimeter. The result was almost the same as subjective perimetry under the same conditions. I would like to discuss the conditions of measurement and demonstrate several clinical applications.

METHOD

The characteristics of the recording system have been previously described in detail. The photic stimulus was obtained from a modified Goldmann's perimeter (Fig. 1). This apparatus consisted of light source, electric shutter, fiber opticus (light guide) and Goldmann's perimeter (TAKATA, MT-40). The light source and electric shutter were set on the outside of the electrical shielded room and connected to the perimeter by the fiber opticus. The light source was the halogen electric bulb (D.C. 21V, 150W) and the electric shutter was driven by a Pulse Stimulator (NIHON-KODEN, SEN-1101), which also produced the trigger pulse. Durations of the photic stimulus were examined by the Photo Transister (NEC, PT8). The delay in time between the trigger pulse and the photic stimulation was 6.25 msec. The output of the fiber optics was fitted up to the lamp box of Goldmann's perimeter. The light source of the background illumination was replaced as Fig. 1. In stimulating fovea, subjects gazed at four small dots arranged in the shape of a lozenge which were 15° in distance from the hole of the telescope and the target was projected to the center of the lozenge. In a stimulation of the

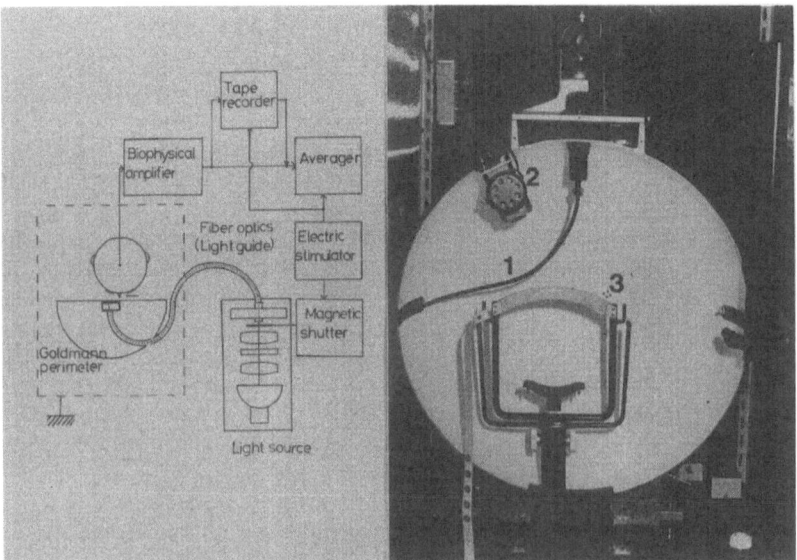

Fig. 1. 1. Fiber opticus. 2. Light source for the background illumination 3. Fixation targets in stimulating fovea.

462

peripheral parts of the retina, the fixation point was the hole of the telescope.

In the present study, the conditions of measurement were as follows: 10 asb background, 1000 asb target, the target size of 64 mm^2 (V spot of Goldmann's perimeter), target on duration of 1000 msec excepting in the study of interstimulus interval and random stimulus from 2 to 6 sec interval excepting in the study of the interstimulus interval. In the examination of the interstimulus interval (ISI), the duration of the photic stimulus was 10 msec.

The EEG was recorded with the biophysical amplifier (NIHON-KODEN, AVB-1. hi-cut 100H$_z$ and time constant 0.3 sec). The active electrode was at the Vertex (C$_z$) in the 10-20 international system and the reference electrode was on either ear lobe. The EEG was continuously monitored on the oscilloscope. 50 responses were summated on-line with the data processing computer (NIHON-KODEN, ATAC 350) and these were plotted by the X-Y plotter (YOKOKAWA, BW-201B). Occasionally, however, the record was made off-line, using the 4 channel FM tape recorder (TEAC, R400).

The subjects were 15 persons with normal vision and 4 patients respectively with optic nerve atrophy, glaucoma, traumatic optic nerve damage and malingering.

RESULTS

1. Spatial difference of VERs elicited by focal retinal stimulations is demonstrated in fig. 2.

In my previous reports, I confirmed that there was no effect of artifacts such as EOG and Auditory Evoked responses with regard to this apparatus (Maruo 1977). In stimulating fovea, the responses were recorded over the occiput to the vertex. In the stimulation of a peripheral part of the retina as temporal 50°, however, the responses at the Vertex were more dominant than those at the occiput. In other words, the responses by the stimulating fovea could be recorded over the diffused scalp, but the responses by stimu-

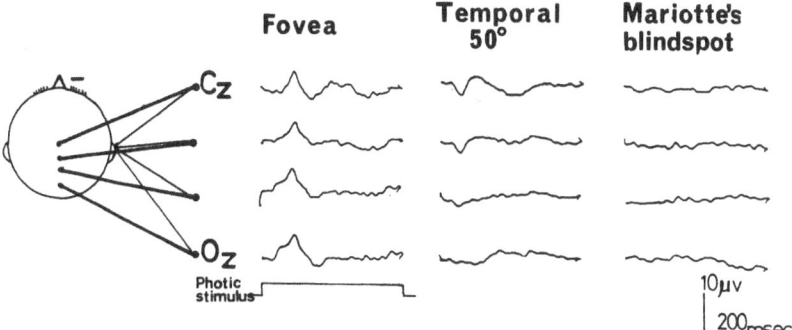

Fig. 2. Negativity at the labeled electrode results in downward deflection in this and the following records.

463

lating a peripheral part of the retina was only recorded at the central region of the scalp (Cz). No response was elicited by stimulating Marriotte's blind spot.

The response at the vertex which was elicited by stimulating a peripheral part of the retina consisted of several components. I considered that it was called Vertex Potential. These positive and negative waves were labeled p_1, N_1, P_2 and N_2, according to Davis designation (Davis, Mast, Yoshie & Zerlin 1966).

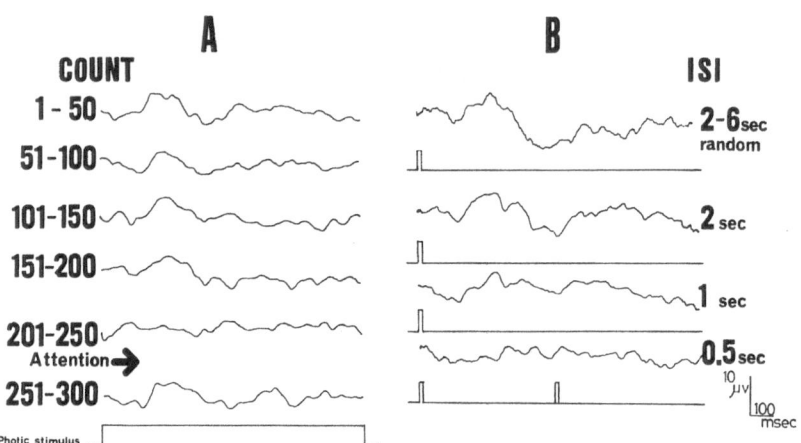

Fig. 3.

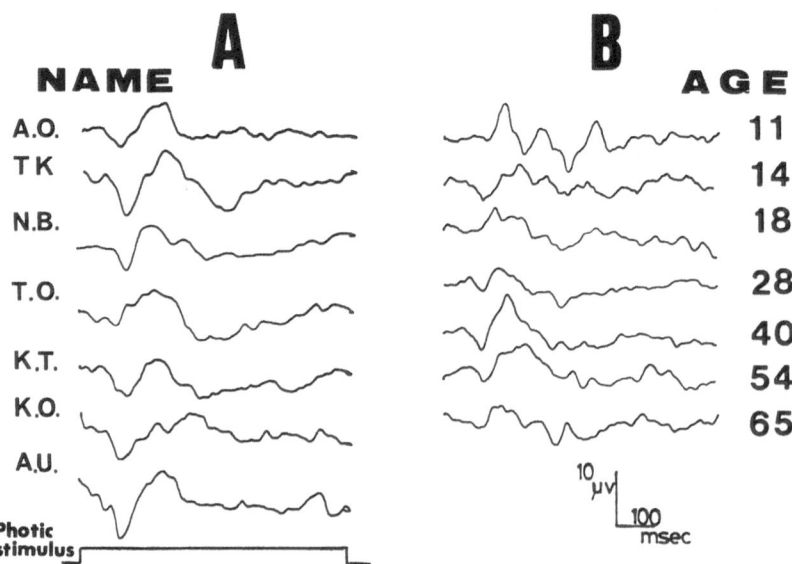

Fig. 4.

2. Characteristics of Vertex Potentials elicited by focal retinal stimulations (Fig. 3) (Fig. 4).

No Vertex Potential could be elicited when ISI was short. If the intervals between the stimuli were shorter than 1 sec, it was scarcely possible to pick up the responses. The amplitude of the response at 2-6 sec intervals was clearly larger than that at 1 sec intervals (Fig. 3B).

Fig. 3A shows the phenomenon of habituation. Vertex Potentials averaging from 1 to 50 counts were larger than that from 151 to 200 counts. No response could be measured by stimuli from 201 to 250 times. By diverting the subject's attention or resting a few minutes, the response cound be evoked again. Fig. 4A and B show the individual difference and disparity in age. The N_1 latency of seven subjects of the same age; (m ± 2s = 156 ± 22 msec), and age discrepancy of N_1 latency between 11 and 65 years old; (m ± 2s = 171 ± 50 msec). The waves of the Vertex Potential were more stable figure than those of occipital VER using a xenon flash.

3. EEG Perimetry: Normal data (Fig. 5).

A case of the objective perimetry using Vertex Potentials is indicated at Fig. 5 with subjective kinetic perimetry under the same conditions. By stimulating the Fovea, temporal 30°, 50°, 70° and nasal 30°, 50°, the response could be evoked, but it was impossible to measure the response from temporal 90° and nasal 70°. This result is almost equal to the subjective kinetic perimetry under the same conditions.

4. EEG Perimetry: Clinical data (Fig. 6)

Case 1: 40-year-old male with optic atrophy. He had a central scotoma of about ten degrees at the subjective kinetic perimetry with 64 mm². From 1 in the central scotoma, the response could not be elicited, but at 2 the clear response could be gained.

Case 2: 20-year-old male with traumatic optic damage. The kinetic perimetry shows the nasal depression of the affected eye. By stimulation at 1, no response can be evoked. It shows that N_1 latency of the response at 2 is more prolonged than that at 3.

Case 3: 35-year-old female with open angle glaucoma. The kinetic perimetry shows a concentric contraction. By stimulating at 1 and 2, the responses could be elicited, but at 3 no response could be seen.

Case 4: The author thinks this case is a malingering after the trauma, because this patient can easily walk in a dark room. He insisted that he could not see the target at 1, but from this point the Vertex Potential could be evoked.

DISCUSSION

Since Copenhaver and Beinhocker, various experiments concerning the objective perimetry by using VER have been done but we cannot say that these attempts have been successful enough.

Van Lith (1976) said that an objective perimetry by means of VER was even more hopeless than that of ERG, and also Henkes (1974) and Adachi (1977) described this attempt was impossible.

On the other hand, it is well known that VER consists of specific and non-specific components, and the latter can be measured on a wide area of the scalp. The Vertex Potential comes within the category of non-specific response. Up to the present, only occipital VER had been used for the objective perimetry, however the author made use of this Vertex Potential.

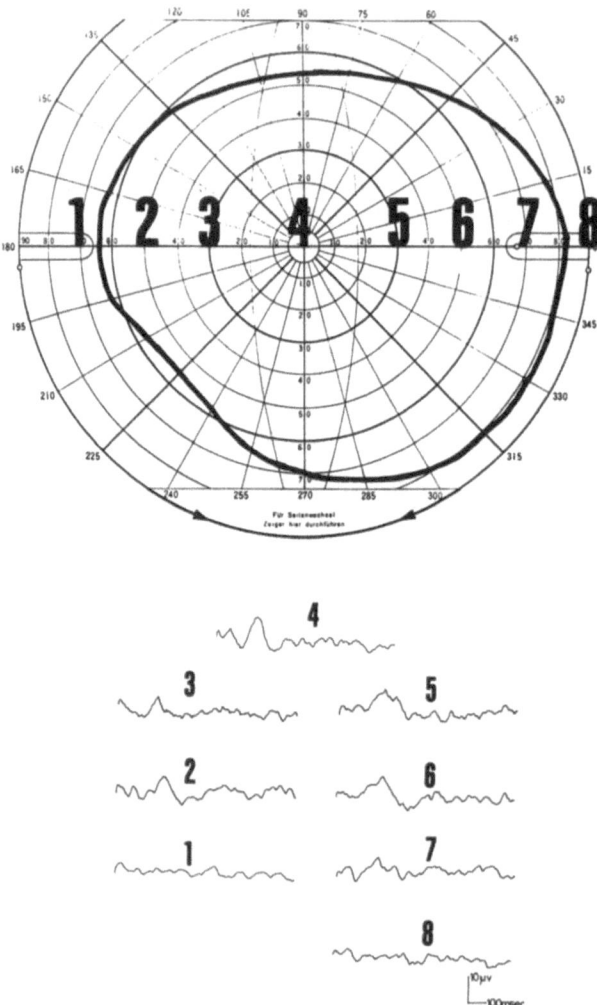

Fig. 5. Upper columm; kinetic perimetry under the same conditions and the stimulus points were indicated.

Regarding the characteristics of the Vertex Potential, very similar waves are evoked by stimuli in different modalities such as light, tone etc.. Because of this, it became very important to exclude the artifact of the AER. As regards this apparatus, the AER was not elicited because the electric shutter which made a noise was set outside the electrically shieled room. Also there was no problem in the fixation of a subjective eye for using the Goldmann's perimeter.

In stimulating fovea, the responses were recorded over the occiput to the vertex, however in a stimulation of a peripheral part of retina as temporal 50°, the responses at the vertex were more dominant than those at the occiput. The responses elicited by stimulating fovea were not only occipital VER but also Vertex Potential and could be picked up from the occiput to the vertex as the wave patterns that these two responses combined. But the response elicited by stimulating the peripheral part of the retina, was only Vertex Potential.

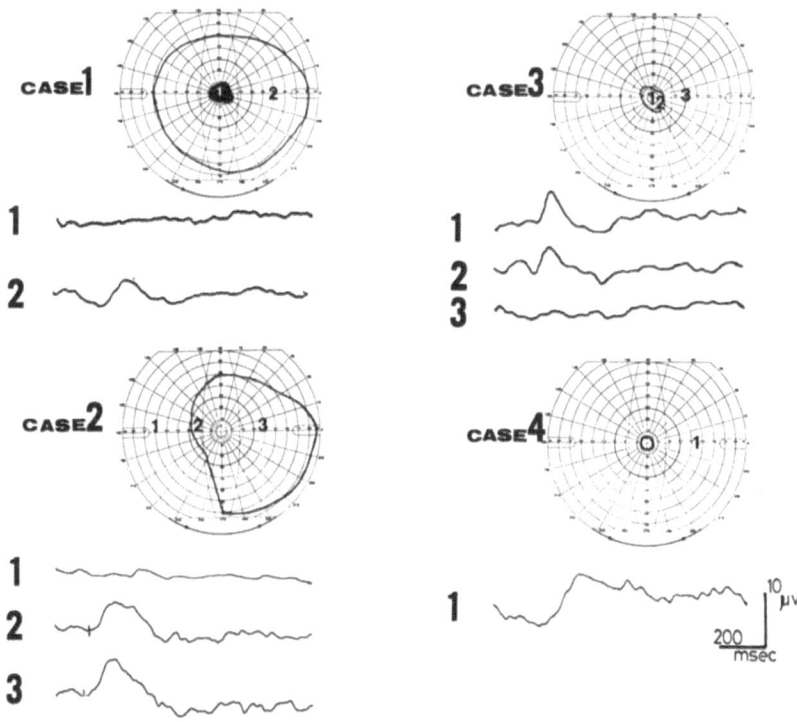

Fig. 6. Case 1. Optic atrophy; Case 2. Traumatic optic damage; Case 3. Chronic open angle glaucoma; Case 4. malingering.

467

In this experiment, the Vertex Potentials elicited by the focal retinal stimulations did not show the effect of individual differences or age discrepancies. For clinical use, the above characteristics of the Vertex Potential were advantageous, but the following points are disadvantageous. The serial measurement for many hours descreased the amplitude of the response. I supposed this phenomenon was based on habituation, and it was limited to measure at 4 or 5 points of the visual field. And also the function of the interstimulus interval had to be considered. Davis explained that for maximal amplitude the intervals between stimuli had to be over 6 sec and probably at least 10 sec and if the intervals were regular the average amplitude was about $\frac{1}{2}$ maximal at 3 sec, $\frac{1}{4}$ at 1 sec and $\frac{1}{6}$ at 0.5 sec. In my experiment, no response could be evoked at an interstimulus shorter than 1 sec. Because of these faults, it is difficult to measure at many points of the visual field, but I would farther improve this technique.

I considered that the EEG perimetry by this method was almost the same as the subjective kinetic perimetry under the same conditions in a normal person and in clinical cases. In the case of traumatic optic nerve damage (Case 2), the N_1 latency of the response stimulating at the border of the depression was longer than that at the intact part. From this result, I would expect the difference of the sensitivity of the visual field can be indicated by the latency of the Vertex Potential. And also the EEG perimetry is useful to diagnose malingering (Case 4).

REFERENCES

Adachi, E. Perimetry by the human scotopic visual evoked cortical potential *Acta Soc. Ophthalm. Jap.* 81: *340* (1977).

Copenhaver, R.M. & Beinhocker, G.D. Objective visual field testing. J.A.M.A., 186: *107* (1963).

Copenhaver, R.M. & Beinhocker, G.D. Evoked occipital potentials recorded from scalp electrodes in response to focal visual illumination. *Invest. Ophthalmol.* 2: *393* (1963).

Davis, H., Davis, P.A., Loomis, A.L., Harvey, E.N. & Hobart, G. Electrical reactions of the human brain to auditory stimulation during sleep. *J. Neurophysiol.* 20: *500* (1939).

Davis, H., Mast, T., Yoshie, N. & Zerlin, S. The slow response of the human cortex to auditory stimuli. Electtroencephal. *Clin. Neurophysiol.* 21: *105* (1966).

Henkes, H.E. VanLith, G.H.M. Electroperimetry. Ophthalmol. 169: *151* (1974).

Lith, G.H.M.,van Perimetry and electrophysiology. *Docu. Ophthalmol. Proceeding series*, 14: *169* (1976) Tübingen.

Maruo, T. Electroencephalographic perimetry. Part 2 *Acta Soc. Ophthalm. Jap.* 81: *1360* (1977).

Maruo, T. Electroencephalographic perimetry. Part 3 *Acta Soc. Ophthalm. Jap.* 82: *226* (1978).

Maruo, T. Electroencephalographic perimetry. Part 1 *Jpn. Rev. Clin. Ophthalmol.* 71: *533* (1977).

Author's address:
Department of Ophthalmology
School of Medicine
Kobe University
Japan

RELATION BETWEEN CENTRAL AND PERIPHERAL VISUAL FIELD CHANGES WITH KINETIC PERIMETRY

TETSURO OGAWA & RYUJIRO SUZUKI

(Tokyo, Japan)

INTRODUCTION

The most serious disturbance in visual function is primarily deterioration of central visual acuity, followed by visual field changes. Furthermore, it is also important to detect visual field changes for diagnostic and therapeutic purposes.

From our experience, central visual field (CVF) examination is the prime visual field measurement in the detection of visual field changes. Many reports have dealt with early glaucomatous visual field changes, Aulhorn (1967) Drance (1964) and many other authors stressed the importance of CVF changes. However, the only report concerning a clinical comparative study of CVF and peripheral visual field (PVF) appears to be that of Blum (1959) almost 20 years ago. His data indicated that PVF examinations were of little value in detection, diagnosis and therapy.

The present authors undertook to study the relation between CVF and PVF changes in cases examined with kinetic perimetry by the Goldmann perimeter, and their results confirmed the significance of CVF examination in the detection of visual field changes, and the relative insignificance of PVF examination.

MATERIALS AND METHODS

Materials

The present study includes the results of kinetic perimetry by the Goldmann perimeter of 1296 eyes examined from January to October 1976 at our clinic.

Methods

As standard procedure V/4, I/4, I/3, I/2, I/1 isopters were measured, out of which I/2 and V/4 isopters were respectively selected as representative of CVF and PVF. In this study, the lower normal limits of I/2 and V/4 isopters were standardized as the standard boundary isopters utilizing Furuse's work (1964) which contained a list of mean values and 5% rejection limits of I/2 and V/4 isopters of each 15 degree meridian.

Abnormal CVF changes can be categorized as follows; 1. I/2 with defects or I/2 smaller than I/2 standard boundary isopter. 2. central or paracentral scotoma deeper than I/2, enlargement of blind spot. PVF changes were defined as; 1. V/4 with defects or V/4 smaller than V/4 standard boundary isopter.

1,296 eyes were divided into the following 4 groups; I. CVF negative, PVF positive. II. CVF positive, PVF negative. III. both positive. IV. both negative.

RESULTS

729 eyes (56.3%) had visual field changes, 567 eyes (43.7%) had no changes in either CVF or PVF. Table 1 shows the classification of diseases, distribution of visual field changes and the numerical relation between CVF and PVF changes.

In the glaucoma group, CVF changes were found in early stage cases and both CVF and PVF changes were found with more advanced cases, but there was no case in which only PVF changes were detected. In Group IV, 17 eyes out of 131 eyes with glaucoma had extremely slight changes showing so little depression (of I/1) that they would be judged normal by our criteria. CVF changes were demonstrated by Friedmann visual field analyser in 45 eyes. The remainder which did not show visual field changes at that time were considered to be so-called tonometric and tonographic glaucoma.

In the chorioretinal diseases group, visual field changes coincided with the location and the size of focus.

An extremely low number of only 6 eyes in 6 patients out of 1296 eyes showed isolated PVF changes. Apart from these cases, the visual field

Table. 1.

	I CVF negative PVF positive	II CVF positive PVF negative	III CVF positive PVF positive	IV CVF negative PVF negative	Total
Chorioretinal diseases	5 eyes	117	120	141	283
Diseases in visual pathways	1	104	111	46	262
Glaucoma	0	90	157	131	378
Others	0	15	9	27	51
Normal	0	0	0	322	322
Total (%)	6 (0.5%)	326 (25.2%)	397 (30.6%)	567 (43.7%)	1296

changes could be detected without PVF examinations. The following case reports serve as examples.

Case 1. 24-year-old male; right eye status, post retinal detachment operation.

About 30 days prior to the first visual field examination, he underwent cryocautery and the chorioretinal atrophy which was found ophthalmoscopically at the upper equatorial region corresponded to the inferior PVF defect and the detachment was well repaired. (Fig. 1.)

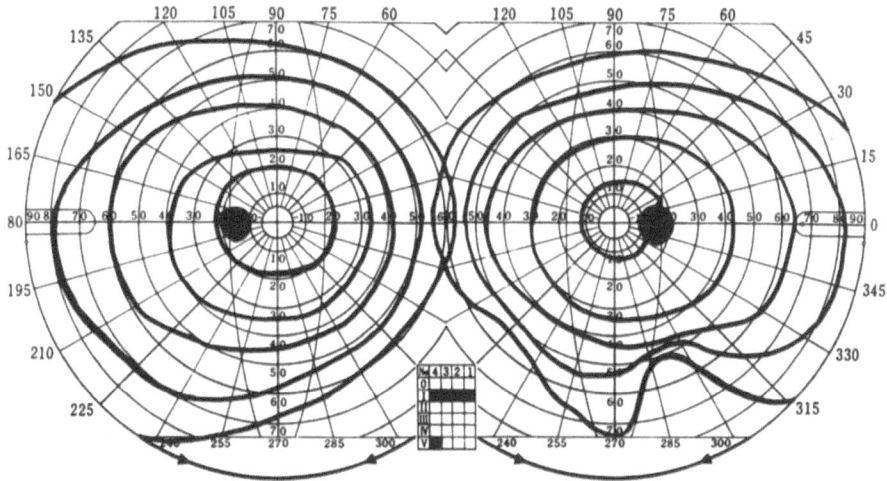

Fig. 1. Visual fields of Case 1.

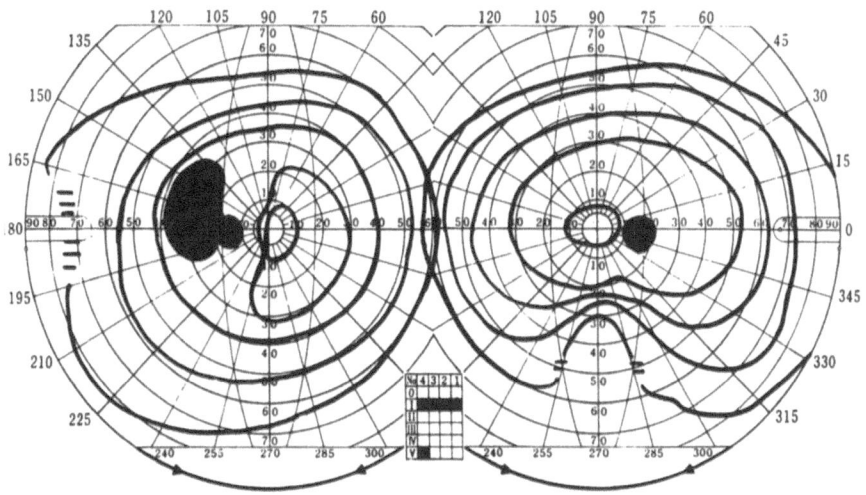

Fig. 2. Visual fields of Case 2.

471

Case 2. 52-year-old female, status: post pituitary tumor operation.

The inferior PVF defect in right eye was examined with similar results 9 times pre- and post-operatively. (Fig. 2.) There were no remarkable findings in the right eye and it was estimated that this inferior PVF defect was the result of localized nerve fibers damage. The visual field of the left eye showed temporal hemianopsia, regressing after the operation.

Case 3. 28-year-old female; admitted for detailed examinations for glaucoma.

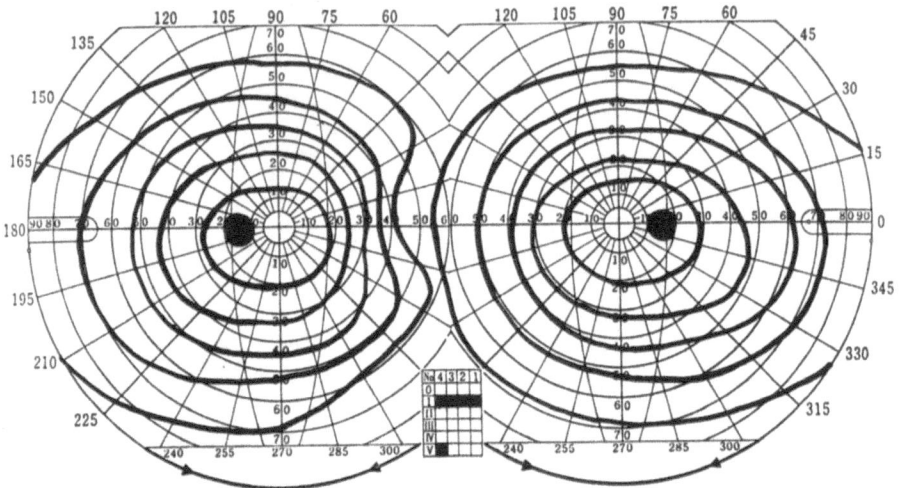

Fig. 3. Visual fields of Case 3.

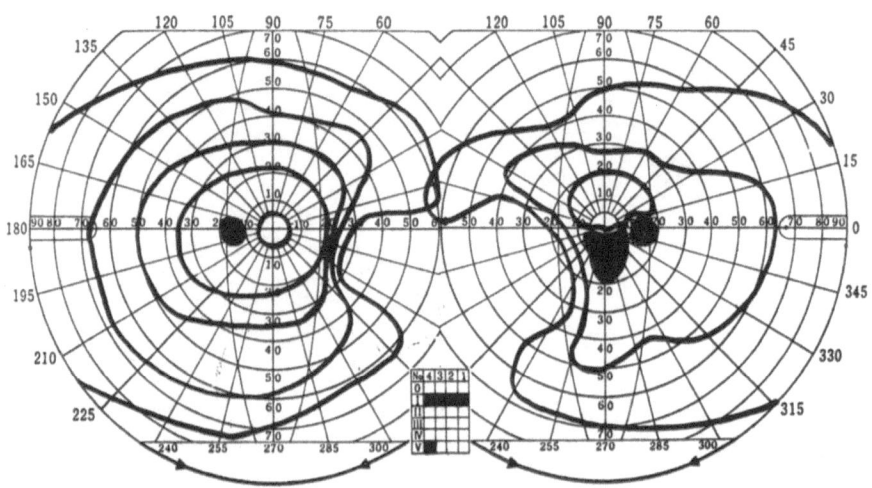

Fig. 4. Visual fields of Case 4.

An isolated nasal PVF defect in the left eye was observed, therefore glaucomatous visual field changes was suspected. (Fig. 3.)

However, glaucoma was not indicated by the results of other examinations. Ophthalmoscopic findings showed a large area of lattice degeneration in the temporal equatorial retina and retinal degeneration extending to about 3 o'clock, these changes being consistent in location and size with PVF defect.

Case 4. 34-year-old male; complaining of diplopia and decreased visual acuity of the right eye.

Right orbital apex syndrome was diagnosed, and in the left eye, retinal degenerations were found. These were the results of photocoagulation therapy for occlusion of the retinal branch vein 3 years ago, and corresponded with the PVF defect of the left eye. (Fig. 4.)

DISCUSSION

In kinetic perimetry by the Goldmann perimeter, usually V/4, I/4, I/3, I/2, I/1 isopters are measured. The isopter obtained by V/4 stimulus indicates the basic area of the island of vision, and when V/4 isopter is affected, two types of visual field changes are theoretically considered, general constriction and only peripheral constriction including the type of partial peripheral field defects. However peripheral constriction alone is very rare, and most cases are accompanied by CVF changes.

Harrington (1971) stated that 90% of visual field changes could be detected either wholly or in part by only CVF examinations with a tangent screen, because most visual field changes detected in PVF extended inward to CVF.

The report of Blum on the visual field changes in 3078 eyes in 1892 patients indicated that only 25 eyes (0.812%) in 22 patients had PVF changes without CVF changes. He contended that PVF examinations did not contribute to diagnosis, prognosis or treatment, and questioned the value of routine PVF examinations, but admitted that such conditions as retinal detachment and cerebrovascular accident may cause partial PVF defects.

From analysis of this series of 1296 eyes, only 6 eyes (0.5%) were in Group I, if CVF alone had been examined, these 6 cases would have been overlooked as showing no significant changes.

Of these 6 cases with negative CVF and positive PVF findings, 5 were considered due to retinal degenerations which were detected ophthalmoscopically before the visual field examinations and the remaining case of post pituitary tumor operation displayed CVF changes at the preoperative stage.

Therefore, from a clinical point of view, it can be argued that it would not have mattered, had PVF examinations not been performed. It is also obvious that in the overwhelming majority of cases, CVF examination yields much more information, in addition to being economical in terms of time. However, this does not mean that PVF examinations are valueless; they are important in providing information on the entire visual field which is essen-

473

tial in grasping the condition of diseases or therapeutic effectiveness.

Greve (1973) divides the perimetry for glaucoma into two phases, detection and assessment. According to this philosophy, and considering the fact that of the 1296 eyes examined on the suspicion of visual field changes, 567 eyes (43.7%) showed no abnormality and only 6 eyes (0.5%) were CVF negative and PVF positive, it would appear that CVF examination alone is fully sufficient for the detection phase. Of course PVF examinations should be performed in the assessment phase, if necessary.

SUMMARY

We studied the incidence of visual field changes in 1296 eyes with kinetic perimetry by the Goldmann perimeter for a comparative study of CVF and PVF changes.

6 eyes (0.5%) out of 1296 eyes showed CVF negative and PVF positive findings. With the exception of those 6 eyes, all diseases accompanied by visual field changes had CVF changes, indicating that only CVF examination should be employed for initial screening.

REFERENCES

Aulhorn, E. & Harms, H. Early visual field defects in glaucoma. Basel, S. Karger A.G. 151-186 (1967).

Blum, F.G., Gates, L.K. & James, M.R. How important are peripheral fields? Arch. Ophthal. 61: 1-8 (1959).

Drance, S.M. The early field defects in glaucoma. Invest. Ophthal. 8: 84-91 (1964).

Furuse, M. Clinical study on the photometric harmony in the visual field. Report I. Normal eyes. Acta Soc. Ophthalm. Jpn. 68: 1208-1223 (1964).

Greve, E.L. Single and multiple stimulus static perimetry in glaucoma; the two phases of visual field examination. Docum. Ophthal. 36: 98-108, 158-202 (1973).

Harrington, D.O. The visual fields. 3rd ed. St. Louis, Mosby, 14-47 (1971).

Author's address:
Department of Ophthalmology,
Tokyo Medical College Hospital
6-7-1 Nishishinjuku, Shinjuku-ku,
Tokyo, 160, Japan

DISCUSSION ON THE FREE PAPERS SESSION

CHAIRMAN: J.M. ENOCH

Enoch: The paper by A. Dubois-Poulsen is to be discussed by Dr. Aulhorn.
Aulhorn: I have to speak about a very interesting paper of Dubois-Poulsen. The subject is the enlargement of the blind spot in binocular investigation. His findings are: in monocular measurement, the diameter of the blind spot has 6 degree in the horizontal meridian and 7 degree in the vertical meridian, but in binocular measurement the diameter is 9 degree. It means in the vertical and horizontal meridian 2 degrees more in binocular measurement. This phenomenon is absent in the darkness.

Then the diameter is the same in monocular and binocular measurements. The results are the same whatever their experimental conditions are. Polarized filters, coloured filters, temporal differences, it is always the same result. The fact that the phenomenon is absent in darkness indicates to us that the reason for the difference in monocular and binocular investigation can be only an inhibition of the function in the immidiate surrounds of the blind spot in binocular vision.

These phenomena are without doubt of great importance in strabismus. I think it is a new phenomenon.

Enoch: The second of the non-read papers was presented by the female half of Frisen team. "The evaluation of perimetric procedures, a statistical approach". Dr. Frankhauser will be the discussor.

Frankhauser: This paper has all the characteristics typical of those prepared by statistical mathematicians, namely clarity of expression and precision of definitions.

Basic quantities, which are essential for every visual field examination procedure, such as notions of sensitivity, specificity and predictive value of the diagnosis 'normal' or 'abnormal' are analysed in this paper.

Implicitly, the author deals with probabilities involved in Baye's theorem. The forward probabilities (sensitivity and specificity) can be deduced from a model analysis of the method, taking the measurement error into account. As pointed out by the author, the predictive values (backward probabilities), however, also depend on the prevalence of abnormal states in a given population; usually, in practice, these a priori probabilities are not known, and hence the probability whether an apparently pathological feature has a pathological meaning is not known either. This applies to differences observed in follow-up studies as well.

The paper expresses the spirit of a rational thinking in terms of well-defined quantities.

Drance: I have not had the opportunity of reading the paper but from what Dr. Fankhauser has just said I am sure that we will find this paper extremely usefull in tomorrow's discussion. It is this type of probability or relative risk (as it is used in epidermiological terms) which becomes quite crucial to definitions and the importance which one attaches to certain findings that occur in normal and diseased individual before one can in fact decide who is more likely to have disease and with what certainty.

This whole area is something which I would completely endrose for clinicians, unfortunately, we are only beginning to realize this true meaning of these problems and this paper will, if nothing else, invite further discussions in the years to come.

Enoch: The third of the non-read paper is by Dr. Honda, A. Nigi, M. Miki of Kyoto. "Eyemovements during peripheral field tests, monitored by electro-oculogram". I shall discuss the paper. These able authors have taken a rather straight forward and in some ways very simple approach. They have measured gross eye movements during a perimetric examination. They find in substantial populations, in particular among children, older individuals, and people with central defects, that there is poor fixation and therefore a lack of reliability in many of the individual determinations during the testing of the visual fields. While in essence a simple discussion, it is a crucial discussion.

This research points to the very profound need for routine monitoring of fixation during perimetric testing. Some of our finer instruments provide that capability, but few do so among many other instruments available. Further, this kind of research points up the desirability of limiting static target presentations to about 200 milliseconds. That is to a duration shorter than the latency for a saccadic eye movement. This paper very strongly supports the position taken in the standard wherein we recommend that the duration of presentation be limited to a period of time of less than the latency for a saccadic eye movements.

Fankhauser: When a fixation monitoring device of high efficiency is used, rejecting all answers coinciding with a fixation deviation, the detrimental effect of fixation instability upon threshold stability is not observed. (Bähler, H.: Untersuchung über die Streuung perimetrischer Kontrastschwellen in Funktion der Expositionszeit. Doctoral thesis. Faculty of Medicine, University of Bern).

Enoch: The next paper is presented by H. Kitahara, K. Kitahara, H. Matsuzaki of Tokyo with "Trial of a colour perimeter". Dr. Verriest.

Verriest: It is with great pleasure that I will comment the paper of Kitahara etc. Because a few years ago these authors and myself worked exactly along the same research lines. We independently calibrated the Tübingen perimeter, and it is also at the same moment that we established some foundations of a new movement in clinical colour perimetry based on the

476

determination of the achromatic increment threshold for monochromatic targets. But with this new paper Kitahara et al. are now much more advanced than myself, because they effectively realized the wish that I shall present in my chairman's report for the IPS RG on Colour Perimetry. They in fact constructed a prototype of a perimeter in which the unfiltered background luminance level reaches 2000 cd.m^{-2} (I asked just the same figure), while the unfiltered target luminance reaches 22000 cd.m^{-2} (The RG asked only 10.000 cd.m^{-2}). No less than 16 well spaced narrow-band interference filters are available, and the authors carefully determined which background selective filters best isolate the tricolour vision mechanisms. I'm really full of admiration for the technical achievement of what I considered to be only a dream. This achievement is even more complete than the dream, as I never expected that the exposure times could also be varied between 10 msec. and 10 sec. My congratulations for this outstanding realization.

Enoch: The next paper is by Dr. Kubota, of Tokyo. "Video-pupilographic perimetry. Report 4 on the technique how to operate the revormed device and perimetric findings on the rabbits eyes". Prof. Harms will discuss the paper.

Harms: Dr. Kubota reports on an improvement of the video-pupilographic perimeter of *Nayasaki*. With this modification a central visual field down to 7 degree can be obtained. — The possibilities of this apparatus are tested in human subjects. The blind spot could be accurately detected. — The apparatus is used for objective perimetry in pigmented rabbits. The results in 2 animals were as follows:
1) In the central field the sensitive area of pupillary light reflex in the retina was a band 15 degrees wide extending horizontally below the disc and medullary nerve fibers. This area corresponds to the so-called visual streak. streak.
2) For the measurement of peripheral field the threshold of light reflex on the ventral side was lower than on the dorsal side of the disc and medullary nerve fibers.

I believe this is an interesting and important method for the examination of visual functions in animal experiments, perhaps the single simple method available today. It seems to me that there is a little problem: the luminance of the background is different in different parts of the field. That is not an optimal situation for perimetry. But we know the technical genius of our Japanese colleagues. Therefore I am sure that in a near future they will solve this difficult technical problem in a satisfying manner.

Enoch: The next paper is by E. Shinatzo and H. Matsuo from Tokyo "Clinical experiences with a new meridian dot target". Dr. Friedmann will discuss this manuscript.

Friedmann: This was a very interesting paper. These authors have developed what they call a meridian multiple dot plate which consists of two dots equi-distant from fixation and then they can make another two dots allowing them to go out to 25 degrees. They can do the profiles in any meridian they like. They compare results with the kinetic Goldmann and also with the Tübingen perimeter and they find interesting variations between profiles. They measured normal people with their instrument, and repeated the study on the Tübingen perimeter.

There is about 1.3 log. unit difference between results which they account for theoretically in terms of summation. As has been reported before, summation of very short stimuli, certainly does not behave at all like summation with longer stimuli. They show differences in early glaucoma field defects, that is where most of the function is still present, between the two instruments. When the scotoma is dense the difference not longer exists. A paper using short stimuli this afternoon commented on the fact that the location of early defects in the visual field does not agree with the publication of Dr. Aulhorn. We have analysed our figures from many cases (but I haven't got them with me) and we also have to disagree with Dr. Aulhorn. I think that these disagreements are really interesting; we are just showing differences in technique and I think one of the things we have to look forward to the future is to use both techniques to get further information, not one or the other.

Enoch: The next paper is by T. Maruo of Kobe. "Electroencephalographic perimetry".

Ernest: I don't want to discuss this paper but I have a couple of questions about it. Were the patients given tasks requiring concentration during testing? And two: Were power spectrum analyses carried out on any of the recordings?

Maruo: I think the Vertex Potential represents the excitation of the cortex, and it is related to the function of recognition. It is possible to conduct objective perimetry using the Vertex Potential.

Enoch: The next paper is by T. Ogawa, R. Suzuki of Tokyo. "Relation between central and peripheral field changes with kinetic perimetry". Dr. Bynke is the discussant.

Bynke: Dr. Ogawa and Dr. Suzuki have conducted a comparative study of the frequency of central and peripheral visual changes in a large sample of 1926 eyes and they have used Goldmann's kinetic perimeter for these studies. Visual field defects were found in more than 700 eyes. And in most cases there were changes not only in the peripheral field but also in central field. But one group was the most interesting i.e., where the central field was normal but the peripheral field was positive. This was the case in 6 eyes, that is a very small number. These cases had glaucoma or retinal detachment or retinal disease and in one case there was a puititary adenoma. This last case had central defects in one eye and peripheral defects in the other one. This paper is of great importance because not much has been done on this field before, and my comment is that many of our examination methods are based on the fact that most visual field defects are central, for example the tangent screen examination, Mr. Friedmann's analyser examines the central field and also other methods, for example, Krakau's automatic perimeter does so. We know that we can continue with these methods. They are sufficient in most cases but there are in fact some cases which exhibit only peripheral defects. But we don't miss them very often.

Greve, E.L. & Verduin, W.M. In 1972 when we were considering to use an oscilloscope for automated perimetry we conducted a similar study. The results have not yet been published so far, except in reports for the Institute for Perception and Health Organization. Our findings were as follows and they confirm the findings of Ogawa and Suzuki (see this volume).

The VF of 600 patients with VF defects were analysed. The question was whether the defect or part of the defect would have been found if only the VF up to 20° eccetricity has been examined. It turned out that 96% of all defects would have been detected by an examination limited to a 20° radius VF. This does not imply that the defects were entirely within 20°. In 55% of the cases, part of the VF defect was also located outside the 20° area, and in many of these cases interesting topographical information was found outside the 20° area.

However if one is only concerned with detection of defects, 4% of defects will be missed by an examination limited to the 20° radius visual field.

Frisen: I would like to raise the question that applies not only to this paper but many papers that have been presented this morning.

And that is the utility of the V/4. This target was used for testing the peripheral limits of the visual field in this paper and also in many of the other papers. But in my mind this is a disservice to the testing of the peripheral visual field because a measure of the normal periphery can usually be obtained with a I/4 or possible II/4 target and the V/4 in my mind is much to supraliminal. You cannot indentify early defects or any early depressions of visual function by using such a target.

Would anybody care to comment on the utility of the V/4 except for delinating absolute visual field defects?

Drance: I adress myself to this problem. First, not in terms that Dr. Frisen asked, but in terms of the paper which was written I want to adress this problem from the glaucoma point of view, not from the neuro-ophthalmological point of view.

I think that even in Dr. Harms and Dr. Aulhorn's tremendous study of over 2000 glaucomatous eyes they found that there was somewhere between 1 or 1.5% of their material who showed isolated nasal steps without any of the other characteristic findings. So if one accepted that finding alone one would say that when one examined 100 potential glaucoma patients for a visual field defect. $1\frac{1}{2}$ out of hunderd, a 3 out of every 200 in approximate terms would have their early visual field defects missed. That is a very small number if one is the minister of health who has to decide whether one is going to employ a particular testing which costs ten minutes and so many dollars. One can make that sort of decision and work out the risks and the costs. But when one is a physician who has the responsability

479

to face a patient across the examination table who is interested not in the other 197 patients but himself, he has a right to have his early visual field defects discovered and therefore the appropriate measurements to be undertaken. It is clear that one is looking for and the figure of 1.5% is probably a very conservative one. A large number of patients show a peripheral visual field defect in glaucoma as their only early visual field defect. It still is not the majority.

We are still looking at 5%, 10%. It is a small number relatively speaking but a very important group of people. I would therefore say that any paper that puts the situation as an either/or proposition, does no service to the individual patient allthough it certainly will benefit the manufacturer and the minister and all these very important people. But let me go back to Dr. Frisen's point because I think he makes a very important point and that is the peripheral visual field is really plotted in the majority of people who see 6/6 and have clear media on the Goldmann perimeter with a target size which is infinitely smaller than the V/4 and that with the I/4 or II and a little bit one will get way out to the periphery in most people (except for the lids and the nose). Therefore the important thing really is not that we should get stuck on V/4 or IV/4 or anything less, but that we should in fact measure the peripheral visual field with whatever target is required for that purpose and in patients who have cataracts and media that are not clear one sometimes has to go to the V/4 in order to get way out to the peripheral field.

Enoch: The last of the non-read paper is by Lars Frisen. "Relationship between perimetric eccentricity and retinal locus in a human eye."

I shall discuss this paper. Frisen and his co-worker placed markers on the retina of an eye about to be removed. Then they tested the linearity of the displacement of those markers with the distribution of points in the visual field after the eye was removed. This paper is actually a brief abstract of one paragraph and my comments are: *first:* the question is terribly important particularly in terms of the kinds of treatment that many of us are doing these days when we try to relate lesions or points on the retina to various functional tests. One of the critical issues is the linearity of the conversion, or if you will the registration between the point tested and the retinal point assigned to the test point that has been established functionally. What Frisen is trying to do here is to relate the two, i.e., he is try to determine how good the match is out to many degrees from the fovea. My single critism of this paper is that he has not provided enough details relative to the technique used. However much of this material has appeared in an earlier publication in Acta Ophthalmologica.

REPORT OF THE IPS RESEARCH GROUP ON STANDARDS

May 3, 1978

1. On May 3, 1978 at the Keio Plaza Hotel in Tokyo, the Research group on Standards of the IPS, made final modifications upon, voted on, and approved the third draft on the International Perimetric Society: Perimetric Standards, 1978.
The vote was unanimous.

Prior to this vote, a draft standard was prepared in Bonn, Bundesrepublik Deutschland on Nov. 11, 12, 1977 by an Ad Hoc Drafting Committee of the Research Group. That committee was elected by the IPS R.G. on Standards at its meeting in Tübingen on Sept. 19, 1976. The draft standard was circulated to all members of the organization for critism as well as other interested parties. Over thirty detailed sets of comments were received. Comments were collated, modifications were made, and the revised standard was presented to the research group. Individuals were encouraged to petition the Research Group on Standards at its meeting on May 3, 1978 if they had unresolved concerns. Three individuals took advantage of this opportunity. The points they raised were resolved to the satisfaction of all parties.

2. On May 4, 1978 the revised glossary to this standard was approved by the R.G. on Standards.

3. On May 4, 1978 the International Perimetric Society Committee voted unanimously to approve the document titled *International Perimetric Society: Perimetric Standards, 1978*. It agreed to publish this document, less glossary in the proceedings of this meeting. The IPS Committee requested Prof. Dubois-Poulsen to submit the approved draft standard to the Concillium Ophthalmologicum Universale for approval and subsequent publication in the Acta of the Tokyo meeting. That document will include both standard and approved glossary.

4. The R.G. on Standards unitiated discussion of new goals for consideration by this committee.

5. Lastly, the Chairman wishes to thank Dr. Greve, Dr. Matsuo and their staffs, the members of the Research Group and the many interested members and others who have contributed to the formulation of the standard.

Jay M. Enoch

Chairman
R.G. on Standards, IPS

REPORT ON COLOUR PERIMETRY

GUY VERRIEST

(Ghent, Belgium)

ABSTRACT

There are big differences between the means and goals of colour perimetry as it was done in the past and that of the actually determined static achromatic increment threshold spectral sensitivity curves for monochromatic targets. Even when a white background is used, such curves present normally three peaks corresponding to three different opponent colour vision mechanisms.

Pathological conditions can be characterized or by the reduction of a given mechanism, or by loss of opponent function, or by increased opponent function etc. The method requires a.o. sufficient background and target luminances, and also the knowledge of the radiance of the target.

I will first emphasize that there are very big differences between the means and goals of colour perimetry as it was done in the past, before the introduction of the quantitative bowl perimeters, and the means and goals of contemporary colour perimetry, as it is developped today by the vast majority of the members of the IPS RG on Colour Perimetry.

Colour perimetry of the past was performed by means of photometrically and colorimetrically not or ill defined pigmentary objects, with as goals (1) either to provide less intense objects for measurements of central isopters and of relative defects, or (2) to recognize acquired colour vision defects in periphreal vision. For (2) the subject was generally asked to name the perceived colours; this method has been improved in different ways; it had a great diagnostic usefulness and is actually again advocated by some authors, as Ohta, Frisén and Dannheim.

However, the major stream in the actual trends in colour perimetry is entirely different from old colour perimetry. Instead of pigmentary objects, only monochromatic or nearly monochromatic objects of known wavelengths and energies are used. Instead of colour namings and of assessments of photochromatic intervals, only the achromatic increment thresholds are determined: thus now the subject has only to say when he perceives the object, disregarding his eventual colour perception. Instead of using the old kinetic methods, the increment thresholds are now nearly always determined in the modern static way, but at each studied retinal location such static increment thresholds are determined for a series of well chosen object wavelengths. And as the energies of the objects are known, the results for white or colour perimetry. Lakowski's modified Goldmann perimeter and the prototype presented by Kitahara at this symposium will surely help to determine the ideal parameters.

Author's address:
Dienst Oogheelkunde, Akademisch Ziekenhuis,
De Pintelaan 135, B-9000 Gent, Belgium.

CLOSING SPEECH

A. DUBOIS-POULSEN

My Dear Colleagues.

The third symposium of the International Society of Perimetry is over. Like its precedent ones it was a great success. It is acknowledged by all that the idea of exploring the visual field as completely as possible in all its modalities is becoming more fruitful than ever.

If we consider the road behind us, how long is the way we did travel over. It was on the occasion of the last International Congress in Paris, during the first International Symposium on visual field that we thought to lay the foundation of a society which would perpetuate the idea of the first meeting, would bring together the perimetrists of the whole world and would give life to an idea which in truth was not recognised everywhere. Our colleagues will always prefer the anatomical proceedings to the functional ones, because they think that these are more objective and because they have a correlation with surgery. They are so putting into practice an incomplete clinical work in which the functional understanding is absent. We endeavoured to demonstrate that this is a mistake and I think we succeeded very well.

We all remember the brilliant sessions of the first symposium in Marseille where we were so generously received by Professor Jayle, who could not be among us because of his health.

We remember with appreciations the Symposium of Tübingen which was held under the chairmanship of Mrs. Aulhorn.

It was a great performance of good work and friendship. The books which were published on these occasions, even if the first is contestable, are confirming the importance of our efforts and vitality of our thoughts.

The third Symposium is not less important than the others. The chairman, my dear friend Professor Matsuo, organized it in a masterly manner with his collaborators.

As usual, the main force in this affair was Erik Greve who supervised everything from Amsterdam. Our society owes to him the high point of development which it has actually reached.

Our Japanese friends have imposed in this symposium the great qualities which we know to them: courtesy, gentleness, cordially, artistical sense allied to precision in the organization of the least detail.

I would like to say how deeply I was personally touched by all I saw and heard. I am not a neophyte in Japan. I came here seventeen years ago. This journey had been a wondering astonishment and I kept here good friends whom I have been meeting again with great emotion and pleasure for they remained faithful to me. Professor Umazume whom I was glad to see so young in spite of the years; my dear friend Matsuo, who stayed so long a time in my laboratory who initiated himself to perimetry in my own service and who is nowaday addicted to this disciplin. I have today the great joy to compliment him for this magnificient success, to see that he is one of the masters of the Japanese comtemporary ophthalmology and to hartily thank him for the faithfulness and friendship he shows to me in every circumstance. I found again everything I knew in my first journey and nevertheless my wonder is still greater. The traditional Japanese receptions are splendid and marvelous feasts for the eyes and at the same time the celebration of good humor and of friendship.

On a scientific point of view our meeting was a great success. If we compare it with the preceding ones we can say that we considered more limited perimetrical subjects in a more exhaustive manner. The first years have made us more aware of the extent of the problems and do not treat them as a whole but one by one.

In this symposium we acquired a more precise knowledge of the perimetric signs in glaucoma. We must be aware that glaucoma is for a long while a very silent disease, so the methods of detection must be very accurate. They have been improved. We must remember of the technic of supraliminal stimuli which is very interesting. The idea to study the receptive field-like functions localized in the inner retina is new and it has been shown that they are unequivocally altered in open angle glaucoma. The early signs of glaucoma have been precised. In confirmed glaucoma the relative value of the different signs has been well established. A great question has been discussed. The glaucomatous scotoma, are they reversible? In general the loss of visual field in this disease is permanent. There are some known exceptions, the so-called pressure amaurosis, which is for a time reversible and the defects caused by elevation of pressure due to corticosteroids. Nevertheless a proportion of scotomas is reversible, especially if the tension has been lowered by surgical means, if the patient is young, if the disc is not too altered. We must remember the importance of the fiber bundles in this disease and we heard of many technical procedures to deal with them.

In spite of all these efforts glaucoma is still a very mysterious disease. The visual field defects are not only dependent on intra ocular pressure. Compensation mechanisms have been put in evidence. The loss of these mechanisms is very important. But we must be modest and say 'We don't know' and work.

As to the neurogical aspects of perimetry it was stated that the aspect of the chiasmal lesions, which seemed so confusing may be classified in symmetric type, asymmetric type and atypical aspects, and that the compression of the optic pathways is not the only factor causing visual field defects.

It was demonstrated that the funduscopic aspect of the papilla and specially of the peripapillary fibers is essential in the interpretation of perim-

486

etric results. In automation technic we went further than the mechanical and electronic aspects and considered the physiological methods. The thresholds fluctuations have a detrimental effect. The remedy is in application of overaging methods. The technic based on the distribution of scanning points in a rectangular grid is better than the method of the points aligned along a meridian. It is very important to measure the retinal sensitivity at the exact point of the ophthalmoscopically seen lesion. The new equipments for performing qualitative perimetry observing the fundus by means of infrared television ophthalmoscopy are very interesting and I think that the Japanese school has presented to us a prominent contribution to our general knowledge of the field. Our Japanese colleagues may be proud of their technical ability.

I don't forget the considerable work of standardization which has been carried out by our colleague Enoch. He attached himself to the ungrateful task of standardizing and precising the perimetric methods. It is a huge and hard work. You saw the results and I am sure they will be very usefull.

We may therefore congratulate ourselves about the work which has been performed. On the other hand we are very sad for after a glorious reign of four years our queen is abdicating. We know what we owe to her. Good luck, charm and gentleness have been the characteristics of her reign. We are grateful to her and we regret her very deeply. But as in all kingdoms after the queens departure there is another king. To Elfriede the first is succeeding Stephen the first. I wish to our colleague Drance happiness and good authority to rule over us.

It is now time to say good bye. I say to you all Sayonara. To the next time in Bristol. Many and many thanks again to you my japanese friends, to Professor Harutake Matsuo and to his collaborators. There are only few words in French to express my feelings: Merci, merci de tout coeur. Aligato, Aligato gozaï Maïta.

LIST OF CONTRIBUTORS

T. Aoyama, 265
M.F. Armaly, 177
E. Aulhorn, 73, 363
I. Azuma, 261
H. Bebie, 295
H. Bynke, 87, 101, 109, 319
G. Calabria, 273
E.C. Campos, 137, 381
F. Dannheim, 43, 151
G.R. Douglas, 119
S.M. Drance, 119, 159, 279, 292
A. Dubois-Poulsen, 423, 485
P. Dunn, 411
N. Endo, 167
J.M. Enoch, 137, 381, 475
J.T. Ernest, 205
M. Fairclough, 119
F. Fankhauser, 295
C.R. Fitzgerald, 381
A.J. Friedman, 263
L. Frisén, 5, 81, 409
M. Frisén, 427
F. Furuno, 127, 197, 247
E. Gandolfo, 273, 327
E.L. Greve, 1, 127, 197, 371
J. Hamazaki, 311
S. Hamazaki, 311
T. Hara, 403
K. Harasawa, 351
H. Harms, 363
S.S. Hayreh, 53
A. Heijl, 319
T. Hohki, 95
C. Holmin, 319
Y. Honda, 433
I. Iinuma, 229
A. Inatomi, 359
Y. Isayama, 27, 241
K. Iwata, 233
K. Kani, 341
H. Karmeyer, 363
G. Kikuchi, 311
H. Kitahara, 439
K. Kitahara, 439
Y. Kitazawa, 211

S. Koike, 311
H. Kosaki, 255
S. Kubota, 447
D. Kuehne, 43
R. Lakowski, 159, 411
P.R. Lichter, 111
D. Lüedecke, 43
T. Maruo, 461
K. Matsudaira, 395
H. Matsuo, 247, 311, 333, 340, 417, 421, 453
H. Matsuzaki, 439
H. Mieno, 311
M. Miki, 433
T. Miyamoto, 351
K. Mizokami, 241
Y. Nakao, 95
A. Negi, 433
T. Ogawa, 469
Y. Ogita, 341
Y. Ohiwa, 211
Y. Ohta, 351
T. Otori, 95
C.D. Phelps, 187
P. Podhajsky, 53
G. Schöldström, 409
E. Shinzato, 453
C.L. Standardi, 111
R. Susanna, 119
R. Suzuki, 369, 395, 469
M. Taga, 311
Y. Tagami, 17, 241
V. Tagliasco, 327
O. Takahashi, 211
M. Tanzil, 73
B. Thomas, 119
M. Tomonaga, 369
W.M. Verduin, 127, 197
G. Verriest, 483
L. Vestergren-Brenner, 87
E.B. Werner, 223
K. Yamasowa, 261
S. Yamazi, 261
T. Yokota, 311
M. Zingirian, 273, 327